THE NEUROTRANSMITTER ERA IN NEUROPSYCHOPHARMACOLOGY

Edited by
Thomas A. Ban and Ronaldo Ucha Udabe

CINP

Library of Congress Cataloging-in-Publication Data
Ban, T.A., Ucha Udabe, R. (Eds.)
The Neurotransmitter Era in Neuropsychopharmacology
Includes bibliographical references and indexes.
ISBN: 987-9165-68-3

1.Neurotransmitters. 2.Neuropsychopharmacology.
3.Neuropharmacology. 4.Psychopharmacology.
5.Collegium Internationale Neuro-Psychopharmacologicum.

Publisher: International College of Neuropsychopharmacology (CINP)
CINP Central Office
Glenfinnan Suite,
Braeview House 9/11, Braeview Place,
East Kilbride G74 3XH,
Scotland, UK
E-mail: cinp@cinp.org
Website: http://cinp.org

CONTENTS

PART FOUR

EFFECT OF DRUGS ON NEUROTRANSMITTERS

PART FIVE

REFLECTIONS

PART SIX

HISTORICAL PERSPECTIVE

PREFACE

This is the first volume of what may become the third series of publications of the history committee of the Collegium Internationale Neuro-Psychopharmacologicum (CINP). The origin of this committee was in an informal collaboration between Ole Rafaelsen, Hanns Hippius and Tom Ban that started in 1986 at the end of Rafaelsen's presidency (1984-1986) during the 15th CINP congress in San Juan, Puerto Rico. The purpose of the collaboration was to reconstruct the history of the organization from eyewitness records before time had narrowed the witnesses. Rafaelsen died shortly after, but Hippius and Ban continued with the work; from 1986 to 1996 they prepared a series of four booklets, the last one in collaboration with Oakley Ray, reviewing events that led to the founding of CINP and the first 30 years in the history of the organization (Ban and Hippius, 1988, 1992, 1994; Ban and Ray, 1996; Ban, Ray and Hippius, 1996).

By the time the first series on the history of CINP was published, the history committee became one of the 12 constitutional committees of the organization and Ban was appointed as chairman. The mandate of the committee was reviewing and continuously updating the history of the organization, documenting events, and reporting the history of the organization to the membership.

In 1996 the history committee was strengthened by the appointments of Edward Shorter, a social historian with the background in the history of psychiatry, and David Healy, a psychiatrist with special interest in the history of psychopharmacology. The new team extended the scope of the mandate of the committee from the history of the organization to the history of the field. In a period of eight years it published a series of four volumes on The History of Psychopharmacology and the CINP, As Told in Autobiography (Ban, Healy and Shorter, 1998, 2000, 2002, 2004). In this second series the history of neuropsychopharmacology and the organization unfolds through personal accounts written primarily by members and fellows of CINP.

In 2004 at the 24th CINP Congress in Paris (France), Ronaldo Ucha Udabe succeeded Ban as chairman of CINP's history committee. Members of the newly appointed committee included: Nancy Andreasen (vice-chair), Frank Ayd, Tom Ban, Arvid Carlsson, Alec Coppen, David Healy, Hanns Hippius, Juan Lopez-Ibor, Alfred Pletscher, Herman van Praag, Oakley Ray, and Pedro Tellez-Carrasco. Andrea Tone, a social historian was appointed consultant to the committee; and Philippe Robert and Nina Schooler became liaisons with the executive committee and the council of CINP respectively.

The committee decided to complement the memoirs of the second series with reviews prepared by basic scientists and clinicians involved in different areas of neuropsychopharmacology which are focused on one or another particular period in the development of the field. On the recommendation of Pletscher, the neurotransmitter era in neuropsychopharmacology was chosen as the first period to be reviewed. The collection of these reviews is presented in this volume. Several members of the history committee participated in the project: Healy, Pletscher, and van Praag contributed chapters, and Ban and Ucha Udabe co-edited the book.

We should like to acknowledge the encouragement of CINP President Brian Leonard (2004-2006) in pursuing this project. It is fair to say that without his support this book would not have seen the light of day.

We owe a debt of gratitude to Claudia Antonelli for her conscientious editorial assistance. We wish to thank Gabriela Patterson and Ignacio Portes for the many hours of secretarial work. We also wish to express our appreciation to Edward Shorter for his editorial suggestions. Christopher Ban was of great help in the final editorial work.

Thanks are due to Juan Carlos Stagnaro, president of Polemos Editorial, for his assistance in publishing this book, and to Dr. Gregers Wegener for the preparation of the second edition.

REFERENCES
1. Ban, T.A., Hippius, H. (Eds.), 1988. Thirty Years CINP. A Brief History of the Collegium Internationale Neuro-Psychopharmacologicum. Springer-Verlag, Berlin/ Heidelberg/ New York/ London/ Paris/ Tokyo, pp. 1-138.
2. Ban, T.A., Hippius, H. (Eds.), 1992. Psychopharmacology in Perspective. A Personal Account by the Founders of the Collegium Internationale Neuro-Psychopharmacologicum. Springer-Verlag, Berlin/ Heidelberg/ New York/ London/ Paris/ Tokyo, pp. 1-94.
3. Ban, T.A., Hippius, H. (Eds.), 1994. Towards CINP. From the Paris Colloquium to the Milan Symposium. JM Productions, Bremtwood (Tennessee), 1-54.
4. Ban, T.A., Ray, O.S. (Eds.), 1996. A History of the CINP. JM Productions, Brentwood (Tennessee), pp. 1-457.
5. Ban, T.A., Ray, O.S., Hippius, H. (Eds.), 1996. The Early Years. From the Inaugural Meeting to the Third Congress in Munich. In: Ban, T.A., Ray, O.S. (Eds.), A History of the CINP. JM Productions, Brentwood (Tennessee), pp. 311-457.
6. Ban, T.A., Healy, D., Shorter, E. (Eds.), 1998. The Rise of Psychopharmacology and the Story of CINP. Animula, Budapest, pp. 1- 448.
7. Ban, T.A., Healy, D., Shorter, E. (Eds.), 2000. The Triumph of Psychopharmacology and the Story of CINP. Animula, Budapest, pp. 1- 375.
8. Ban, T.A., Healy, D., Shorter, E. (Eds.), 2002. From Psychopharmacology to Neuropsychopharmacology in the 1980s and the Story of CINP As Told in Autobiography. Volume 3 of the series The History of Psychopharmacology and the CINP, As Told in Autobiography. Animula, Budapest, pp. 1- 408.
9. Ban, T.A., Healy, D., Shorter, E. (Eds.), 2004. Reflections on Twentieth-Century Psychopharmacoloy. Volume 4 of the series The History of Psychopharmacology and the CINP, As Told in Autobiography. Animula, Budapest, pp. 1- 896.

INTRODUCTION

In this volume on the neurotransmitter era, the first epoch in the history of neuropsychopharmacology is reviewed by a group of basic scientists and clinicians who actively contributed to the development of the new field. Neuropsychopharmacology is the scientific discipline dedicated to the study and treatment of the pathophysiology of mental syndromes with centrally acting drugs. The neurotransmitter era represents a period in the history of neuropsychopharmacology in which the study of the pathophysiology and the treatment of mental illness are based on knowledge derived from the effect of drugs on neurotransmitter dynamics.

The book is divided into six parts. Part One (two chapters) deals with research that set *the foundation of neuropsychopharmacology* primarily in Bernard Brodie's laboratory at the National Heart Institute and in other laboratories (e,g., Julius Axelrod's, Seymour Kety's) of the National Institutes of Health (NIH) of the United States. The authors are Alfred Pletscher, a collaborator of Brodie in the mid-1950s and Irwin Kopin, a collaborator of Axelrod and Kety in the late 1950s and early 1960s. Pletscher was a member of the team that demonstrated the relationship between reserpine's sedative and serotonin depleting effects; Kopin was a member of the team that contributed significantly to .the understanding of catecholamine metabolism.

The focus in Part Two (three chapters) is on the three *neurotransmitters* that are at the core of the neurotransmitter era: norepinephrine, serotonin and dopamine. The history of these neurotransmitters is reviewed and their role in mental pathology as well as in the mode of action of psychotropic drugs, is discussed by Fridolin Sulser (norepineprine), David Grahame-Smith (serotonin) and Philip Seeman (dopamine). Sulser became interested in norepinephrine in the early 1960s while working with desipramine, a metabolite of imipramine that was to become the first selective norepinephrine re-uptake inhibitor antidepressant; his research contributed to the understanding of the action mechanism of antidepressants. Grahame-Smith became interested in serotonin in the early 1960s while studying the carcinoid syndrome, a syndrome caused by argentaffin cell tumor that produces an excess of serotonin; his research contributed to understanding the synthesis and function of serotonin in the central nervous system. Philip Seeman became interested in dopamine in the early 1970s while studying the action mechanism of haloperidol; his research contributed to the understanding of the action mechanism of neuroleptics.

Part Three (three chapters) covers research with drugs, such as levodopa, monoamine oxidase inhibitors and reserpine, that was instrumental in establishing relationships between *pharmacological actions and clinical effects.* Oleh Hornykiewicz reviews research with levodopa, the precursor of dopamine; Moussa Youdim looks at work with monoamine oxidases and monamine oxidase inhibitors;

and Silvio Garattini surveys research with reserpine. Hornykiewicz, in the early 1960s, helped understand the importance of dopamine in Parkinson's disease; his research opened the path for neurotransmitter replacement therapy. Youdim, in the late 1960s, played a role in the recognition of different forms of monoamine oxidases in the brain; his research opened the path for the development of selective monamine oxidase inhibitors. Garattini, in the late 1950s was involved in research with reserpine; he was part of the team that developed the reserpine reversal test used in pharmacological screening for antidepressants.

Part Four (four chapters) is dedicated to the *effect* of psychotropic *drugs on neu - rotransmitters* In three of the four chapters the relationship between the mechanism of action of these drugs and their therapeutic and adverse effects are discussed. John Davis deals with tricyclic antidepressants, Elliott Richelson with neuroleptics and Gordon Johnson with lithium salts. In the fourth chapter Herman van Praag reviews the neurotransmitter era in psychiatry. Davis in the mid-1960s co-authored one of the first papers on the catecholamine hypothesis of depression; he was first to conduct meta-analysis with psychotropic drugs. Richelson in the late 1970s became interested in the interaction of psychotropic drugs with neurotransmitter receptors and transporters; his research contributed to the understanding how the receptor and the transporter affinity profile of a psychotropic drugs relates to its adverse effects and to some of its pharmacodynamic interactions.with other drugs. Johnson became interested in lithium in the late 1960s while working in the research unit of Arnold Friedhoff at Bellevue Hospital in New York; he was part of the team that demonstrated the superiority of lithium to chlorpromazine in the treatment of mania. Van Praag was one of the first psychiatrists to correlate the concentration of neurotransmitter metabolites in the cerebrospinal fluid with clinical psychopathology; he was also one of the first in the mid-1960s to propose a serotonin hypothesis of depression.

Part Five (three chapters) is devoted to *reflections* on neuropsychopharmacology by Norbert Matussek, a neuropsychopharmacologist, Joseph Knoll, a pharmacologist, and Oldřich Vinař, a psychiatrist. Matussek was one of the firsts (and the first in Europe) in the mid-1960s to propose a norepinephrine hypothesis of depression; he was also among the firsts to suggest biological (endocrinological) markers of endogenous depression. Knoll, in the mid-1960s developed the first selective monoamine oxidase inhibitor to be used in the treatment of Parkinson's disease and depression; his research during the past 40 years opened the path for mesencephalic enhancer regulation. Vinař was involved in the introduction of the first set of psychotropic drugs in the former Czechoslovakia; he contributed to the clinical development of numerous psychotropic drugs for well over 40 years.

In Part Six (two chapters), the final part of the volume, the place of the neurotransmitter era in the history of neuroscience is delineated by Kjell Fuxe and Luigi Agnati; and the neurotransmitter era is discussed in a *historical perspective* of brain research by David Healy. Fuxe in the mid-1960s participated in the mapping of central dopamine, norepinephrine, and serotonin neurons in the brain of various species' of animals with the employment of the Falck-Hillarp technique; his research during the past 30 years in collaboration with Luigi Agnati has focused on the demonstration of communication in the brain outside the synapse that supplements *wiring (synaptic) transmission*, based on neurotransmitters, with *volume transmission*, based on high affinity G-protein coupled receptors. Healy, in the late 1990s published a series of 78 interviews with leading psychopharmacologists of the neurotranmitter era, including 8 contributors of this volume; he was first to review the "the creation of psychopharmacology" and the history of "the antidepressant era" (Healy, 1996, 1997, 1998, 2000, 2002).

The Neurotransmitter Era in Neuropsychopharmacology also includes a *Prologue* on *Fifty years of psychopharmacology* by Brian Leonard, the president of CINP (2004-2006); an *Epilogue On specificity and communication: Reflections on the place of languages in psychopharmacology* by Joel Elkes, A CINP-Pfizer, Pioneer in Neuropsychopharmacology, and *Concluding remarks* on *The neurotransmitter era in neuropsychopharmacology* by Thomas Ban and Ronaldo Ucha Udabe, the editors of this volume. Leonard developed a basic curriculum across all areas of psychopharmacology aimed specifically at the need of third-world countries, including Tanzania, Uganda and Zimbabwe; the third edition of his Fundamentals of Psychopharmacology was published in 2003 (Leonard, 2003). Elkes was first in the late 1950s to provide some evidence and provisional formulations of drug effects in relation to receptor specificity; his selected writings were published as the first volume in the Pioneers in Neuropsychopharmacology series of CINP (Ban, 2001). Ban, one of the editors of this volume, was first in the 1960s to develop a conditioning test battery for the study of psychopathological mechanisms and psychopharmacological effects; his Psychopharmacology, published in 1969, was the first comprehensive text to cover general, systematic and applied psychopharmacology (Ban, 1969). Ronaldo Ucha Udabe, the other editor of this volume has contributed to the clinical development of numerous psychotropic drugs during the past 40 years; he co-authored Psicofarmacologia, one of the first such textbooks in the world (and the first in the Latin Americas) to review the first 10 years in the development and clinical use of psychotropic drugs (Fisher, Poch and Ucha Udabe, 1965).

The book is complemented with a comprehensive Index of drugs, names and subjects.

REFERENCES
1. Ban, T.A., 1969. Psychopharmacology. Williams & Wilkins, Baltimore, pp. 1-485.
2. Ban, T.A. (Ed.), 2001. Selected Writings of Joel Elkes. Animula, Budapest, pp. 1-532.
3. Fisher, E., Poch, G., Ucha Udabe, R., 1965. Psicofarmacología. López Echegoyen, Buenos Aires, pp. 1-464.
4. Healy, D., 1996. The Psychopharmacologists. Altman, London, pp. 1-633.

5. Healy, D., 1997. The Antidepressant Era. Harvard University Press, Cambridge, pp. 1-317.
6. Healy, D., 1998. The Psychopharmacologists II. Altman, London, pp. 1-640.
7. Healy, D., 2000. The Pssychopharmacologists III. Arnold, London, pp.1-580.
8. Healy, D., 2002. The Creation of Psychopharmacology. Harvard University Press, Cambridge, pp. 1-469.
9. Leonard, B., 2003. Fundamentals of Psychopharmacology. Wiley, Chichester.

LIST OF CONTRIBUTORS

AGNATI, Luigi, MD, Professor, Department of Biomedical Sciences, Section of Human Physiology, University of Modena and Reggio Emilia, Modena, Italy.

BAN, Thomas A., MD, Emeritus Professor, Department of Psychiatry, Vanderbilt University, Nashville, Tennessee, USA.

DAVIS, John M., Gilman Professor, The Psychiatric Institute, Department of Psychiatry, University of Illinois at Chicago, Chicago, Illinois, USA.

ELKES, Joel MD, Distinguished Service Professor Emeritus, Department of Psychiatry, The Johns Hopkins University, Baltimore, Maryland, USA; Distinguished University Professor Emeritus, Department of Psychiatry, University of Louisville, Louisville, Kentucky, USA; Emeritus Professor, Department of Psychiatry, McMaster University, Hamilton, Ontario, Canada; Senior Scholar-in-Residence, Fetzer Institute, Kalamazoo, Michigan, USA.

FUXE, Kjell, MD, Professor, Department of Neuroscience, Karolinska Institute, Stockholm, Sweden.

GARATTINI, Silvio, MD, Director, Mario Negri Institute for Pharmacological Research, Milano, Italy.

GRAHAME-SMITH, David G., MB, PhD, Emeritus Professor, Department of Clinical Pharmacology, University of Oxford, UK; Emeritus Fellow, Corpus Christi College, Oxford, UK.

HEALY, David T., MD, Director, North Wales Department of Psychological Medicine, University of Wales, Bangor, Wales, UK; Professor, Department of Psychological Medicine, Cardiff University, Bangor, Wales, UK.

HORNYKIEWICZ, Oleh, MD, Emeritus Professor, Division of Biochemistry and Molecular Neurobiology, Institute of Brain Research, University of Vienna, Austria.

JOHNSON, Gordon F., MBBS, Emeritus Professor, Department of Psychiatry, University of Sydney, Australia; Director, Mood Disorders Unit, Northside Clinic, Greenwich, Sydney, Australia.

KNOLL, Joseph, MD, PhD, DSc, Emeritus Professor, Department of Pharmacology, Semmelweis University, Budapest, Hungary.

KOPIN, Irwin, J., MD, Emeritus Scientist, National Institute of Neurological Disorders and Stroke, Bethesad, Maryland, USA; Emeritus Scientist, National Institute of Health, Bethesda, Maryland, USA.

LEONARD, Brian, PhD, Emeritus Professor, Department of Pharmacology, National University of Ireland, Galway, Ireland.

MATUSSEK, Norbert, J., MD, Emeritus Professor, Department of Psychiatry, Ludwig-Maximilians-University, Munich, Germany.

PLETSCHER, Alfred, MD, PhD, Emeritus Professor, Department of Pharmacology, University of Basle, Switzerland.

RICHELSON, Elliott, MD, Professor of Psychiatry and Pharmacology, Mayo College of Medicine, Rochester, Minnesota, USA; Distinguished Investigator, Mayo Foundation for Medical Education and Research, Rochester, Minnesota, USA; Consultant in Psychiatry and Pharmacology, Mayo Clinic, Jacksonville, Florida, USA.

SEEMAN, Philip, MD, Emeritus Professor, Departments of Pharmacology and Psychiatry, University of Toronto, Ontario, Canada.

SULSER, Fridolin, MD, Emeritus Professor, Department of Psychiatry and Pharmacology, Vanderbilt University, Nashville, Tennessee, USA.

UCHA UDABE, Ronaldo, MD, PhD, Professor of Postgraduate Education in Psychopharmacology, National University of Buenos Aires, Argentina; Professor of Postgraduate Education in Psychopharmacology, Argentine Catholic University, Buenos Aires, Argentina.

VAN PRAAG, Herman, M., MD, PhD, Emeritus Professor, Department of Psychiatry, University of The Netherlands at Maastricht, Maastricht, The Netherlands; Emeritus Professor, Department of Psychiatry, Albert Einstein College of Medicine, New York City, New York, USA; Scientific Adviser, Academic Hospital Maastricht, Maastricht, The Netherlands.

VINAŘ, Oldřich, MD, DSc, Emeritus Associate Professor, Department of Psychiatry, Charles University, Prague, Czech Republic.

YOUDIM, Moussa B.H., PhD, Finkelstein Professor Life Sciences and Pharmacology, Technion-Rappaport Family Faculty of Medicine, Haifa, Israel; Director, Eva Topf and US National Parkinson Foundation Center of Excellence for Neurodegenerative Diseases, Technion-Rappaport Family Faculty of Medicine, Haifa, Israel.

ABBREVIATIONS

A	adenosine receptor
Aβ	amyloid ß
AC	adenylate cyclase
ACTH	adrenocorticotrope hormone
AD	Alzheimer's disease
AGN 1135	N-propargyl-l-aminoidan
AMP	adenosine monophosphate
ANS	autonomous nervous system
APP	amyloid precursor protein
AR	amine re-uptake
Arg	arginine
Asp	aspartate
ATF	activating transcriptor factor
ATP	adenosine triphosphate
BDNF	brain derived neurotrophic factor
B_{max}	maximal binding capacity
C	carbon
CA	catecholamines
cAMP	cyclic adenosine monophosphate
cDNA	cyclic deoxyribonucleic acid
CCK	cholecystokinin
cGMP	cyclic guanosine monophosphate
CGP 3466	N-methyl-N-propargyl-10-aminomethyl-dibenzo [b,f]oxepin
Ci/mMole	Curie per millimole
CINP	Collegium Internationale Neuro-Psychopharmacologicum
CMI	clomipramine, chlorimipramine
CNS	central nervous system
Compound 4560	chlorpromazine
CRE	cyclic adenosine monophosphate response enhancer elements
CREB	cyclic adenosine monophosphate response element binding
CRF	corticotropin-releasing factor
CSF	cerebrospinal fluid
β-CTF	β-C-terminal fragment
D	dopamine receptor
DA	dopamine

DAergic	dopaminergic
DAO	diamine oxidase
DATATOP	deprenyl and tocopherol antioxidative therapy of Parkinson's disease
DDC	dopa decarboxylase
DHMA	dihydroxymandelic acid
DHPG	3,4-dihydroxyphenylglycol
DLB	Lewy body disease
D-dopa	dextrodopa
DMI	desipramine, desmethylimiparmine
DMT	dimethyltryptamine
DNA	deoxyribonucleic acid
DOPA	3,4 dihydroxyphenylalanine
DOPAC	dihydroxyphenylacetic acid
DOPS	dihydroxyphenylserine
DRN	dorsal raphé nucleus
DT	dopamine transporter
E-250	phenylisopropylmethyl propylamine
ECF	extracellular fluid
ECS	extracellular space
ECT	electroconvulsive therapy
EEG	electroencephalography
EPI	epinephrine
ERK	extracellular signal regulated Kinase (s)
FDA	Food and Drug Administration
FGF	fibroblast growth factor
μg	microgram
GABA	γ-aminobutyric acid
GalR	galanin receptor
GAP	growth-associated protein
GDNF	glial neurotrophic factor
GH	growth hormone
GMP	guanosine monophosphate
GNNF	glia derived neurotrophic factor
GPCRs	G-protein coupled receptor (s)
G protein	guanine nucleotide regulatory protein
GR	glycocorticoid receptor
GTP	guanosine triphosphate
5-HIAA	5-hydroxyindoleacetic acid
HMN	horizontal molecular networks
HPLC	high-pressure-liquid-chromatography
5-HT	5-hydroxytrypatmin, serotonin

5-HTergic	serotonergic
5-HTP	5-hydroxytryptophan
5-HTT	5-HT transporter protein
HVA	homovanillic acid
IC_{50}	half of maximal inhibition concentration
I.R.E.	National Institut Voor Radio-Elementen
K	potassium
Kd	dissociation constant
Ki	dissociation constant
Km	Michaelis constant
l allel	long allele
L-dopa	levodopa
levodopa	3,4-dihydroxy phenylalanine
LC	locus coeruleus
LCS	Laboratory of Clinical Science
LH	luteinising hormone
M 30	5-(N-methyl-N-propargylaminomethyl)-8-hydroxyquinoline
MA	monoamine (s)
MAergic	monoamineregic
MAO	monoamine oxidase
MAOI	MAO inhibitor
MAP	mitogen activated protein
MAPkinases	mitogen activated protein kinases
MCPP	m-chlorophenylpiperzine
5MeODMT	5-methoxy-N,N-dimethyltrypatmine
mg	milligram
Mg	magnesium
MHPG	3-methoxy-4-hydroxyphenylglycol
MN	metanephrine
MPP+	dihydropiridine ion
α-MPT	α-methyl-para-tyrosine
MPTP	1-methyl-4-phenyl-1,2,3,6-tetrahydropyridine
MRC	Medical Research Council
m-RNA	messenger RNA
α-MTrp	α-[^{11}C]methyl-L-tryptophan
N 7001	melitracene
N 7049	litatracen
Na	sodium
NA	noradrenaline
NAergic	noradrenergic
NE	norepinephrine

NGF	nerve growth factor
NIDDK	National Institute of Diabetes and Digestive and Kidney Diseases
NIH	National Institutes of Health
NIMH	National Institute of Mental Health
NINDS	National Institute of Neurological Disorders and Stroke
nM	nanomole
NMDA	N-methyl-D-aspartic acid
NMN	normetanephrine
NO	nitrous oxide
NPY	neuropeptide Y
NPYR	neuropeptide Y receptor
OCD	obsessive-compulsive disorder
P-2565	2-hydroxy-3-(N,N-diethylcarbamyl)-9,10-dimethyl-1,2,3,4,6,7-hexahydrobenzoquinolizine
PC	pheochromocytom
PCP	phencyclidine
PCPA	p-chlorophenylalanine
PD	Parkinson's disease
PEA	phenylethylamine
PET	positron emission tomograp
PHS	Public Health Service
PK	protein kinase
PMA	phorbolester phorbol 12 - myristate 13 acetate
PNMT	phenylethanolamine-N-methyl transferase
PP	protein phosphatase
(-)-PPAP	(-)-1-phenyl-2-propylaminopentane
PrBCM	propylbenzilylcholine mustard
QNB	3-quinuclidinyl benzilate
REC	receptor (s)
RIMA	reversible MAO-A inhibitor
RM	receptor mosaic
RNA	ribonucleic acid
Ro	Roche
Ro 4-1284	2-ethyl-1,3,4,4,7,11b hexahydro-3-isobutyl-9, 10-dimethoxy-2H-benzo [a] quinolizin-2-ol hydrochloride
RP	Rhone Poulenc
RP 4560	chlorpromazine
RRI	receptor-receptor interaction
SAME	S-adenosylmethionine
sAPPα	soluble amyloid precursor protein α

s allele	short allele
SAS	sub-arachnoid space
SHSY-5Y	human dopaminergic neuroblastoma cells
SOD	superoxide dismutase
SPECT	single photon emission tomography
SSRI	selective serotonin re-uptake inhibitor
SU 5171	methyl-18-0-(3-dimethylamonobenzoyl) reserpate
SV	synaptic vesicles
SWS	slow wave sleep
t 1/2	half-time
TCA	tricyclic antidepressant
TES	treatment emergent symptoms
TGACGTCA	thymine, guanine, adenine, cytosine, guanine, thymine, cytosine, adenine
TH	tyrosine hydroxylase
THC	tetrahydrocannabinol
TM	transmembrane
TPH	tryptophan hydroxylase
TRKB	tyrosine Kinase receptor B
TSH	thyrotropin stimulatig hormone
UCP	uncoupling of proteins
US-DHEW	United States Department of Health, Education and Welfare
VAT	vesicular amine transporter
VMA	vanillylmandelic acid
V_{max}	maximum velocity
VT	volume transmission
WT	wiring transmission

PROLOGUE

Fifty years of psychopharmacology

Brian E. Leonard

In 1957, a group of 32 pharmacologists and psychiatrists met in Zurich, Switzerland to discuss the establishment of an international society for psychopharmacology. This meeting led to the organisation of the first congress of the Collegium Internationale Neuro-Psychopharmacologicum (CINP) in Rome the following year. At this congress, E. Rothlin was elected as president with J.Delay, P.H.Hoch, H.Hoff and D.M. Shepherd as vice presidents. Many of the great names in psychopharmacology were associated with the formation of the CINP. Several of them are still alive. Clearly a career in psychopharmacology is good for both physical and mental health!

My first contact with the CINP came in 1964 when Philip Bradley, one of the founder members, organised the 4th international congress in Birmingham University, England, where I had obtained my undergraduate and postgraduate training. By present standards, the 1964 congress was a very small, but friendly, affair in which youngsters at the start of their careers could easily interact with the senior researchers who were contributing to the rapid advance of this relatively new field. This proved to be a major turning point in my own career that, as a result of the congress, moved from pharmacology and neurochemistry to psychopharmacology and an interest in the biology of psychiatric disorders.

The present volume, produced as part of the excellent series of monographs by the history committee, is an occasion for reflection on the tremendous strides that been made in psychopharmacology since the CINP was founded. As a young lecturer, I remember the excitement generated by the discovery of the mechanism of action of the depressogenic antihypertensive drug reserpine and the monoamine re-uptake inhibitory properties of the first tricyclic antidepressant imipramine. For the first time it was possible to provide a reasonable explanation not only for the mode of action of monoamine oxidase inhibitor and tricyclic antidepressants but also for the psychopathology of depression. The amine theory of depression, that still forms the basis of drug development today despite its many limitations, arose from these early discoveries. At that time, the first neuroleptic, chlorpromazine, had been shown to effectively control the positive symptoms of schizophrenia. The later discovery that chlorpromazine blocked the dopamine receptor (there was only one dopamine receptor in those halcyon days!) in the brain opened up a new era of schizophrenic research. The discovery that meprobamate, an analogue of the muscle relaxant mephenesin, was an effective anxiolytic at doses that did not cause marked sedation, soon revolutionised the treatment of anxiety. Thus by the mid-1960s major advances had been made in the effective treatment of the three major types of psychiatric disorder. For the first time in the history of psychiatry, it was possible not only to control the symptoms of these disorders with drugs but also to begin to establish the biochemical basis of the disorders.

Such revolutionary changes did not occur purely by chance. They were related to the development of sensitive techniques for the detection and quantification of biologically active molecules by paper and column chromatography, and by spectrophotometry and fluorimetry, in brain tissue. High-speed centrifuges enabled the preparation of synaptosomes and the elucidation of sub-cellular mechanisms controlling the synthesis, release and metabolism of monoamine neurotransmitters. Electrophysiological techniques, such as patch clamping and the recording of evoked potentials enabled a more dynamic appreciation of drug-induced changes in the rodent brain to be explored. These technical advances acted as a trigger to the development of psychotropic drugs. The establishment of the first neuroscience courses in many universities in Europe, North America and elsewhere coincided with the increasing impact of psychopharmacology. This was a very exciting time for any young researcher who had an interest in brain function. More importantly, the discovery of reasonably safe and effective psychotropic drugs changed the clinical management of psychiatric disorders to such an extent that the lifetime incarceration of severely mentally ill patients in psychiatric hospitals became a thing of the past. Psychotropic drugs brought hope to millions of patients and their families, a situation that has become even more apparent in recent years.

Having spent a professional lifetime in psychopharmacology, both in academia and in the pharmaceutical industry, and having witnessed the phenomenal progress that has been made in experimental and clinical neuroscience over the past 40 years, I am frequently astounded by the negative attitude of the mass media, public commentators and even some psychiatrists to the advances that have been made. Of course, there have been, and are, problems that result from overenthusiastic use of potent psychotropic drugs that necessitate effective legislation to ensure the safety and efficacy of all drugs. Yes, pharmaceutical companies have frequently been found wanting in terms of the safety and efficacy of the drugs they have marketed. The Food and Drug Administration in the United States, and the corresponding Medicines Review Boards elsewhere, were established in response to the public concerns over the safety of drugs marketed by the pharmaceutical industry. But the fact remains that the development of psychotropic drugs over the past 50 years has contributed more to the effective treatment of psychiatric disorders than any other a rea of psychiatry.

The history of psychopharmacology for the past 50 years has been a reflection of the history of the CINP. I am confident that the impact of this organisation on both basic and clinical research will be even greater in the future. The present monograph of the history committee, chaired by Ronaldo Ucha Udabe, will serve to illustrate the outstanding contributions to the field and especially to the neurotransmitter era by some of our senior members. I am certain that the coming 50 years will more than vindicate my optimism regarding the importance of the CINP and its role in the development and application of drugs for the treatment of the mentally ill.

PART ONE

THE FOUNDATION

OF NEUROPSYCHOPHARMACOLOGY

CHAPTER 1

THE DAWN OF THE NEUROTRANSMITTER ERA IN NEUROPSYCHOPHARMACOLOGY

Alfred Pletscher

The middle of the twentieth century can be considered as the starting point of a new era in the pharmacotherapy of psychiatric disorders. At its origin were members of two new classes of drugs, namely the neuroleptics reserpine and chlorpromazine, and the antidepressants iproniazid and imipramine. These drugs had the advantage of being more effective and specific than the then available drugs (e.g., barbiturates, opiates, phenylethylamines) and seemed to exert a new quality of action in combating mental disorders like schizophrenia and depression. The indications of the drugs for these conditions were all discovered by serendipity in the course of clinical practice. In fact both, reserpine submitted to clinical trials for its blood pressure-lowering effect (Bein, 1956), and chlorpromazine prepared for use as antihistaminic (Charpentier, 1947), found unexpected application as neuroleptics. Also both, iproniazide synthesized as an agent against tuberculosis (Fox and Gibas, 1953), and imipramine thought to act as a hypnotic (Kuhn, 1957), surprisingly revealed antidepressant activity in man. (Lithium, whose psychotropic effect had also been discovered in the clinic, was not included in this paper, because it did not have a relevant role in neurotransmitter research, at least in the early period). However, the mechanisms of action of the new drugs were not known. Certainly not many psychiatrists at the time would have predicted that their psychotropic effects were connected with changes of low molecular weight chemicals, such as aromatic amines, in the central nervous system. This situation began to change when pharmacologists and biochemists discovered that some of the new drugs caused profound alterations in the dynamics of aromatic monoamines (also called biogenic amines) in the brain. These amines, in particular serotonin, norepinephrine and (later on) dopamine had been found to be normal constituents of the brain, where they were suspected to exert a specific function. The first indications that psychotropic drugs interfered with cerebral monoamines were based on experiments with reserpine and iproniazid. Subsequently other neuropsychotropic compounds were observed to affect these amines and the findings, which finally extended beyond the realm of aromatic monoamines, contributed essentially to the establishment of the neurotransmitter hypothesis of neuropsychotropic drug action.

In this chapter the early contributions of basic research to the neurotransmitter hypothesis of neuropsychotropic drug action, based on the available scientific literature and personal experience, will be summarized.

SEMINAL FINDINGS

The first experiments with reserpine and iproniazid will be reported in some detail, because they are considered to be important for initiating the new era of neuropsychopharmacology.

RESERPINE

Reserpine, an indole alkaloid, is a constituent of the plant Rauwolfia serpentina, which was traditionally used in Indian folk medicine for its psychosedative properties. The alkaloid had been isolated and prepared by chemical synthesis in the Swiss pharmaceutical company Ciba S.A. (now merged in Novartis S.A.). Reserpine was introduced in the treatment of hypertension because in animal experiments it lowered blood pressure (Bein, 1956). When used in clinical practice, quite unexpectedly, the substance also showed antipsychotic activity. The psychotropic effect of reserpine stimulated the interest of Bernard B. Brodie at the National Institutes of Health (NIH), Bethesda, Maryland in the USA. In his laboratory, reserpine was found to exert some pharmacological effects similar to those of serotonin, a biogenic monoamine that had been previously reported to occur in the brain (Amin et al., 1954; Twarog and Page, 1953), and to have a physiological function in the central nervous system (Gaddum, 1953a; Wooley and Shaw, 1954). In Brodie's laboratory both reserpine and serotonin were shown to exhibit sedative effects and potentiate the hypnotic action of hexobarbital in mice by a central mechanism (Shore et al., 1955a). The potentiation caused by either of these two substances was antagonized by lysergic acid diethylamide (LSD) (Shore et al., 1955b), a substance previously reported to block the effects of serotonin on smooth muscles (Gaddum, 1953b), and to produce psychotic states in man (Stoll, 1947). These findings led to the hypothesis that reserpine might exert its psychotropic action by interfering with serotonin in the brain. Further experiments with dogs confirmed this hypothesis. In fact, reserpine increased the urinary excretion of 5-hydroxyindolacetic acid (5-HIAA) (Shore et al., 1955b), the major metabolite of serotonin (Udenfriend et al., 1956).

The direct proof that reserpine can release serotonin from body stores was obtained by direct measurements of the amine in the tissues. Since the available colorimetric assay method for serotonin was not sensitive enough for measuring the amine in the brain, the first experiments were perfomed in the intestine of rabbits, because this tissue exhibits a high concentration of the amine (localized in the enterochromaffine system). The results showed that parenteral application of reserpine caused a dose-dependent, rapid and almost complete depletion of the amine and that several days were required for repletion of the stores (Pletscher et al., 1955). This motivated research to measure serotonin in the brain of rabbits, where serotonin concentration is more than ten times lower than that in the intestine. Determinations of serotonin in the brain became possible because the prototype of a highly sensitive spectrophoto-fluorimeter (developed at the NIH of USA) became available (Bowman et al., 1955). The results obtained with reserpine corresponded to those found in the intestine: the drug caused a rapid, dose-dependent depletion of cerebral serotonin, with a very slow recovery of the amine stores. Simultaneously with the serotonin depletion the animals became sedated and showed symptoms of cholinergic stimulation (e.g., miosis) (Pletscher et al., 1956). Among the diff e rent available Rauwolfia alkaloids only those with a sedative action caused depletion of cerebral serotonin (Brodie et al., 1956a). These experiments indicated that reserpine, concomitantly with its psychotropic action, released serotonin from its stores in the brain and other tissues in which the amine was protected from its metabolizing enzyme monoamine oxidase (MAO). The liberat-ed serotonin becomes accessible to MAO and is degraded, leading to the formation of 5-HIAA and increased urinary excretion of this metabolite of serotonin. The findings in brain supported the hypothesis that the psychotropic effect of reserpine might be mediated through interf e rence with the cerebral dynamics of serotonin. The reason why changes in serotonin metabolism led to the tranquillizing effect of reserpine was not clear. According to a later hypothesis it was assumed that the tranquillizing effect results from neuronal depletion of monoamine transmitters and the consequent inter-fe rence with neurohumoral transmission (Pletscher, 1965).

IPRONIAZID

The hydrazide derivative iproniazid, a derivative of the tuberculostatic drug isoni-azid, was prepared by Hoffmann-La Roche S.A., U.S.A. (Fox and Gibas, 1953) in o rder to improve the tuberculostatic effect of the parent compound. In clinical tri-als, iproniazid showed therapeutic activity in patients with tuberculosis, but in addi-tion, surprisingly it also exhibited mood-elevating activity in various clinical condi-tions (Pletscher et al., 1960). Therefore the drug was introduced as a therapeutic agent for mental depression. At the same time (i.e., in the early 1950s), but inde-pendent of the clinical findings in tuberculosis, other investigators discovered that iproniazid was a potent irreversible inhibitor of MAO (Zeller and Barsky, 1952; Zeller et al., 1952). In animals, a single dose of iproniazid caused a moderate ele-vation of cerebral serotonin, which lasted for several days. No overt behavioral or autonomic effects of the drug were observed. However, pre t reatment of the animals with iproniazid attenuated the reserpine-induced decrease of cerebral serotonin (Pletscher, 1956). Thereby reserpine no longer caused sedation and miosis, but the animals showed arousal and sympathetic stimulation (e.g., mydriasis) (Besendorf and Pletscher, 1956; Brodie et al., 1956b). Iproniazid administered after reserpine, i.e., when the cerebral serotonin depots were exhausted, had no influence on the reserpine-induced behavioral and autonomic effects. Isoniazid, which caused no marked inhibition of MAO, neither affected cerebral serotonin levels nor influenced the reserpine-induced serotonin depletion, and had no effect on the behavioral and autonomic alterations induced by reserpine.

The counteraction of the biochemical and behavioral effects of reserpine by the antidepressant iproniazid was of interest since reserpine was known to occasionally produce mental depression in patients. The results with the combined administration of iproniazid and reserpine led to a tentative hypothesis on the mechanism of action of iproniazid. In animals pretreated with iproniazid, the relatively high amounts of serotonin released by reserpine from the presynaptic stores were thought to accumulate in the synaptic cleft due to MAO-inhibition, inducing arousal and sympathetic stimulation by serotonin's action on postsynaptic receptors. Iproniazid, given alone, was thought to increase the synaptic serotonin released by physiological nerve impulses in the course of neurohumoral transmission. This (relatively minor) accumulation of synaptic serotonin would lead to the antidepressant action in man. In animals such an effect of iproniazid alone could not be detected by gross observation.

The findings with iproniazid, especially those with the combined administration of iproniazid and reserpine, provided additional evidence that alterations of the serotonin dynamics in brain might be connected with the psychotropic action of drugs.

EARLY DEVELOPMENT

The initial hypothesis that changes in serotonin dynamics might be related to mental effects of neuropsychotropic drugs was subject to criticism by psychiatrists and pharmacologists. Nevertheless, it was an important starting point for the neurotransmitter hypothesis and stimulated further research. However, it needed corrections and additions. Thereby new findings with neuroleptics and antidepressants as well as developments with levodopa have been at the center of interest.

NEUROLEPTIC DRUGS

RESERPINE-TYPE DRUGS

Serotonin-depletion was soon shown not to be the only effect of reserpine on neurotransmitter dynamics. Biological and spectrophotofluorimetric methods for catecholamine determinations revealed that the drug also depleted noradrenaline and dopamine from the animal brain (Carlsson et al., 1957a; Holzbauer and Vogt, 1956) and that the time course of this decrease was similar to that of serotonin. Therefore, catecholamines (and serotonin) had to be considered as candidates involved in the behavioral effects of reserpine, although the role of the individual amines for the psychotropic effect of reserpine remained to be elucidated. The "serotonin hypothesis" became the "aromatic monoamine (biogenic amine) hypothesis".

Experiments with a new chemical class of compounds, i.e., the benzo(a)quinolizines, confirmed this view. In fact, several derivatives of this class, e.g., tetrabenazine and Ro 4-1284 caused a marked but relatively short-lasting (8-12 hours) decrease of cerebral serotonin, an increase of urinary 5-HIAA and, as later found, also a depression of noradrenaline and dopamine in brain (Pletscher, 1957; Pletscher et al., 1962). The effects of benzoquinolizines on the amines were paralleled by reserpine-like sedation. In addition, both the amine-lowering and behavioral actions of the new compounds were counteracted by pretreatment with iproniazid. These experiments showed that a connection between reserpine-like sedation and amine depletion was not confined to reserpine, but also existed for a different class of chemical compounds (i.e., the benzoquinolizines). This confirmed the biogenic amine hypothesis. It was only later, by other investigators, that the mechanism of action of reserpine-type of drugs at the cellular level, i.e., their interference with the vesicular amine transporter (VAT), was clarified. However, the role of the individual amines (serotonin and catecholamines) for the behavioral effects of the drugs remained unclear.

PHENOTHIAZINE-TYPE DRUGS

Chlorpromazine (a phenothiazine) and haloperidol (a butyrophenon) showed neuroleptic action in man, but in contrast to reserpine, did not markedly influence the brain concentration of biogenic amines, including dopamine. However, they increased the cerebral levels of catecholamine- and especially dopamine-metabolites, e.g., 3-methoxytyramine and homovanillic acid (Anden et al., 1963; Carlsson and Lindqvist, 1963; Laverty and Sharman, 1965). This was taken as evidence, that neuroleptics blocked dopamine receptors that, by a feedback mechanism, led to an enhancement of dopamine turnover. Blockade of dopamine receptors provided also an explanation for some of the beneficial effects of neuroleptics in schizophrenia and for some side effects of the drugs, e.g., tardive dyskinesia.

ANTIDEPRESSANTS

The first two classes of modern antidepressants, the MAO-inhibitors and tricyclic antidepressants were shown to interfere with cerebral monoamine dynamics. Their effect on biogenic amines was found to be due to different mechanisms of action.

MAO-INHIBITORS

As described before, the pioneer of this class is iproniazid. Further experiments showed that antidepressant activity was not restricted to compounds of the hydrazide type, but also occurred with MAO-inhibitors (e.g. tranylcypramine, parg y-line) of other chemical classes. On the other hand, hydrazides without relevant MAO-inhibitory action (e.g. isoniazid) did not show antidepressant effect (Pletscher et al., 1960, 1965). These findings supported the hypothesis, that the antidepressant action was causally related to MAO-inhibition and alterations of monoamine dynamics. The question which of the individual biogenic amines was responsible for the clinical action of MAO-inhibitors (MAOIs) could however not be solved (as in the case of reserpine-type drugs), because the drugs interf e red with the metabolism of s e rotonin as well as of catecholamines.

TRICYCLIC COMPOUNDS

The first re p resentative of this class was imipramine, a tertiary amine dibenzazepine. It showed antidepressant effect in man, but did not relevantly inhibit MAO. However, it antagonized the behavioral syndrome elicited by reserpine and the benzoquinolizine Ro 4-1284 in animals. This antagonism depended on the level of the imipramine metabolite desmethylimipramine in the brain and also on the release of s to red noradre n a l i n e. In fact, the anti-reserpine action was blunted after depletion of cerebral noradrenaline by αmethyltyrosine, an inhibitor of noradrenaline synthesis (Sulser et al., 1961, 1964). Other experiments clarified the cellular mechanism of action of tricyclic antidepressants. They showed that these drugs blocked the uptake of noradrenaline (Axelrod et al., 1961) and serotonin into the brain neurons. Secondary amine antidepressants (e.g., desipramine, DMI) were more potent than the tertiary amine antidepressants (e.g., imipramine) in inhibiting the transport of noradrenaline, whereas the tertiary amine antidepressants were more selective in inhibiting this transport of serotonin (Carlsson et al., 1969).

Thus, tricyclic compounds, similar to MAOIs, seemed to enhance the synaptic concentrations of monoamines released from presynaptic stores. This probably explained the antidepressant effect, although the mechanisms of action of the two classes of drugs differed (inhibition of monoamine uptake and MAO respectively).

MONOAMINE PRECURSORS

Interest in levodopa, the biological precursor of dopamine, was raised by the discovery that dopamine occurs in relatively high concentrations in the brain centers responsible for the control of extrapyramidal movements (e.g., the striatum) (Carlsson et al., 1958). Also, levodopa antagonized the motor depression and the decrease of cerebral dopamine induced by reserpine (Carlsson et al. 1957b). This led to the assumption that dopamine was involved in the regulation of extrapyramidal motor activity. Indeed, in the striatum of deceased patients with Parkinson's disease dopamine concentration was markedly lower than that in controls (Ehringer and Hornykiewicz, 1960), and in patients suffering from Parkinson's disease the urinary excretion of dopamine was found to be diminished, indicating a dopamine deficiency (Barbeau et al., 1961a). Administration of levodopa (which in contrast to dopamine does cross the blood-brain barrier leading to an increase of cerebral dopamine by its decarboxylation) caused symptomatic improvement in Parkinson patients (Barbeau et al., 1961b, Birkmayer and Hornykiewicz, 1961; Cotzias et al., 1967). This action of levodopa was improved by simultaneous administration of an inhibitor of extracerebral decarboxylase (i.e., benserazide), which protected the amino acid from further metabolism and inactivation in the extracerebral tissues (Bartholini et al., 1967). These findings supported the hypothesis that dopamine itself was a neurotransmitter, whereas up to then the amine had been considered to be a mere intermediate in the biosynthesis of noradrenaline and adrenaline. In addition, the results with exogenous levodopa provided further support for the involvement of aromatic monoamines in neuropsychotropic drug action.

CONSEQUENCES OF THE SEROTONIN HYPOTHESIS

Early developments extended the original serotonin hypothesis, since they showed, that amines other than serotonin (i.e., catecholamines) were involved in neurotransmission. Furthermore, the neurotransmitter hypothesis was confirmed by the findings, that numerous neuropsychotropic drugs of different pharmacological classes interfered with the cerebral dynamics of aromatic monoamines. It was thought that this interference is causally connected with the clinical action of the drugs although the functional role of the individual monoamines was not entirely clear for all the drug classes.

IMPLICATIONS FOR NEUROPSYCHIATRY

In the course of its development, the neurotransmitter hypothesis has extended far beyond the effects of its original "actors", the aromatic monoamines. Numerous other neurotransmitters and neuromodulators, including peptides, have been discovered. In addition, an impressive knowledge of other elements of the neurotransmitter system has been acquired, e.g., receptors, receptor subtypes, transport systems, signaling molecules, transfer factors, genetic elements. The neurotransmitter hypothesis of neuropsychopharmacology, i.e., the hypothesis that the clinical effects of psychotropic drugs are causally related to alterations in neurotransmitter dynamics, now has a firm basis. However, many problems remain to be solved, e.g., the question of the mechanisms by which neurohumoral changes lead to psychotropic effects. Also, the functional roles of the individual transmitters and their mutual interactions are still not yet clear in all aspects. Even the physiopathology of the neurotransmitter "pioneers" serotonin and catecholamines has not yet been fully elucidated. Nevertheless, the introduction of the transmitter concept added a new dimension to psychiatry, namely biological neuropsychopharmacology. For many psychiatrists and pharmacologists the dawn of the neurotransmitter era has initiated a change or introduced a new paradigm in their understanding of the mechanisms of action of neuropsychotropic drugs.

The increasing knowledge of the neurotransmitter systems had also practical consequences for drug research. Thus, already in the early period, the various elements of the monoaminergic system could be used as targets for the development of new, potentially useful drugs. For instance, determinations of amine release from the animal brain helped to screen for reserpine-like drugs, and estimations of dopamine turnover by measurements of dopamine metabolites in vivo were helpful for the development of neuroleptic drugs. Also, MAO-inhibition in vivo and in vitro was a lead for the development of antidepressants of the iproniazid type, and interference with amine uptake in brain slices, synaptosomes and blood platelets as well as the reserpine and benzoquinolizine reversal was used to screen for potential new imipramine-like antidepressants. A special case is levodopa whose discovery as a therapeutic agent in Parkinson's disease was based on biochemical research, which led to successful clinical trials in man. Subsequent to these early developments, in which random screening played an important role, pharmaceutical research has gained considerable further momentum. For instance, the progress in the physico-chemical sciences enabled the exact elucidation of the molecular nature and configuration of neurotransmitter elements, such as receptor- and transport proteins. This has opened new possibilities for a more rational and hopefully more efficient design of novel types of drugs, interacting with these structures.

In conclusion, the dawn and early success of the neurotransmitter hypothesis, which resulted from an attentive interaction between clinical observation and basic research, opened a new paradigm in neuropsychopharmacology and promoted the development of modern neuropsychotropic drugs.

ABSTRACT

The neurotransmitter hypothesis in neuropsychopharmacology originated from the aromatic monoamine hypothesis. Its protagonists were drugs of the neuroleptic and antidepressant class, whose novel type of clinical action had been discovered by serendipity in the course of clinical application. Subsequent basic research revealed that the drugs interfered with neurotransmitters. Reserpine and iponiazid were the first modern psychotropic drugs shown to change the cerebral dynamics of aromatic monoamines (i.e., serotonin and catecholamines) by affecting neuronal amine storage and inhibition of MAO respectively. Similar biochemical changes occurred with drugs of other chemical classes, exerting reserpine- and iproniazid-like clinical actions. Also, imipramine-type antidepressants and chlorpromazine-type neuroleptics were found to affect cerebral monoamines, i.e., by interfering with their uptake at the neuronal membrane, and by enhancing dopamine turnover respectively, the latter as a consequence of blockade of dopamine receptors. The changes in monoamine dynamics paralleled the clinical action of the drugs.

The original monoamine hypothesis initiated the neurotransmitter era in neuropsychopharmacology, introducing a new paradigm in psychiatry. Also, it provided novel screening tests and new leads (e.g., levodopa) in the search for modern neuropsychotropic drugs.

REFERENCES
1. Amin, A.H., Crawford,T.B., Gaddum, J. H., 1954. The distribution of substance P and 5-hydroxytryptamine in central nervous system of the dog. J. Physiol. 126, 596-618.
2. Andén, N.E., Roos, B.E., Werdinius, B., 1964. Effect of chlorpromazine, haloperidol and reserpine on the level of phenolic acids in rabbit corpus striatum. Life Sci. 3, 149-158.
3. Axelrod, J., Whitby, L.B., Hertting, G., 1961. Effect of psychotropic drugs on the uptake of ^{3}H-norepinephrine by tissues. Science 133, 383-384.
4. Barbeau, A., Murphy, G.F., Sourkes, T., 1961a. Excretion of dopamine in diseases of basal ganglia. Science 133, 1706-1707.
5. Barbeau, A., Sourkes, T. L., Murphy, G.F., 1961b. Les catécholamines dans la maladie de Parkinson. In : De Ajuriaguerra J., (Ed.), Monoamines et système nerveux central. Symposium Bel-Air/Genève 1961. Georg, Genève et Masson, Paris, pp. 247-262.
6. Bartholini, G., Burkard, W.P., Pletscher, A., Bates, H.M., 1967. Increase of cerebral catecholamines caused by 3,4-dihydroxyphenylalanine after inhibition of peripheral decarboxylase. Nature 215, 852-853.
7. Bein, H.J., 1956. Pharmacology of Rauwolfia. Pharmacol. Rev. 8, 435-483.
8. Besendorf, H., Pletscher, A., 1956. Beeinflussung zentraler Wirkungen von Reserpin und 5-Hydroxytryptamin durch Isonikotinsäurehydrazide. Helv. Physiol. Acta 14, 383-390.
9. Birkmayer W., Hornykiewicz, O., 1961. L-3-4-Dihydroxyphenylalanin (=Dopa)-Effekt bei Parkinson Akinese. Wien. Klin. Wschr. 73, 787-788.
10. Bowman, R.L.,Caulfield, P.A., Udenfriend, S., 1955. Spectrophotometric assay in the visible and ultraviolet. Science 122, 32-33.
11. Brodie, B.B., Shore, P.A., Pletscher A., 1956a. Limitation of serotonin-releasing activity to those alkaloids possessing tranquilizing action. Science 123, 992-993.
12. Brodie, B.B., Pletscher, A., Shore, P.A., 1956b. Possible role of serotonin in brain function and in reserpine action. J. Pharmacol. Exp. Therap. 116, 9.
13. Carlsson, A., Lindqvist, M., 1963. Effect of chlorpromazine on formation of 3-methoxytyramine and normetanephrine in mouse brain. Acta pharmacol. (Kbh.) 20, 140-144.
14. Carlsson. A., Rosengren, E., Bertler, A., Nilsson, J., 1957a. Effect of reserpine on the metabolism of catecholamines. In: Garattini, S., Ghetti, V. (Eds.), Psychotropic Drugs. Elsevier, Amsterdam, pp.363-372.
15. Carlsson, A., Lindqvist, M.. Magnusson, T., 1957b. 3,4-Hydroxyphenylalanine and 5-hydroxytryptophan as reserpine antagonists. Nature 180, 1200-1201.
16. Carlsson, A., Lindqvist, M., Magnusson, T., Waldeck, B., 1958. On the presence of 5-hydroxytyramine in brain. Science 127, 471-473.
17. Carlsson, A., Corrodi, H., Fuxe, K. Höckfelt, T., 1969. Effect of antidepressant drugs on the depletion of intraneuronal 5-hydroxytryptamine stores caused by 4-a-ethyl-meta-tyramine. Eur. J. Pharmacol. 5, 357-366.
18. Charpentier, P., 1947. Sur la constitution d'un diméthylamino-N phenothiazine. C.R. hebd. Séance Acad. Sci. 225, 306-308.

19. Cotzias, G.C., van Woert, M.H., Schiffer, L.M., 1967. Aromatic amino acids and modification of Parkinsonism. New Engl. J. Med. 276, 374-379.
20. Ehringer, H., Hornykiewicz, O., 1960. Verteilung von Noradrenalin und Dopamin (3-Hydroxytyramin) im Gehirn des Menschen u. ihr Verhalten bei Erkrankungen des extrapyramidalen Systems. Klin. Wschr. 38, 1236-1239.
21. Fox, H.H., Gibas J.T., 1953. Synthetic tuberculostats. VII. Monoalkyl derivatives of isonicotinylhydrazine. J. org. Chem. 18, 994-1002.
22. Gaddum, J.H., 1953a. Drugs antagonistic to 5-hydroxytryptamine. In: Ciba Foundation Symposium on Hypertension. Churchill, London.
23. Gaddum J.H., 1953b. Antagonism between lysergic acid diethylamide and 5-hydroxytryptophan. J. Physiol. 121, 15.
24. Holzbauer, M., Vogt, M., 1956. Depression by reserpine of the noradrenaline concentrations in the hypothalamus of the cat. J. Neurochem. 1, 8-11.
25. Kuhn, R., 1957. Die Behandlung depressiver Zustände mit einem Iminodibenzylderivat (G 22355). Schweiz. Med. Wschr. 87, 1135-1140.
26. Laverty, R., Sharman, D.F., 1965. Modification of drugs of the metabolism of 3,4-dihydroxyphenylethylamine, noradrenaline and 5-hydroxytryptamine in the brain. Br. J. Pharmacol. 24, 759-772.
27. Pletscher, A., 1956. Beeinflussung des 5-Hydroxytryptamin-stoffwechsels im Gehirn durch Isonikotinsäurehydrazide. Experientia 12, 479-480.
28. Pletscher, A., 1957. Release of 5-hydroxytryptamine by benzoquinolizine derivatives with sedative action. Science 126, 507.
29. Pletscher, A., 1965. Biogenic amines. In: Bente, D., Bradley P.B. (Eds.), Neuro-psychopharmacology, volume 4. Elsevier Publishing Company, Amsterdam, pp. 16-23.
30. Pletscher, A., Shore, P. A., Brodie, B.B., 1955. Serotonin release as a possible mechanism of reserpine action. Science 122, 374-375.
31. Pletscher, A., Shore, P.A., Brodie, B.B., 1956. Serotonin as a modulator of reserpine action in brain. J. Pharmacol. Exp. Ther. 116, 84-89.
32. Pletscher, A., Gey, K.F., Zeller, P., 1960. Monoaminooxydase-Hemmer: Biochemie, Chemie, Pharmakologie, Klinik. In: Jucker, E. (Ed.), Progress in Drug Research, vol.2. Birkhäuser Verlag, Basel/Stuttgart, pp. 417-590.
33. Pletscher, A., Brossi, A., Gey, K.F., 1962. Benzoquinolizine derivatives: a new class of monoamine decreasing drugs with psychotropic action. Internat. Rev. Neurobiol. Volume 4. Academic Press Inc., New York, pp. 275-306.
34. Pletscher, A., Gey, K.F., Burkard, W.P., 1965. Inhibitors of monoamine oxidase and decarboxylase of aromatic amino acids. In: Eichler, O., Farah, A. (Eds.), Handbook of Experimental Pharmacology, Volume 19. Springer Verlag, Berlin/Heidelberg/New York, pp. 593-735.
35. Shore, P.A., Silver, S.L.,Brodie, B.B., 1955a. Interaction of serotonin and lysergic acid diethylamide (LSD) in the central nervous system. Experientia 11, 272-273.
36. Shore, P.A., Silver, S.L., Brodie, B.B., 1955b. Interaction of reserpine, serotonin and lysergic acid diethylamide in brain. Science, 122, 284-285.
37. Stoll, W.A., 1947. Lysergsäurediaethylamid, ein Phantasticum aus der Mutterkorngrouppe. Schweiz. Arch. Neurol. Psychiat. 60, 279.
38. Sulser, F., Watts, J., Brodie, B.B., 1961. On the mechanism of antidepressant action of imipramine-like drugs. Ann. N.Y. Acad. Sci.96, 270-296.
39. Sulser, F., Bickel, M.H., Brodie, B.B., 1964. The action of desmethylimipramine in counteracting sedation and cholinergic effects of reserpine-like drugs. J. Pharmacol. Exp. Therap. 144, 321-330.
40. Twarog, B.M., Page, I.H., 1953. Serotonin content of some mammalian tissues and urine and its determination. Am. J. Physiol. 175,157-161.
41. Udenfriend, S., Titus, E., Weissbach, H., Peterson, R.E., 1956. Biogenesis and metabolism of 5-hydroxyindole compounds. J. Biol. Chem. 219, 335-344.
42. Woolley, D.W., Shaw, E., 1954. A biochemical and pharmacological suggestion about certain mental disorders. Science 119, 587.
43. Zeller, E.A., Barsky, J.,1952. In vivo inhibition of liver and brain monoamine oxidase by 1-isonicotinyl-2-isopropyl hydrazine. Proc.exp.biol. N.Y. 81, 459-461.

44. Zeller, E.A., Barsky, J., Berman, E.R., Fouts, J.R., 1952. Action of isonicotinic acid hydrazide and related compounds on enzymes involved in the autonomic nervous system. J. Pharmacol. Exp. Ther. 106, 427-428.

CHAPTER 2

MY FIRST TEN YEARS AT NIH:
THE DAWN OF PSYCHOPHARMACOLOGY

Irwin J. Kopin

I arrived at the National Institute of Health (NIH) of the United States in 1957, at the dawn of a new age that saw the birth and early development of biological psychiatry and neuropsychopharmacology. I had completed two years of internship and residency training in internal medicine at Boston City Hospital and entered the US Public Health Service to fulfill my military service obligation. I was hired by Dr. Philippe Cardon as a clinical associate to select and care for relatively healthy schizophrenic patients that had been screened for either a strong family history of schizophrenia or complete absence of any first-degree relative with schizophrenia. These patients were to be subjects that were to be studied for biochemical abnormalities in a protocol that was designed by Dr. Seymour Kety, who many regard as the father of biological psychiatry. Kety had recently stepped down from being the scientific director of the National Institute of Mental Health (NIMH) to head the Laboratory of Clinical Science (LCS) in that Institute.

Kety saw the opportunities opened by the recent discoveries that indicated that chemicals could alter mind and behavior and that furthering understanding of brain function and therapeutic approaches to the treatment of psychiatric disorders would be derived from biochemical studies of psychoses. He fostered the growth of the research program in the LCS by following an approach to "directing" science that is best expressed in his own words, quoted from an interview with Phil Holzman, then professor of psychiatry at McLean Hospital in Belmont, Massachusetts: "I had confidence that the best way to direct people's interest toward mental illness was by having it directed by themselves. One could hope that this could be accomplished in a consortium of scientists working in their own field but getting together once in a while at lunch, at conferences, learning a little bit about mental illness and perhaps finding out how something they were interested in might fit into the picture" (Personal communication).

There were weekly seminars in which recent findings and reviews of developments that had sewn the seeds of a veritable therapeutic revolution in psychiatry. Until the early 1950s, psychiatrists were limited in their ability to treat patients with major psychosis. Psychotherapy and shock treatment, with insulin-induced hypoglycemia or electrical current, were the main therapeutic interventions. In the early 1950s the realization that chemicals could alter brain function and possibility that drugs might be used to treat psychoses emerged. There was a confluence of evidence that biogenic amines were implicated in the pathogenesis of the major psychoses, schizophrenia and depression. The awakening of interest in hallucinogens and the discovery of the effects of drugs such as chlorpromazine, monoamine oxidase inhibitors (MAOIs) and reserpine, provided strong indications that chemical alterations could affect brain function.

In 1952, Humphrey Osmond and John Smythies, who had recently immigrated to Canada from England, thought that the hallucinations produced by lysergic acid diethylamide (LSD) and mescaline would provide clues about thought abnormalities in schizophrenia and were studying their effects in normal subjects, including themselves (see Hoffer et al., 1954). Osmond had read about how LSD had been accidentally discovered by Hofmann in Switzerland. The compound was first synthesized in a search of ergot-like compounds that might be useful in the treatment of migraine headaches. Hofmann had discovered, by self-administration of the drug, that it caused "dizziness, feeling of anxiety, visual distortions, symptoms of paralysis, desire to laugh" as he later recounted his early description of the hallucinogenic effects of the drug (Hofmann, 1979). Mescaline had been found to be the most potent component of peyote, a cactus plant used for centuries in Mexico to induce a "mystic state" with hallucinations (Heffter, 1897). It was Osmond (1957) however, who called attention to the structural similarity of mescaline to adrenaline. Also, there had been anecdotal reports that, during World War II, when supplies of fresh adrenaline ran short and adrenaline from old stock that had turned slightly pink was used, presumably due to spontaneous oxidation to adrenochrome, some patients had experienced temporary hallucinations. In 1954, Abraham Hoffer, Osmond and Smythies promulgated the theory that adrenochrome was an endogenous hallucinogen that was responsible for the development of schizophrenia (Hoffer et al., 1954). In 1953, Osmond had provided English author Aldous Huxley with a dose of mescaline, and one-year later Huxley's book "*The Doors of Perception*" detailed his hallucinatory experiences after taking this drug (Huxley, 1954). The title comes from a quote from William Blake: "If the doors of perception were cleansed everything *would* appear to man as it is, infinite." (Blake, 1792). But most psychiatrists did not adhere to the notion in this new culture that the hallucinatory experiences from mescaline and LSD were "mind expanders." Based on observations that LSD could antagonize the peripheral effects of the recently discovered amine, serotonin, and the structural similarity between these two indole-containing structures, Wooley and Shaw (1954) suggested that the hallucinogenic effects of LSD might result from an antagonism or mimicking of the actions of serotonin in the central nervous system.

Chlorpromazine was developed as a potentially better antihistamine, but was found to have a strong sedative effect. When Henry Laborit, a French surgeon, tried it as a pre-anesthetic sedative, he found that the patients developed a "euphoric quietude." (Laborit et al., 1952). A fellow surgeon described this remarkable effect to his brother-in-law, Pierre Deniker, an assistant to Jean Delay, head of the psychiatry department at Sainte Anne Hospital in Paris. Delay and Deniker (1952a, b) were the first to report the therapeutic efficacy of chlorpromazine in psychotic patients and introduced the term "neuroleptic" to describe the actions of this drug. Unmanageable patients became manageable, catatonic patients became mobile and other schizophrenic symptoms abated. The US Food and Drug Administration (FDA) approved the use of chlorpromazine in 1954 and although patients were not completely symptom-free, mental hospitals retained fewer patients and the field of psychopharmacology was born.

Another fortuitous series of events began with the discovery in 1945 by Chorine that nicotinamide had a bacteriostatic effect on the tuberculosis bacillus (Chorine, 1945). This prompted a search for related drugs that might be useful to treat tuberculosis and isonicotinylhydrazine (isoniazid) and its isopropyl derivative, 1-isonicotinyl-2-isopropyl hydrazine (iproniazid, Marsilid) emerged as candidates for clinical trials (Bloch et al., 1954). Since all bases had been reported to inhibit bacterial diamine oxidase, Albert Zeller and his colleagues examined the mode of action of these two hydrazine derivatives by studying their effect on amine oxidases *in vitro* and found that they inhibited monoamine oxidase (MAO). Iproniazid, the more potent of these agents, inhibited liver and brain MAO when administered to animals (Zeller et al., 1952). Meanwhile, in the clinical trials with tubercular patients, it was noted that some of the patients treated with iproniazid felt too good (Bloch et al., 1954). Their general behavior belied the lack of improvement of their X-rays; they overexerted themselves, generally ignored appropriate medical safeguards, and were inappropriately elated. Some patients became clearly manic. These observations prompted the initiation of studies of iproniazid in psychiatric patients. Jean Loomer and Nathan Kline, who was the research director at Rockland State Hospital, first reported the usefulness of iproniazid as a "psychic energizer" in the treatment of depression (Loomer et al., 1957). The potential market for an effective antidepressant and need for an alternative drug necessitated by the hepatotoxic and other side effects of iproniazid fueled the search for more specific and less toxic MAOIs. During the next few years, over 100 hundred other compounds were reported to inhibit MAO and iproniazid was replaced by other MAOIs (Zeller and Fouts, 1963).

After Ulf von Euler had definitively identified norepinephrine (NE) as the sympathetic neurotransmitter in peripheral tissues (Euler, 1948), in 1954, Marthe Vogt showed that NE was not only also present in brain, but was distributed in a manner that indicated it was likely a neurotransmitter in specific brain regions (Vogt, 1954). Serotonin was first isolated from blood in 1948 in Irving Page's laboratory (Rapport et al., 1948) and in 1953 was reported by Betty Twarog and Page to be present in the central nervous system (Twarog and Page, 1953).

The introduction of reserpine provided the final link implicating brain amines to mental disorders. For many centuries, the root of the snakeroot plant, Rauwolfia serpentina, was used in India for treating snakebites, but it came to be used for treating anxiety, insomnia, and "general insanity" (Gupta et al., 1943) and high blood pressure (Bhatia, 1942). Dr. Rustom Vakil's report that *serpina,* made from dried root of

Rauwolfia serpentina "has a definite place in the treatment of cases of high blood pre s-sure," brought this first successful treatment for hypertension into Western medicine (Vakil, 1949). This prompted Ciba to put reserpine on the market as an antihypertensive agent (Wilkins and Judson, 1953). It was soon found to cause depression in some patients (Achor et al., 1955; Harris, 1957). When reserpine was discovered to deplete brain amines (serotonin, NE and dopamine) another link of brain function to amines was established (Brodie et al., 1957; Carlssson, 1959; Holzbauer and Vogt, 1956).

At about the time I arrived at NIH, results of a series of studies of LSD were being completed by collaborative efforts of investigators from several institutes. Lou Sokoloff, Seymour Perlin, Conan Kornetsky and Kety studied the effects of LSD on cerebral circulation and overall metabolism in human (Sokoloff et al., 1957). Julius Axelrod, Roscoe Brady, Bem h a rd Witkop and Ed Evarts examined the distribution and metabolism of LSD in animals (Axelrod et al., 1957). In an electrophysiologic study that addressed the visual system, Ed Evarts and Wade Marshall looked at the effects of LSD on the excitability cycle of the lateral geniculate in cats (Evarts and Marshall, 1957) while Conan Kornetsky (1957) examined the relationship of physiological and psychological effects of LSD in humans. In the National Heart Institute, Albert Sjoerdsma was studying patients with malignant carcinoid, tumors that secrete serotonin and with K o rnetsky and Evarts, he examined the effects of LSD in these patients with excess s e rctonin (Sjoerdsma et al., 1957). Finally, the antidiuretic effect of LSD in humans was the subject of investigation by Marian Kies and others (Kies et al., 1957).

The studies on LSD having been mostly completed, the research focus shifted to studies of catecholamines and serotonin. Since I was obtaining spinal fluid samples for diagnostic purposes from these patients, I was able to use a portion of the fluid in an attempt to find 5-hydroxyindoleacetic acid (5-HIAA), the metabolite of serotonin. As indicated above, Al Sjoerdsma's group, in the Heart Institute, had recently described serotonin as the biogenic amine secreted by malignant carcinoid tumors (e.g., Sjoerdsma and Udenfriend, 1955). Because brain also had been shown to contain serotonin, it appeared reasonable to try to determine if 5-HIAA was present in spinal fluid. Dr. Marian Kies, Chief of the Section on Biochemistry in the LCS, was writing a book on experimental allergic encephalitis and allowed me to use her space. I tried to desalt the spinal fluid and perform paper chromatography, but there was too little 5-HIAA to detect using this method. I attended Kety's seminars and because of the interest that I had shown and the laboratory work that I was doing, Dr. Kety asked me to join the research associate program that had been started that year; he became my mentor and that changed the course of my professional career.

The discussions in the seminars encouraged testing of the reports of biological abnormalities in schizophrenia. Lauer et al. (1958) in Zeller's laboratory reported that after ingestion of 5 grams "load" of tryptophan, schizophrenics, unlike normal subjects, failed to excrete higher urinary concentrations of 5-HIAA. Kety asked me to confirm that finding. I repeated the study, but collected 24-hour urine specimens. In agreement with Lauer et al. (1958), I found that the concentrations of 5-HIAA in urine from schizophrenics were indeed lower than in normal subjects, but the volumes of urine from the schizophrenics were 3-fold greater. The increases in amounts of 5-HIAA, however, were the same (Kopin, 1959). The difference in urine volumes was the result of the enthusiasm of the nursing staff encouraging the patients to drink large amounts of water to ensure adequate urine flow to facilitate the collection of the specimens, whereas this was not necessary in normal subjects.

The 1952 Nobel Prize in Chemistry was awarded to Martin and Synge for their development of partition chromatography and paper chromatography had become a staple in biochemistry laboratories as a means of separating and identifying substances in urine. Jay Mann and Elwood LaBrosse applied this method to examine the excretion of phenolic acids, known to be the metabolites of amines, since there had been reports of the appearance in the urine of schizophrenics a "spot" that was absent in the urine of no mal subjects (Mann and Labrosse, 1959). I remember the initial excitement in the laboratory when they found such a spot; the spot was present in the urine in 9 of 10 schizophrenics and absent from the urine in 9 of 10 of the normal volunteer subjects. The one schizophrenic patient who did not excrete that compound was younger than the other patients and behaved differently. The one normal volunteer who did excrete the compound was older that the others and also had different habits than the younger Mennonite volunteers. It was soon determined that the compound was derived from coffee, which the Mennonites did not drink. Also, all the schizophrenic subjects drank coffee, except for the younger patient whose urine did not contain the compound. Number of other "spots" that seemed to distinguish schizophrenic from normal subjects also were found to have a dietary origin (see e.g., Closs et al., 1967).

Julius Axelrod, who had been investigating the metabolism of drugs, attempted, unsuccessfully, to identify adrenochrome in blood, but he and Stephen Szara found none (Szara et al., 1958). A breakthrough came when Marvin Armstrong and his coworkers reported that 3-methoxy-4-hydroxy-D-mandelic acid (vanillylmandelic acid, VMA) was a major urinary metabolite of NE (Armstrong, et al., 1958). The metabolite was identified and quantified using paper chromatography; large amounts of VMA were found in the urine of patients with phaeochomocytoma, a catecholamine-producing tumor, usually of the adrenal medulla. The results of studies from Schayer's laboratory on the effects of iproniazid on the excretion of metabolites of ^{14}C-labeled epinephrine (EPI) and NE had provided convincing evidence that MAO was involved in the metabolism of these catecholamines (Schayer and Smiley, 1953). Armstrong had found the orally administered dihydroxymandelic acid (DHMA) resulted in the enhanced excretion of VMA and thought that the catecholamines were deaminated and subsequently O-methylated. Axelrod, however, examined the possibility that O-methylation preceded deamination. He discovered catechol-O-methyltransferase, showed that, as for all methylations, the methyl donor was S-adenosylmethionine and presented evidence that direct O-methylation of the catecholamines was the major route of metabolism of administered catecholamines (Axelrod et al., 1958, Axelrod and Tomchick, 1958). His identification of the O-methylated metabolites was dependent upon obtaining the authentic compounds. Shiro Senoh, the first Japanese visiting scientist to come to the NIH, working in Bernhard Witkop's Laboratory of Chemistry in the National Institute of Arthritis and Metabolic Diseases, now NIDDK, was assigned the task of synthesis of these compounds and three days later he delivered the O-methylated products, which had been named metanephrine (MN) and normetanephrine (NMN) (Axelrod et al., 1958).

About one year earlier, as a result of the increasing number of research grant proposals to the NIH that involved measurement of catecholamines, the Pharmacology and Experimental Therapeutics Study Section in the NIH Division of Research Grants decided that it was necessary to sponsor a Symposium on Catecholamines. This symposium was held in the Clinical Center at NIH in October of 1958, but at the time that the symposium was planned, the metabolites of the catecholamines had not been clearly demonstrated. From his discovery of DOPA decarboxylase, Blaschko described how he deduced correctly the biosynthetic pathway for formation of catecholamines. EPI, NE and dopamine had been shown to be substrates for MAO and, as indicated above, from early studies of the metabolism of ^{14}C-EPI, it was generally assumed that MAO metabolized catecholamines. However, relatively little else was known about the processes involved in chemical neurotransmission. Little or nothing was known about regulation of the formation of the neurotransmitter, mechanisms for its storage and release in response to a stimulus, the sequence of events that were involved in producing responses, or processes for inactivation of the released transmitter.

That first Catecholamine Symposium was remarkable. Five of the participants subsequently received Nobel prizes! Ulf von Euler, who was awarded the Prize in 1970, described the methods that were then being used for the assay of catecholamines in plasma, tissue and urine (Euler, 1959). Robert Furchgott, recipient of the Prize in 1998 for his discovery of nitric oxide as a signaling molecule, discussed receptors and how drugs acted at those sites (Furchgott, 1959). Rall and Sutherland (1959) presented for the first time the discovery of cyclic adenosyl monophosphate (cAMP), for which Sutherland received the 1971 Prize. Julius Axelrod, who shared the 1970 Prize with von Euler and Bernard Katz, reviewed his work on the discovery of O-methylation as the major route of catecholamine metabolism (Axelrod, 1959) and Arvid Carlsson, Nobel Laureate of 2000, showed the evidence that brain dopamine, which is present in high concentration in the striatum is involved in control of motor functions and that the parkinsonian-like syndrome produced by reserpine in rabbits could be reversed by treatment with L-dopa (Carlsson, 1959).

George Koelle, one of the organizers of the symposium, emphasized the importance of understanding how non-metabolic mechanisms may be involved in terminating the actions of NE released at nerve terminals. Koelle (1959) listed five such mechanisms, but could offer no experimental evidence to support any of these and none turned out to be correct. It was the introduction of isotopically labeled catecholamines that allowed further understanding of the metabolism and disposition of the endogenous catecholamines.

To better study the metabolism and disposition of catecholamines in humans, Kety arranged for the custom synthesis of tritium-labeled catecholamines of sufficiently high specific activity to allow administration of doses that would not elicit excessive physiologic responses. In 1959, I joined Julius Axelrod in the efforts to study catecholamine metabolism using some of the ^{3}H-NE that Kety made available to us. When given to rats, the major urinary metabolite was not VMA. We knew that its formation was blocked in animals treated with iproniazid and that the ^{3}H remained in the same site. After enzymatic hydrolysis with glusulase (sulfatase plus glucuronidase), but not glucuronidase, the radioactivity could be extracted into an organic solvent at neutral pH. To identify this compound, I synthesized 3-methoxy-4-hydroxyphenylglycol (MHPG) and we showed with paper chromatography in two solvent systems that it had the identical mobility as the hydrolysed tritiated metabolite (Axelrod et al., 1959). We also identified MHPG-sulfate as a minor catecholamine metabolite in human urine (Labrosse et al., 1961). 3,4-Dihydroxyphenylglycol (DHPG) was then found in the urine of rats that had been treated with pyrogallol to inhibit O-methylation (Kopin and Axelrod, 1960). At that time, we thought that the difference between humans and rats in the major urinary metabolite of the catecholamines was due to a species difference in the ratio of oxidation vs. reduction of the aldehyde formed by the deamination of the catecholamines. To study the magnitude of O-methylation vs. deamination as the initial metabolic inactivation of administered EPI in humans, I used a double label protocol that required ^{14}C-MN as well as ^{3}H-EPI (Kopin, 1960). I synthesized ^{14}C-methyl-S-adenosylmethionine (^{14}C-SAME) to use for the enzymatic preparation of the required labeled O-methylated EPI and used the product for studies in both animals (Kopin et al., 1961a) as well as in humans. That ^{14}C-SAME, and later ^{3}H-SAME, was used by Axelrod to discover a number of other methylating enzymes, including phenylethanolamine-N-methyl transferase (PNMT), which converts NE to EPI in the adrenal medulla (Axelrod, 1962). Axelrod and Weissbach (1961) discovered the melatonin-synthesizing enzyme, hydroxyindole-O-methyltransferase. We used that enzyme and the ^{14}C-SAME to make ^{14}C-melatonin and established that 6-hydroxymelatonin was the major melatonin metabolite (Kopin et al., 1961b).

When Julie Axelrod and his colleagues examined the tissue content of ^{3}H-NE after its intravenous administration, they found that much of the compound was retained in the tissues, particularly in the heart, long after the actions of the catecholamine had dissipated. This led Julie to speculate that the catecholamine was taken up into the sympathetic nerves. George Herttting, a visiting scientist from Vienna, suggested that removing the superior cervical ganglion of a cat and allowing the sympathetic nerves in the salivary gland and nictitating membrane to degenerate could test the idea (Hertting et al., 1961a). Julie's desk was at the far end, near the window, of his 12'x 24' laboratory. There was a 3' wide work bench on the right, a doorway to a second laboratory on the left, then work bench bearing a mechanical shaker for solvent extractions, and then a sink where Julie washed his own glassware. (He told a number of us that he got his best ideas while cleaning his glassware). Beyond that there was a blackboard that was set on the wall behind Julie's back when he sat at his desk. It was on that blackboard that the next experiments were outlined and I clearly remember the discussions and the diagram that outlined the experiment we were to perform to remove the superior cervical ganglion of cat and administer ^{3}H-NE. We found that uptake and retention of ^{3}H-NE in the excised tissues were markedly reduced after chronic, but not after acute, denervation (Hertting et al., 1961a). Furthermore, cocaine and other drugs known to potentiate the action of NE and nerve stimulation interfered with the uptake process (Whitby et al., 1960). Axelrod then instituted a series of experiments designed to determine the ability of various drugs to either inhibit the uptake into the heart of ^{3}H-NE or promote its release. The results of these studies, published in 1961, established the importance of reuptake of neurotransmitters as a means for terminating their action and as a site for the action of psychoactive drugs (Hertting et al., 1961b). These discoveries were the basis for Axerod's 1970 Nobel Prize.

During my first five years at NIH I had worked closely with Julie and we were co-authors on over a dozen papers, (e.g., many are cited in the references of this paper). In 1962, I was appointed a Section Chief and began independent research, although still collaborating with Julie on several projects. In subsequent studies with ^{3}H-NE administration, I found that there were differences in the metabolic products of the substance recovered in the urine during its initial metabolism or after tyramine-induced release of the retained ^{3}H-NE, and the metabolites excreted at later times or during reserpine-induced depletion of the tissue stores of retained ^{3}H-NE (Kopin and Gordon, 1962). We found that the predominant pathway when NE was in an active form, outside the neuron, was by O-methylation, whereas deamination predomimnated when the catecholamine was being metabolized intraneuronally, without having become active.

These and other important developments that were being contributed by basic scientists and clinicians around the world made clear the need for better communication among basic scientists and clinicians. It was against this background that during these fomative years of 1957-1967 that both the Collegium Internationale Neuropsychopharmacologicum and the American College of Neuropsychophamacology were founded and saw their early development and growth.

During my first ten years at NIH, a host of extremely talented young scientists came to NIH to work with Dr. Axelrod or with me, often with both. George Hertting, Lincoln Potter and Lionel Whitby had been among the first and participated in the earliest experiments. Among the many that followed were Sol Snyder, Richard Wurtman, Jacques Glowinsky, Leslie Iversen, Ross Baldessarini, Jose Musacchio, Joseph Fischer, Joseph Schildkraut, Saul Schanberg, George Breese, Tom Chase and Goran Sedvall. Glowinsky brought to the laboratory a method for intracysternal injection of ^{3}H-NE to study brain catecholamine metabolism (Glowinsky and Axelrod, 1964, 1965, Glowinsky et al., 1965). With Dick Wurtman, studies were expanded to include melatonin and the diurnal rhythm of pineal gland function (Wurtman and Axelrod, 1966). Others helped to initiate studies of false transmitters and their role in the hypotensive e ffects of MAOIs (Kopin et al., 1964). The brain amine metabolism studies continued and other investigations further contributed to our understanding the mechanisms of actions of sympathomimetic amines and other psychoactive drugs, tachyphylaxis, e ffects of neuronal activity on NE synthesis, etc (Axelrod et al., 1962; Potter et al., 1962). The investigations of biogenic amines were not confined to our laboratory or even the NIMH. For example, Toshi Nagatsu with Sid Udenfriend in the National Heart Institute discovered and characterized *tyrosine hydroxylase* (Nagatsu et al., 1964). Pletscher, Shore, Spector, Costa and others in Bern a rd Brodie's laboratory discovere d and investigated many aspects of reserpine's amine depleting effect, psychoactive drug metabolism and influence on biogenic amines, etc. (Brodie et al., 1957; Carlsson, 1959; Pletscher et al., 1956; 1957; Shore et al., 1957). The NIH was rapidly expanding, funding was generous and new ideas, concepts, and discoveries poured forth.

While Seymour Kety continued his research on the cerebral circulation, he also kept abreast of the developments relating brain amines reflecting a valuable perspective on the implications to psychiatry, particularly with regard to schizophrenia and depression (Kety, 1957, 1959a,b). The occurrence of depressive episodes in patients receiving reserpine that had been reported in the early 1950s and the observations that clinically effective antidepressants, imipramine and desmethylimipramine, inhibit the uptake of NE, led Schildkraut and Kety (1967) to propose, in 1967, the heuristic hypothesis that lack of NE was the fundamental abnormality that was responsible for depression. Kety's impact on understanding of the dynamics and imaging of cerebral blood flow and metabolism (Kety and Schmidt, 1948), his work on the genetics of schizophrenia, (Kety et al., 1968) and his thoughtful critiques, prophesies and heuristic hypotheses (Kety, 1957; 1959a,b) led to his receiving the Lasker Award For a Lifetime of Medical Achievements in 1999, less than one year before his death in 2000 at the age of 84. Julie retired in 1984, but remained active as a Scientist Emeritus at NIH until his death in December, 2004.

I was indeed fortunate to have as mentors two such nurturing and supportive outstanding scientists and will always be grateful that I was able to pursue a career at NIH that was not real work because there was nothing that I would have rather done.

REFERENCES

1. Achor, R.W., Hanson, N.O., Gifford, R.W., Jr., 1955. Hypertension treated with Rauwolfia serpentina (whole root) and with reserpine; controlled study disclosing occasional severe depression. J. Am. Med. Assoc. 159, 841-845.
2. Armstrong, M.D., Shaw, K.N., Gortatowski, M.J., Singer, H., 1958. The indole acids of human urine. Paper chromatography of indole acids. J. Biol Chem. 57, 763.
3. Axelrod, J., 1959. The metabolism of catecholamines in vivo and in vitro. Pharmacol. Rev. 11, 402-408.
4. Axelrod, J., 1962. Purification and properties of phenylethanolamine-N-methyl transferase. J. Biol. Chem. 237, 1657-1660.

5. Axelrod, J., Tomchick, R., 1958. Enzymatic O-methylation of epinephrine and other cate-chols. J. Biol. Chem. 233, 702-705.
6. Axelrod, J., Weissbach, H., 1961. Purification and properties of hydroxyindole-O-methyl transferase. J. Biol. Chem. 236, 211-213.
7. Axelrod, J., Brady, R.O., Witkop, B., Evarts, E.V., 1957. The distribution and metabolism of lysergic acid diethylamide. Ann. N.Y. Acad. Sci. 66, 350-444.
8. Axelrod, J., Inscoe, J.K., Senoh, S., Witkop, B., 1958. O-methylation, the principal pathway for the metabolism of epinephrine and norepinephrine in the rat. Biochim. Biophys. Acta 27, 210-211.
9. Axelrod, J., Kopin, I.J., Mann, J.D., 1959. 3-Methoxy-4-hydroxyphenylglycol sulfate, a new metabolite of epinephrine and norepinephrine. Biochim. Biophys. Acta 36, 576-577.
10. Axelrod, J., Gordon, E., Hertting, G., Kopin, I.J., Potter, L.T., 1962. On the mechanism of tachyphylaxis to tyramine in the isolated rat heart. Bri. Pharm. Chemother. 19, 56-63.
11. Bhatia, B.B., 1942. On use of Rauwolfia serpentina in high blood pressure. J. Indian M.A. 11,: 262-265.
12. Blake, W., 1792. The Marriage of Heaven and Hell. Reprinted Oxford University Press, Oxford, UK, 1975.
13. Bloch, R.G., Dooneieff, A.S., Buchberg, A.S., Spellman, S., 1954. The clinical effect of iso-niazid and iproniazid in the treatment of pulmonary tuberculosis. Ann. Intern. Med. 40, 881-900.
14. Brodie, B.B., Olin, J.S., Kuntzman, R.G., Shore, P.A., 1957. Possible interrelationship between release of brain norepinephrine and serotonin by reserpine. Science 125, 1293-1294.
15. Carlsson, A., 1959. The occurrence, distribution and physiological role of catecholamines in the nervous system. Pharmacol. Rev. 11, 490-496.
16. Chorine, V., 1945. Action de l'amide nicotinique sur les bacilles du genre mycobacterium. C. R. de l'Academie des Sciences (Paris) 220, 150–151.
17. Closs, K., N., Waden, E., Ose, S., 1967. The pink spot in schizophrenia. Nature 214, 483.
18. Delay J, Deniker P., 1952a. 38 cas de psychoses traitées par la cure prolongée et contin-ue de 4560 RP. C.R. Congr.Alién. Neurol. France 50, 503–513.
19. Delay, J., Deniker, P., 1952b. Le traitement des psychoses par une méthode neurolytique dérivée de l'hibernothérapie. C.R. Congr.Alién. Neurol. France 50, 497–502.
20. Euler, U.S., von, 1948. Identification of the sympathomimetic ergone in adrenergic nerves of cattle (sympathin N) with laevo-noradrenaline. Actaphysiol. Scandinav. 16,63-74.
21. Euler, U.S., von, 1959. The development and applications of the trihydroxyindole method for catecholamines. Pharmacol. Rev. 11, 262-268.
22. Evarts, E.V., Marshall, W.H., 1957. The effects of lysergic acid diethylamide on the excitability cycle of the lateral geniculate. Trans. Amer. Neurol. Ass. 80, 58-60.
23. Furchgott, R.F., 1959. The receptors for epinephrine and norepinephrine (adrenergic receptors). Pharmacol. Rev. 429-441.
24. Glowinsky, J., Axelrod, J., 1964. Inhibition of uptake of tritiated-noradrenaline in the intact rat brain by imipramine and structurally related compounds. Nature 204, 1318-1319.
25. Glowinsky, J., Axelrod, J., 1965. Effect of drugs on the uptake, release, and metabolism of H^3-norepinephrine in the rat brain. J. Pharmacol. Exp. Ther. 149, 43-49.
26. Glowinsky, J., Kopin, I.J., Axelrod, J., 1965. Metabolism of H^3-norepinephrine in the rat brain. J. Neurochem. 12, 25-30.
27. Gupta, J.C., Deb, A.K., Kahali, B.S., 1943. Preliminary observations on use of Rauwolfia serpentina Benth. In treatment of mental disorders. Indian M. Gaz. 78, 547-549.
28. Harris, T.H., 1957. Depression induced by Rauwolfia compounds. Am. J. Psychiatry.113, 950.
29. Heffter, A., 1897. Über Pellote. Arch. Exp. Path. Pharmakol. 40, 418-425.
30. Hertting, G., Axelrod, J., Kopin, I.J., Whitby, L.G., 1961a. Lack of uptake of catecholamines after chronic denervation of sympathetic nerves. Nature 189, 66-67.
31. Hertting, G., Axelrod, J., Whitby, L.G., 1961b. Effect of drugs on the uptake and metabo-lism of H^3-norepinephrine. J. Pharmacol. Exp. Ther. 134, 146-153.
32. Hoffer, R.A., Osmond, H,, Smythies, J., 1954. Schizophrenia; a new approach. II. Result of a year's research. J. Ment. Sci. 100, 29-45.

33. Hofmann, A., 1979. LSD: My Problem Child. McGraw-Hill, New York.
34. Holzbauer, M., Vogt, M., 1956. Depression by reserpine of the noradrenaline concentration in the hypothalamus of the cat. J. Neurochem. 1, 8-11.
35. Huxley, A., 1954. The Doors of Perception. Chatto & Windus Ltd, London.
36. Kety, S.S., 1957. The implications of psychopharmacology in the etiology and treatment of mental illness. Ann. N Y. Acad. Sci. 66, 836-840.
37. Kety, S.S., 1959a. Biochemical theories of schizophrenia: a two-part critical review of current theories and of the evidence used to support them. Science 129, 1528–1532, 1590–1596.
38. Kety, S.S., 1959b. Central actions of catecholamines. Pharmacol. Rev.. 11, 565-566.
39. Kety, S.S., Schmidt, C.F., 1948. The nitrous oxide method for the quantitative determination of cerebral blood flow in man: theory, procedure, and normal values. J. Clin. Invest. 27, 484–492.
40. Kety, S.S., Rosenthal, D., Wender, P.H., Schulsinger, F., 1968. The types and prevalence of mental illness in the biological and adoptive families of adopted schizophrenics. In: Rosenthal,D., Kety, S.S. (Eds.), The Transmission of Schizophrenia. Pergamon Press, Oxford,UK, pp 345–362
41. Kies, M.W., Horst, D., Evarts, E.V., Goldstein, N.P., 1957. Antidiuretic effect of lysergic diethylamide in humans. Arch. Neurol. Psychiat. 77, 267-269.
42. Koelle, G.B., 1959. Possible mechanisms for the termination of the physiological actions of catecholamines. Pharmacol. Rev. 11, 381-386.
43. Kopin, I.J., 1959. Tryptophan loading and excretion of 5-hydroxyindoleacetic acid in normal and schizophrenic subjects. Science 129, 835-836.
44. Kopin, I.J., 1960. Technique for the study of alternate metabolic pathways: Epinephrine metabolism in man. Science 131, 1372-1374.
45. Kopin, I.J., Axelrod, J., 1960. 3,4-Dihydroxyphenylglycol, a metabolite of epinephrine. Arch. Biochem. Biophys. 89, 148-149.
46. Kopin, I.J., Gordon, E.K., 1962. Metabolism of norepinephrine-H^3 released by tyramine and reserpine. J. Pharmacol. Exp. Ther. 138, 351-359.
47. Kopin, I.J., Axelrod, J., Gordon, E., 1961a. The metabolic fate of H^3-epinephrine and C^{14}-metanephrine in the rat. J. Biol. Chem. 236, 2109-2113.
48. Kopin, I.J., Pare, C.M., Axelrod, J., Weissbach, H., 1961b. The fate of melatonin in animals. J Biol Chem. 236:3072-3075.
49. Kopin, I.J., Fischer, J.E., Musacchio, J., Horst, W.D., 1964. Evidence for a false neurochemical transmitter as a mechanism for the hypotensive effect of monoamine oxidase inhibitors. Proc. Nat. Acad. Sci. (USA) 52, 716-721.
50. Kornetsky, C., 1957. Relation of physiological and psychological effect of lysergic acid diethylamide. Arch. Neurol. Psychiat. 77, 657-658.
51. Laborit, H., Huguenard, P., Alluaume, R., 1952. Un nouveau stabilisateur végétatif (le 4560 RP). Presse Med. 60, 206–208.
52. Labrosse, E.H., Axelrod, J., Kopin, I.J., Kety, S.S., 1961. Metabolism of 7-H^3-epinephrine-d-bitartrate in normal young men. J. Clin. Invest. 40, 253-260.
53. Lauer, J.W., Inskip, W.M., Bernsohn, J., Zeller, E.A., 1958. Observations of schizophrenic patients after iproniazid and tryptophan. AMA Arch. Neurol. Psychiatry 80, 122-130.
54. Loomer, H.P., Saunders, J.C., Kline, N.S., 1957. A clinical and pharmacodynamic evaluation of iproniazid as a psychic energizer. Psychiatr. Res. Rep. Amer. Psycchiat. Ass. 8, 129-141.
55. Mann, J.D., Labrosse, E.H., 1959. Urinary excretion of phenolic acids by normal and schizophrenic male patients Arch. of Gen. Psychiat. 1, 547-551.
56. Nagatsu, T., Levitt, M., Udenfriend, S., 1964. Tyrosine hydroxylase. The initial step in norepinephrine biosynthesis. J. Biol. Chem. 239, 2910-2915.
57. Osmond, H., 1957. A review of the clinical effects of psychotomimetic agents. Ann N.Y. Acad. Sci. 66, 418-434.
58. Pletscher, A., Shore, P.A., Brodie, B.B., 1956. Serotonin as a mediator of reserpine action in brain. J. Pharmacol. Exp. Ther., 116:84-89.
59. Potter, L.T., Axelrod, J., Kopin, I.J., 1962. Differential binding and release of norepinephrine and tachyphylaxis. Biochem. Pharmacol.11, 254-256.

60. Rall, T.W., Sutherland, E.W., Jr., 1959. Action of epinephrine and norepinephrine in broken cell preparations. Pharmacol. Rev. 11, 464-465.
61. Rapport, M.M., Green, A.A., Page, I.H., 1948. Serum vasoconstrictor (serotonin). IV. Isolation and characterization. J. Biol. Chem. 176, 1243–1251.
62. Schayer, R.W., Smiley, R.L., 1953. The metabolism of epinephrine containing isotopic carbon. J. Biol. Chemi. 202, 425.
63. Schildkraut, J.J., Kety, S.S., 1967. Biogenic amines and emotion. Science 156, 21-37.
64. Shore, P.A., Pletscher, A., Tomich, E.G., Carlsson, A., Kuntzman, R., Brodie, B.B., 1957. Role of brain serotonin in reserpine action. Ann. N. Y. Acad. Sci. 66, 609-615.
65. Sjoerdsma, A., Udenfriend, S., 1955. Studies on indole metabolism in patients with carcinoid (argentaffinoma). J. Clin. Invest. 34, 914-918.
66. Sjoerdsma, A., Kornetsky, C., Evarts, E.V., 1957. Lysergic acid diethylamide in patients with excess serotonin. Arch. Neurol. Psychiat. 75, 488-492.
67. Sokoloff, L., Perlin, S., Kornetsky, C., Kety, S.S., 1957. The effects of d-lysergic acid diethylamide on cerebral circulation and over-all metabolism. Ann. N.Y. Acad. Sci. 66, 468-477.
68. Szara, S., Axelrod, J., Perlin, S., 1958. Is adrenochrome present in blood? Amer. J. Psychiat. 115, 162-163.
69. Twarog, B.M., Page, I.H., 1953. Serotonin content of some mammalian tissues and urine and a method for its determination. Am. J. Physiol. 175, 157–161.
70. Vakil, R.J., 1949. Clinical trial of Rauwolfia serpentina in essential hypertension. Brit. Heart J. 2, 350-355.
71. Vogt, M., 1954. The concentration of sympathin in different parts of the central nervous system under normal conditions and after the administration of drugs. J. Physiol. 123, 451-481.
72. Whitby, L.G., Hertting, G., Axelrod, J., 1960. Effect of cocaine on the disposition of noradrenaline labelled with tritium. Nature 87, 604-605.
73. Wilkins, R.W., Judson, W.E., 1953. The use of Rauwolfia serpentina in hypertensive patients New Eng. J. Med. 248, 8-12.
74. Wooley, D.W., Shaw, E., 1954. A biochemical and pharmacological suggestion about certain mental disorders. Proc. nat. Acad. Sci. 40, 228-231.
75. Wurtman, R.J., Axelrod, J., 1966. A 24-hour rhythm in the content of norepinephrine in the pineal and salivary glands of the rat. Life Sci. 5, 665-669.
76. Zeller, E.A., Fouts, J.R., 1963. Enzymes as primary targets of drugs. Ann. Rev. Pharmacol. 3, 9-32.
77. Zeller, E.A., Barsky, J., Fouts, J.R., Kirschhimer, W.F., Van Orden, L.S., 1952. Influence of isonicotinic acid hydrazide (INH) and isonicotinyl-2- isopropyl hydrazide (IIH) on bacterial and mammalian enzymes. Experientia 8, 349-350.

PART TWO

NEUROTRANSMITTERS

CHAPTER 3

NOREPINEPHRINE AND THE NEUROTRANSMITTER ERA IN NEUROPSYCHOPHARMACOLOGY

Fridolin Sulser

CHEMICAL NEUROANATOMY: LOCALIZATION OF CATECHOLAMINE-CONTAINING NEURONAL SYSTEMS IN BRAIN

Historically, the *norepinephrine (NE) neurotransmitter era in neuropsychophar-macology* was triggered by the discovery of NE in brain (Vogt, 1954), the demonstration of monoamines in nerve cell bodies and nerve terminals in the central nervous system (CNS) (Carlsson et al., 1962) followed by the detailed mapping of monoaminergic neurons by histofluorescence techniques (Dahlstroem and Fuxe, 1964; Hillarp et al., 1966). Briefly, NE terminals in the brain are widely distributed from the spinal cord to the neocortex and are particularly abundant in the hypothalamus. The bulk of the cell bodies of the neurons containing NE are diffusely located in the reticular formation of the lower brain stem with the locus coeruleus containing the most abundant noradrenergic cell population. The axons of these cells ascend via the medial forebrain bundle and terminate as noradrenergic synapses in the hypothalamus, limbic system and cerebral cortex. The basic aspects of the regulation of biosynthesis and turnover of NE, its vesicular storage, its metabolism and reuptake have been extensively reviewed (Bloom and Giarman, 1968; Pletscher, 1973; Weiner, 1970). Evidence for a synaptic transmitter function of NE in the mammalian CNS has been established by electrophysiological and pharmacological criteria (Bloom and Hoffer, 1973; Salmoiraghi, 1966). The synaptic actions of NE were shown to be mimicked by iontophoretic application of cyclic adenosine monophosphate (cAMP) and the effect of both NE and cAMP, are potentiated by phosphodiesterase inhibitors (Hoffer et al., 1971; Siggins et al., 1971).

The development of spectrophotofluorometric methodology (Bowman et al., 1955) made it possible to analyse quantitatively minute amounts of biogenic amines in brain. Using this new methodology, Pletscher et al. (1955) demonstrated for the first time that reserpine's tranquilizing action is associated with a dose - dependent depletion of serotonin in brain. This finding was a historic finding as it catalysed the birth of the neurotransmitter era in neuropsychopharmcology and biological psychiatry.

BRAIN NOREPINEPHRINE AND THE ACTION OF PSYCHOTROPIC DRUGS

Five major classes of psychotropic drugs have been shown to influence central cat-echolaminergic activities: Reserpine – like drugs, monoamine oxidase (MAO) inhibitors, tricyclic antidepressants, amphetamine - like stimulants, phenothiazines and other neuroleptics. Since extensive reviews dealing with the action of these psychotropic drugs on various stages of the life cycle of catecholamines exist (e.g., Carlsson, 1983; Sulser and Sanders - Bush, 1971), this topic will be only briefly reviewed. Reserpine and related natural and semi - synthetic analogues and synthetic benzoquinolizines (e.g., tetrabenazine) deplete catechol - and indolealkylamines because of their interference with the intraneuronal storage of amines (Pletscher et al., 1968) leading to degradation by intraneuronal MAO and to an increase in the deaminated and O - methylated metabolites (e.g., homovanillic acid, 3-methoxy-4-hydroxyphenylglycol). Importantly, all Rauwolfia alkaloids and benzoquinolizine derivatives that cause depletion of NE (and dopamine and serotonin) in brain produce sedation in animals and man. The action of reserpine - like drugs on the vesicular storage of NE can explain the decreased sympathetic tonus (e.g., decrease in blood pressure) but the increased parasympathetic activity of reserpine (miosis, lacrimation) is not simply due to an escape from sympathetic control but rather to an increase in central parasympathetic activity (Bogdanski et al., 1961). A number of pharmacological observations catalysed the introduction of MAO inhibitors (MAOIs) for the treatment of depression: (1) The excitation which occurs in various species following the administration of MAOIs is associated with increased levels of NE in brain (Spector et al., 1960). (2) Pretraetment with MAOIs prevents the decrease in cerebral monoamines by reserpine - like drugs and benzoquinolizines and counteracts or "reverses" the sedative action of reserpine in various species (Carlsson et al., 1957). Experiments utilizing a push - pull cannula have provided data suggesting that the increased levels of NE in brain following MAO inhibition are associated with an increase in extra-neuronal NE. This increase, as measured for example in the perfusate from the hypothalamus (Strada and Sulser, 1972), is assumed to be the consequence of the rise in intraneuronal NE leading to a "spillover" from intraneuronal stores. The pharmacological and therapeutic issues associated with the introduction of MAO subtype-specific and reversible MAOIs are competently reviewed by Robinson and Kurtz (1987).

The clinical efficacy of tricyclic antidepressants could not have been predicted from pharmacological studies conducted prior to Ronald Kuhn's astute clinical observation that imipramine exerts antidepressant activity in patients with major depression (Kuhn, 1957). Then, in 1959, Ernest Sigg observed that imipramine enhanced and prolonged physiological responses to exogenous NE and to NE released by pre - or postganglionic sympathetic nerve stimulation suggesting that tricyclics may also exert their central effects by sensitisation to NE (Sigg, 1959).

This heuristic view was later validated when it was shown that the tricyclic antidepressant desipramine (DMI) failed to antagonize the reserpine- like syndrome in animals whose brain catecholamine stores had been selectively depleted with α - methyl - m-tyrosine, with its antireserpine ("antidepressant") action returning gradually as the levels of NE in brain returned to normal (Sulser et al., 1964). These findings, establishing an important role of NE in the "antidepressant" action of DMI - like drugs coincided with the simultaneous pivotal discoveries in Axelrod's and Brodie's laboratories demonstrating that the biological responses to NE are terminated by inhibition of the catecholamine reuptake at presynaptic noradrenergic nerve endings and that tricyclic antidepressants enhanced noradrenergic activity by blocking this neuronal reuptake of NE in peripheral and central neurons (Axelrod et al., 1961; Dengler et al., 1961). Tricyclic antidepressants act as competitive inhibitors of the high affinity uptake (uptake I) of NE (Berti and Shore, 1967; Maxwell et al., 1969). Uptake I is a saturable process and stereochemically selective for (R) – NE and involves a Na+/K± dependent carrier system (Iversen, 1973). Soon after the discovery of the NE reuptake inhibition by tricyclic antidepressants, it became evident that this class of drugs also inhibited the re-uptake of serotonin (5-HT) into central serotoninergic neurons with tertiary amines of tricyclics being more potent than the corresponding secondary amines in inhibiting the transport of 5-HT whereas the secondary amines were more selective in inhibiting the re-uptake of NE (Carlsson et al., 1969).

Amphetamine and structurally related compounds affect the CNS by releasing preferentially newly synthesized catecholamines (Besson et al., 1969), with dopamine being mainly responsible for stereotyped activity (Randrup and Scheel-Krueger, 1966) whereas dopamine and/or NE appear to be required for locomotor stimulation and aggressive behaviour. In species in which hydroxylation of the aromatic ring of amphetamine is a major metabolic pathway the in vivo formation of the "false transmitter" p-hydroxynorephedrine may be responsible for some of the pharmacological actions of amphetamine. The experimental and clinical aspects of amphetamine and related compounds have been comprehensively reviewed by Costa and Garattini (1970). Since antipsychotic agents including phenothiazines, thioxanthenes and butyrophenones are believed to predominantly affect dopaminergic mechanisms, these drugs will not be reviewed here.

The pharmacological observations - depletion of NE by reserpine-like drugs associated with depressive symptomatology in man (Freis, 1954; Mueller et al., 1955); increased availability of NE by either MAOIs or tricyclics associated with antidepressant activity - provided the experimental rationale for the clinically relevant catecholamine hypotheses of affective disorders (Bunney and Davis, 1965; Schildkraut, 1965). The evolution of these hypotheses reflects the changes over the years in our understanding of the mode of action of antidepressant drugs (Pryor and Sulser, 1991).

THE NORADRENERGIC SECOND MESSENGER CASCADE: SWITCH FROM PRESYNAPTIC TO POSTSYNAPTIC RECEPTOR – MEDIATED EVENTS

While the early studies on the action of psychotropic drugs on NE in brain were focused on *presynaptic* events - synthesis, storage, release, metabolism and reuptake of NE - in the mid 1970's, inspired by the work of Earl W.Sutherland and T.W. Rall (1960), a switch from presynaptic to *postsynaptic* receptor – second messenger mediated events occurred. Catecholamine receptor mediated second messenger cascades and the activation of protein kinases followed by phosphorylation of substrate proteins which serve as up - and down - stream physiological effectors (neurotransmitter receptors, ion pumps, ion channels, transcription factors) were explored. NE activates both protein kinase A (PKA) via the β-adrenoceptor coupled adenylate cyclase - cAMP pathway and protein kinase C (PKC) via the α_1-adrenoceptor coupled phospholipase C - diacylglycerol pathway.

With regards to the action of psychotropic drugs on noradrenergic "post-receptor" events, studies from our laboratory demonstrated that treatment with antidepressants on a clinically relevant time basis - pharmacotherapy with MAOIs and tricyclic antidepressants and also electroconvulsive treatment - caused subsensitivity of the NE-β-adrenoceptor coupled adenylate cyclase system in limbic and cortical structures of the rat brain (Vetulani and Sulser, 1975; Vetulani et al., 1976). This reduced sensitivity was generally accompanied by a decrease in the density of β-adrenoceptors (Banerjee et al., 1977). The desensitisation of the β-adrenoceptor coupled adenylate cyclase system following chronic but not acute administration of antidepressants was quickly confirmed (Bergstrom and Kellar, 1979a, b; Pandey et al., 1979; Schultz, 1976; Wolfe et al., 1978). The desensitisation and/or the down - regulation of β-adrenoceptors following chronic treatment with noradrenergic antidepressants is the consequence of agonist mediated receptor phosphorylation by PKA and possibly by the second messenger independent protein kinase, β-adrenoceptor kinase (Benovic et al., 1986; Premont et al., 1995). The elucidation of the agonist–β-adrenoceptor-coupled second messenger transduction cascade represents one of the highlights of molecular neurobiology. The β-adrenoceptor belongs to the large family of G-protein coupled transmembrane receptors with multiple trans-membrane - spanning domains (Dixon et al., 1988). NE- β-adrenoceptor systems consist of at least 3 separate protein components involved in the transfer of the NE signal: Receptor protein, the enzyme adenylate cyclase and the guanine nucleotide regulatory protein (G protein) with its binding site for GTP. The molecular events leading to the activation of the enzyme and the formation of the second messenger cAMP, the biochemical properties of the three individual components of the system and the role of receptor kinases in G protein coupled receptor regulation have been comprehensively reviewed (Krupnick and Benovic, 1998; Limbirid, 1981; Ostrowski et al., 1992; Rodbell, 1980; Ross and Gilman, 1980). The question arose of whether the de-amplification of the NE– β-adrenoceptor coupled adenylate cyclase system following chronic treatment with antidepressants is reflected beyond the second messenger cAMP or whether the desensitisation reflected a compensatory mechanism to offset the increased synaptic availability of NE (due to either MAO inhibition or blockade of the reuptake of NE) with the overall rate of the NE signal transduction being unchanged. Results from our laboratory demonstrating that chronic administration of the noradrenergic antidepressants desipramine (DMI) and reboxetine down-regulated the biologically active form of the nuclear transcription factor CREB (CREB-P) in the frontal cortex of rats (Manier et al., 2002) - despite the persistent increase in the availability of NE - seem to support the notion of a *net* de-amplification of the NE signal. A number of *in vivo* effects following chronic treatment with antidepressant drugs on the expression of target genes containing cAMP response enhancer elements (CRE) in their promoter region are consistent with this interpretation, [e.g., down-regulation of genes for tyrosine hydroxylase, β_1-adrenoceptors, corticotrophin releasing factor (CRF)]. The results indicating a *net* de-amplification of the NE signal are also consistent with biochemical studies showing a reduction in the NE–β-adrenoceptor-cAMP mediated formation of melatonin in the pineal gland (Heydorn et al., 1982) and a reduction in N–acetyltransferase activity (Friedman et al., 1984) following chronic administration of antidepressants. Since patients with a diagnosis of major depression display a pronounced and sustained central noradrenergic hyperactivity (Wong et al., 2000), it could be argued that the apparent therapeutic superiority of noradrenergic antidepressants over selective 5-HT uptake inhibitors in major depression (Montgomery, 1998) could be due to the slowly developing desensitisation of the NE signal transduction by stabilizing the de-amplification of the NE signal at the level of the β-adrenoceptor coupled adenylate cyclase system. The findings of Stone (1979) demonstrating that chronic foot shock stress desensitises the NE sensitive adenylate cyclase system in the rat cortex and that the loss of β-adrenoceptors correlated positively with the degree of adaptation, are of interest in this regard. Stone has proposed that this decrease in sensitivity to NE may play a role in the adaptation to emotional and physiological stress and that effective antidepressant treatments mimic the desensitising actions of stress on central NE receptor systems.

THE CONVERGENCE OF AMINERGIC NEUROTRANSMITTER AND ENDOCRINE SIGNALS BEYOND THE RECEPTORS

Because all clinically effective antidepressants increase the synaptic availability of NE and/or 5-HT or are converted *in vivo* to metabolites which, in concert with the parent drugs, affect both neurotransmitters, research has focused on the convergence of aminergic signals beyond the GTP-coupled membrane receptors: NE-β-adrenoceptor- cAMP mediated activation of PKA and 5-HT receptor mediated activation of PKC via the second messenger diacylglycerol. Hoefler et al. (1989) have developed a hypothetical model for the convergence of two proteinkinase pathways at the level of transcriptional activation by phosphorylation of hypothetical transcription factors. Using the transcription factor CREB in human fibroblasts, results from our laboratory (Manier et al., 2001) demonstrate the phosphorylation of this transcription factor via both the cAMP - PKA pathway by isoproterenol (β-adrenoceptor mediated) and PKC activation by the phorbolester phorbol 12 - myristate 13 acetate (PMA), leading to the suggestion that this convergence of the neurotransmitter signals at the level of protein kinase mediated phosphorylation may be a critical mechanism of the mode of action of antidepressant drugs.

Perhaps, when one individual neurotransmitter signal is relatively weak, the convergence of signals at the level of protein kinase mediated phosphorylation may overcome such a hypothetical weakness. Some clinical data add support to such a hypothesis. Thus, the addition of the 5-HT uptake inhibitor fluoxetine to the NE uptake inhibitor desipramine has been reported to enhance and hasten therapeutic efficacy (Nelson et al., 1991).

In vitro studies have added an entirely new and exciting perspective to the function of β-adrenoceptors. Thus, using C6 glioma cells in culture as a model system, Yoshikawa and Sabol (1986) have demonstrated that the transcription of the preproenkephalin gene is β-adrenoceptor mediated and synergistically regulated by glucocorticoids. Using the same cell culture it was shown that the transcription of the preproenkephalin gene is regulated via both adrenergic and serotonergic pathways (Eiring et al., 1992). These *in vitro* studies on receptor - receptor interactions are significant as the morphological organization of central monoamine systems have suggested a functional linkage of noradrenergic and serotonergic neurons ever since Dahlstroem and Fuxe (1964) demonstrated the neuronal localization of NE and 5-HT.

Glucocorticoids represent, in addition to NE and 5-HT, the third known physiologically important group of regulators of the β-adrenoceptor coupled adenylate cyclase system in brain (Harelson et al., 1987; Mobley et al., 1983; Roberts et al., 1984). The action of glucocorticoids seems to be mediated via the α_1–adrenergic component of NE receptors (Duman et al., 1985; Stone et al., 1986). The discovery of the regulatory role of glucocorticoids on the central β-adrenoceptor coupled adenylate cyclase mediated signal transduction is significant as glucocorticoid receptors have been identified immunocytochemically in the nuclei of NE and 5-HT cell bodies (Harfstrand et al., 1986). Since glucocorticoid receptor activation regulates gene expression by interaction with specific deoxyribonucleic acid (DNA) sequences in the promoter regions (Ringold, 1985), glucocorticoids may affect the diffusely projecting stress and antidepressant responsive monoamine systems in brain via modulation of transcription of pivotal genes. In this regard, the findings of Pariante et al. (1997) are of psychopharmacological interest. These authors demonstrated in L 929 cells that exposure to desipramine in the presence or absence of the synthetic steroid dexamethasone caused a significant translocation of glucocorticoid receptors from the cytoplasm to the nucleus. Though it is difficult to extrapolate from *in vitro* studies in cell culture to the *in vivo* situation, this action of a predominantly noradrenergic antidepressant (blockade of NE re-uptake) is intriguing as it represents another example of dual signalling. These findings of the convergence of aminergic neurotransmitter and glucocorticoid receptor signals have led to the formulation of the heuristic "Serotonin/NE/gluco-corticoid Link Hypothesis" of affective disorders (Pryor and Sulser, 1991) suggest-ing that the antidepressant - sensitive, 5-HT-linked and glucocorticoid responsive NE-β-adrenoceptor transduction system in brain functions as an amplification/adaptation system of vital physiological functions including mood, sleep, pain, neuroendocrine and central autonomic functions.

PERSPECTIVE

The pursuit of the *functional* implications of the action of NE on the trans-synaptic cascade as depicted in Figure 1 is a major and exciting goal of future research. Phosphorylation of the kinase - inducible domain of the transcription factor CREB is believed to allosterically change the conformation of the trans-activation domain which in turn leads to the transcriptional activation of genes containing the palin-dromic CRE sequence 5' - TGACGTCA - 3' (Hagiwara et al., 1993). The complexity of the biology of transcription factors such as CREB is increased by the demonstration of transcription factor cross - talk at the level of target gene promoters (Goettlicher et al., 1998). As pointed out by these authors, "learning to understand the mechanisms of action of this cross-talk will improve our knowledge on how well a cell fine-tunes its response to a multitude of incoming signals."

Since all currently available antidepressants and mood - stabilizing drugs activate and/or deamplify NE and/or 5-HT mediated receptor - transduction cascades, it is not surprising that these psychotropic drugs have been shown to cause changes in gene expression. We have advanced the heuristic concept of a "Central nervous sys-tem symphony orchestra composed of thousands of instruments (genes), suggesting that the pathogenesis of mental disorders involves a number of instruments (genes) producing dissonance by being played at the wrong times or for the wrong duration or amplitudes, compared with the same genes in a healthy CNS" (Rossby and Sulser, 1997). The identification of these genes and, importantly, the elucidation of their function remain great future challenges. Though this review has primarily been focused on *NE and the Neurotransmitter Era in Neuropsychopharmacology,* future research will have to consider the molecular communications in and between the t h ree major integrative systems, the *nervous,* the *endocrine* and the *immune* system, with their shared languages in receptor-transduction-transcription cascades. A more comprehensive understanding of the *molecular communication* in and between these three integrative receptor mediated transduction-transcription systems will add pertinent functional relevance to *NE and the Neurotransmitter Era in*

Neuropsychopharmacology and the molecular psychopathology of psychiatric disorders. (See Elkes in this volume: pp 2255 - 263).

Figure 1. The cAMP signal transduction pathway. Ligand-receptor (R) interaction activates coupled G proteins (G) which stimulate adenylyl cyclase activity (AC). As a consequence cAMP intracellular levels are increased. cAMP binds to the regulatory subunits of PKA, releasing the active catalytic subunits which migrate into the nucleus and phosphorylate a series of transcriptional activators. Phosphorylated activators bind to CRE in the promoter of responsive genes and modulate their expression. (From Lamas and Sassone-Corsi, 1997).

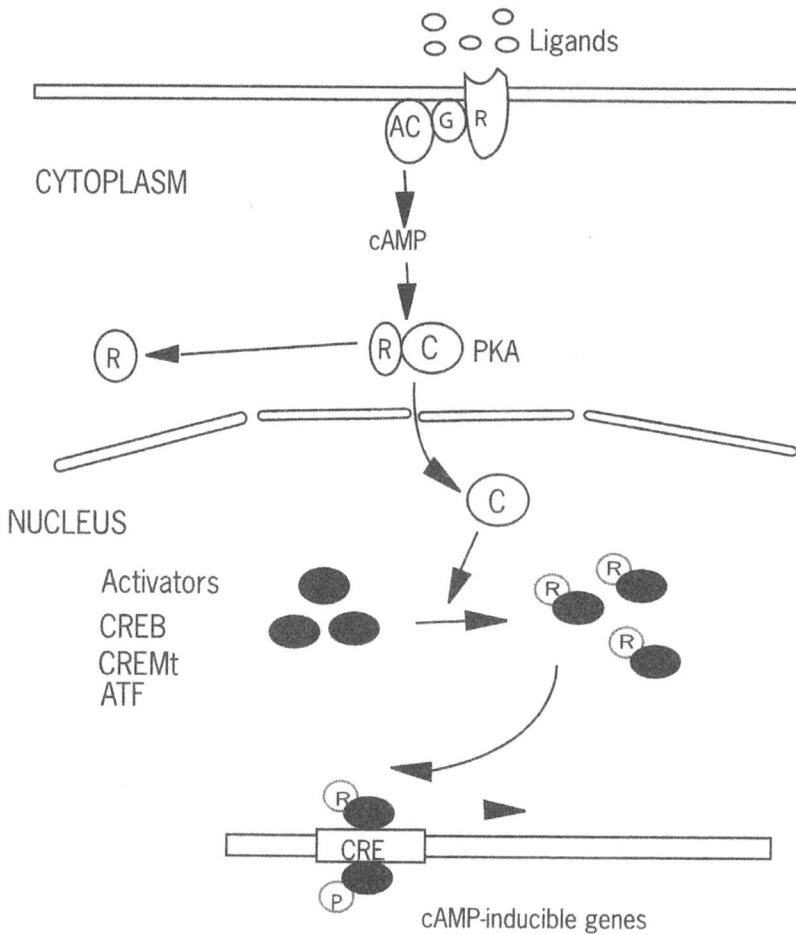

REFERENCES

1. Axelrod, J., Whitby, L.G., Hertting, G., 1961. Effect of psychotropic drugs on the uptake of ^{3}H – norepinephrine by tissues. Science 133, 383-384.
2. Banerjee, L.P., Kung, L.S., Riggi, S.T., Chanda, S.K., 1977. Development of noradrenergic subsensitivity by antidepressants. Nature 268, 455-456.
3. Benovic, J.L., Strasser, R.H., Caron, M.G., Lefkowitz, R.J., 1986. β–Adrenergic receptor kinase: Identification of a novel protein kinase that phosphorylates the agonist-occupied form of the receptor. Proc. Natl. Acad. Sci. USA 83, 2797-2801.
4. Bergstrom, D.A., Kellar, K.J., 1979a. Adrenergic and serotonergic receptor binding in rat brain after chronic desmethyl-imipramine treatment. J. Pharmacol. Exp. Ther. 209, 256-261.
5. Bergstrom, D.A., Kellar, K.J., 1979b. Effect of electroconvulsive shock on monoaminergic receptor binding sites in rat brain. Nature 278, 464-466.
6. Berti, F., Shore, P.A., 1967. A kinetic analysis of drugs that inhibit the adrenergic neuronal membrane amine pump. Biochem.Pharmacol. 16, 2091 - 2094.
7. Besson, M.J., Cheramy, A., Glowinski, J., 1969. Effects of amphetamine and desmethylimipramine on amine synthetis and release in central catecholamine – containing neurons. Europ. J. Pharmacol.7, 111 - 114.
8. Bloom, F.E., Giarman, J., 1968. Physiologic and pharmacologic considerations of biogenic amines in the nervous system. Ann. Rev. Pharmacol. 8, 229-258.
9. Bloom, F.E., Hoffer, B.J., 1973. Norepinephrine as a central synaptic transmitter. In: Usdin, E., Snyder, S. H. (Eds.), Frontiers in Catecholamine Research. Pergamon Press, New York, pp. 637-642.
10. Bogdanski, D.F., Sulser, F., Brodie, B.B., 1961. Comparative action of reserpine, tetrabenazine and chlorpromazine on central parasympathetic activity. J. Pharmacol. Exp. Ther. 132, 176-182.
11. Bowman, R.L. Caulfield, P.A., Udenfriend, S., 1955. Spectrophotofluorometric assay throughout the ultraviolet and visible range. Science 122, 32-33.
12. Bunney, W., Davis, J.M., 1965. Norepinephrine in depressive reactions. Arch. Gen. Psych. 13, 483-494.
13. Carlsson, A., 1983. Antipsychotic agents: Elucidation of their mode of action. In: Parnham, M.J., Bruinvels, J. (Eds.), Discoveries in Pharmacology, Vol 1. Elsevier Science Publishers, Amsterdam, pp. 197-206.
14. Carlsson, A., Rosengren, E., Bertler, A., Nilsson, J., 1957. Effect of reserpine on the metabolism of catecholamines. In: Garattini, S., Ghetti, V. (Eds.), Psychotropic Drugs. Elsevier Publishing Company, Amsterdam, pp. 363 – 372.
15. Carlsson, A., Falck, B., Hillarp, N.A., 1962. Cellular localization of brain monoamines. Acta Physiol. Scand. 56 (Suppl. 196), 1-27.
16. Carlsson, A. Corrodi, H., Fuxe, K., Hoekfelt, T., 1969. Effect of antidepressant drugs on the depletion of intraneuronal brain 5 – hydroxytryptamine stores caused by 4 – ethyl – meta – tyramine. Eur. J. Pharmacol. 5, 357-366.
17. Costa, E., Garattini, S. (Eds.), 1970. International Symposium on Amphetamines and Related compounds. Raven Press, New York, pp. 1- 962.
18. Dahlstroem, A., Fuxe, K., 1964. Evidence for the existence of monoamine containing neurons in the central nervous system. Demonsration of monoamines in the cell bodies of brain stem neurons. Acta Physiol. Scand. 62 (Suppl. 232), 1-55.
19. Dengler, H.J., Spiegel, H.E., Titus, E., 1961. Effect of drugs on uptake of isotopic norepinephrine by cat tissues. Nature 191, 816-817.
20. Dixon, R.A.F., Strader, C.D., Sigal, I.S., 1988. Structure and function of G- protein coupled receptors. Ann.Rep.Med.Chem. 23, 221 -233.
21. Duman, R.S., Strada, S.J., Enna, S.J., 1985. Effect of imipramine and adrenocorticotropin administration on the rat brain norepinephrine - coupled cyclic nucleotide generating system: Alterations in α and β components. J.Pharmacol. Exp. Ther. 234, 409-414.
22. Eiring, A., Manier, D.H., Bieck, P.R., Howells, R.D., Sulser, F., 1992. The "Serotonin/Norepinephrine/Glucocorticoid Link" beyond the β-adrenoceptors. Mol. Brain Res. 16, 211-214.

23. Freis, E.D., 1954. Mental depression in hypertensive patients treated for long periods with large doses of reserpine. N. Engl. J. Med. 251, 1006-1008.

24. Friedman, E.,Yocca, F.D., Cooper, T.D, 1984. Antidepressant drugs with varying pharmacological profiles alter rat pineal β-adrenergic mediated function. J.Pharmacol.Exp.Ther. 228, 545 - 550.

25. Goettlicher, M., Heck, S., Herrlich, P., 1998. Transcriptional cross-talk the second mode of steroid hormone receptor action. J. Molec. Med. 76, 480 - 489.

26. Hagiwara, M., Brindle, P., Harootunian, A., Armstrong, R., Rivier, J. Vale, W. Tsien, R., Montminy, M. R., 1993. Coupling of hormonal stimulation and transcription via the cyclic AMP - responsive factor CREB is rate limited by nuclear entry of protein kinase A. Mol. Cell Biol.13, 4852 - 4859.

27. Harfstrand, A., Fuxe, K., Cintra, A., Agnati, L.F., Zim, I., Wirkstrom, A.,, Okret, S., Yu, Z.L., Goldstein, M., Steinbush, H., Verhofstadt, A., Gustafsson, J.A., 1986. Demonstration of glucocorticoid receptor immunoreactivity in monoamine neurons of the rat brain. Proc. Natl. Acad. Sci. USA 83, 9779-9783.

28. Harrelson, A.L., Rosterre, W., McEwen ,B.S., 1987. Adrenocortical steroids modify neurotransmitter stimulated cyclic AMP accumulation in the hippocampus and limbic brain of the rat. J.Neurochem.48, 1648 – 1655.

29. Heydorn, W.E., Brunswick, F.T., Frazer, A., 1982. Effect of treatment of rats with antidepressants on melatonin concentrations in the pineal gland and serum. J. Pharmacol. Exp. Ther. 222, 534-543.

30. Hillarp, N.A., Fuxe, K., Dahlstroem, A., 1966. Demonstration and mapping of central neurons containing dopamine, noradrenaline and 5 - hydroxytryptamine and their reactions to psychopharmaca. Pharmacol. Rev. 18, 727 - 741.

31. Hoefler, J.P., Deutsch, P.J., Lin, J., Habener, J.F., 1989. Distinct adenosine 3',5' – monophosphate and phorbolester - responsive signal transduction pathways converge at the level of transcriptional activation by the interaction of DNA binding proteins. Molec. Endocrinol. 3, 868-880.

32. Hoffer, B.J., Siggins, G.R., Oliver, A.P., Bloom, F.E., 1971. Cyclic AMP mediation of norephrinephrine inhibition in rat cerebellar cortex: A unique class of synaptic responses. Ann. N.Y. Acad. Sci. 185, 531-549.

33. Iversen, L.L., 1973. Neuronal and extraneuronal catecholamine uptake mechanisms. In: Usdin, E, Snyder, S.H. (Eds.), Frontiers of Catecholamine Research. Pergamon Press, New York; pp. 403-408.

34. Krupnick, J.G., Benovic, J.L., 1998. The role of receptor kinases and arrestins in G protein – coupled receptor regulation. Ann. Rev. Pharmacol, Toxicol. 38, 289 - 319.

35. Kuhn, R., 1957. Über die Behandlung depressives Zustände mit einem iminodybenzylderivat (G 22355). Schweiz. Med. Wochenschr. 87, 1135-1140.

36. Lamas, M., Sassone – Corsi, P., 1997. Coupling transcription to signal transduction: CREM and cAMP. In: Papavissilion, A.G. (Ed.), Transcription Factors in Eukaryotes. Landes Bioscience, Austin, Texas, pp.51-65.

37. Limbird, L.E., 1981. Activation and attenuation of adenylate cyclase. The role of GTP binding proteins as macromolecular messengers, Biochem. J.195, 1-13.

38. Manier, D.H., Shelton, R.C., Sulser, F., 2001. Cross-talk between PKA and PKC in human fibrdlasts: What are the pharmacotherapeutic implications? J. Affect. Disord. 65, 275 -279.

39. Manier, D.H., Shelton, R.C., Sulser, F., 2002. Noradrenergic antidepressants: Does chronic treatment increase or decrease nuclear CREB- P? J. Neural. Transm. 109, 91-99.

40. Maxwell, R.A., Keenan, P.D., Chaplin, E., Roth, B., Eckhardt, S.B., 1969. Molecular features affecting the potency of tricyclic antidepressants and structurally related compounds as inhibitors of the uptake of tritiated norepinephrine by rabbit aortic strips. J. Pharmacol. Exp. Ther.166, 320 – 329.

41. Mobley, P.L., Manier, D.H., Sulser, F., 1983. Adrenal corticoids regulate the norepinephrine sensitive adenylate cyclase system in brain. J. Pharmacol. Exp. Ther. 226, 71 - 77.

42. Montgomery, S.A., 1998. Which antidepressant for which depression? In: Briley, M., Montgomery, S.A. (Eds.), Antidepressant Therapy at the Dawn of the Third Millennium. Martin Dunitz, London, pp.338-348.

43. Mueller, J.C., Pryor, W. W., Gibbons, J.E., Orgain, E.S., 1955. Depression and anxiety occurring during Raunolfia therapy. J.A.M.A. 159, 836-839.

44. Nelson, G.C., Mazure, C.M., Bowers, M.B., Jatlow, P.I., 1991. A preliminary open study of the combination of fluoxetine and desipramine for rapid treatment of major depression. Arch. Gen. Psychiat. 48, 303-307.

45. Ostrowski, J., Kjelsberg, M.A., Caron, M. G., Lefkowitz, RJ., 1992. Mutagenesis of the β_2-adrenergic receptor: How structure elucidates function. Ann.Rev.Pharmacol. Toxicol. 32, 167-183.

46. Pandey, G.N., Heinze, W.J., Brown, B.D., Davis, J.M., 1979. Electroconvulsive shock treatment decreases β-adrenergic receptor sensitivity in rat brain. Nature 280, 234-235.

47. Pariante, C.M., Pearce, B.D., Pisell, T.L., Owens, M.J., Miller, A., 1997. Steroid - independent translocation of the glucocorticoid receptor by the antidepressant desipramine. Molec. Pharmacol. 52, 571 - 581.

48. Pletscher, A., 1973. The impact of monoamine research on drug development. In: Usdin, E, Snyder, S.H. (Eds.), Frontiers of Catecholamine Research. Pergamon Press, New York, pp. 27-37.

49. Pletscher, A., Shore, P.A., Brodie, B.B., 1955. Serotonin release as a possible mechanism of reserpine action. Science 122, 374-375.

50. Pletscher, A., Da Prada, M., Burkard, W.P., Tranzer, J.P., 1968. Effect of benzoquinolizines and ring - substituted aralkyl - amines on serotonin metabolism. Adv. Pharmacol. 68, 55-69.

51. Premont, R.T., Inglese, J., Lefkowitz, R.J., 1995. Protein kinases that phosphorylate activated G protein coupled receptors. FASEB J, 9, 175-182.

52. Pryor, J.C., Sulser, F., 1991. Evolution of the monoamine hypotheses of depression. In: Horta, R, Katona, C. (Eds.), Biological Aspects of Affective Disorders. Academic Press, London, pp.77 - 94.

53. Randrup, A., Scheel - Krueger, J., 1966. Diethyldithiocarbamate and amphetamine stereotype behavior. J. Pharmacol. Pharm. 18, 752-758.

54. Ringold, G.M., 1985. Steroid hormone regulation of gene expression. Ann. Rev. Pharmacol. Toxicol. 25, 529 - 566.

55. Roberts, V.J., Singhal, R.L., Roberts, D.C.S., 1984. Corticosterone prevents the increase in noradrenaline stimulated adenyl cyclase activity in rat hippocampus following adrenalectomy or metopirone. Eur. J. Pharmacol. 103, 235-240.

56. Robinson, D.S., Kurtz, N.M., l987. Monoamine oxidase inhibiting drugs: Pharmacological and therapeutic issues. In: Meltzer, H.Y. (Ed.), Psychopharmacology: The Third Generation of Progress. Raven Press, New York, pp. 1297 - 1304.

57. Rodbell, M., 1980. The role of hormone receptors and GTP regulatory proteins in membrane transduction. Nature 284, 17-22.

58. Ross, E.M., Gilman, A.G., 1980. Biochemical properties of hormone-sensitive adenylate cyclase. Ann. Rev. Biochem. 49, 533-564.

59. Rossby, S.P., Sulser, F., 1997. Antidepressants: Beyond the synapse. In: Skolnick, Ph. (Ed.), Antidepressants: New Pharmacological Strategies. Humana Press, Totowa, NJ, pp. 195-212.

60. Salmoiraghi, G.C., 1966. Central adrenergic synapses. Pharmacol. Rev. 18, 717-726.

61. Schildkraut, J.J., 1965. The catecholamine hypothesis of affective disorders: A review of supporting evidence. Am. J. Psych. 122, 509-522.

62. Schultz, J., 1976. Psychoactive drug effects on a system which generates cyclic AMP in brain. Nature 261, 417-418.

63. Sigg, E. G., 1959. Pharmacological studies with Tofranil. Canad. Psych. Assoc. J. 4, S 75-S83.

64. Siggins, G.R., Hoffer, B.J., Bloom, F.E., 1971. Studies on norepinephrine - containing afferents to Purkinje cells of rat cerebellum. Evidence for mediation of norepinephrine effects by cyclic 3, 5 adenosine monophosphate. Brain Res. 25, 535-553.

65. Spector, S., Kuntzman, R., Shore, P. A., Brodie, B.B., 1960. Evidence for release of brain amines by reserpine in presence of monoamine oxidase inhibitors: implication of monoamine oxidase in noreprinephrine metabolism in brain. J. Pharmacol. Exp. Ther. 130, 256-261.

66. Stone, E.A., 1979. Subsensitivity to norepinephrine as a link between adaptation to stress and antidepressant therapy: A hypothesis. Res. Commun. Psychol. Psychiat. Behav.4, 241 -255.

67. Stone, E.A., Platt, J.E., Herrera, A.S., Kirk, K.L., 1986. The effect of repeated restraint stress, desmethylimipramine, and adrenocorticotropin on the α- and β-adrenergic component of the cyclic AMP response to norepinephrine in rat brain slices. J. Pharmacol. Exp.Ther. 237, 702 - 710.

68. Strada, S. J., Sulser, F., 1972. Effect of MAO inhibitors on metabolism and in vivo release of 3H - norepinephrine from the hypothalamus. Europ. J. Pharmacol. 18, 303-308.
69. Sulser, F., Bickel, M.H., Brodie, B.B., 1964. The action of desmethylimipramine in counteracting sedation and cholinergic effects of reserpine - like drugs J. Pharmacol. Exp. Ther. 144, 321-330.
70. Sulser, F., Sanders - Bush, E., 1971. Effect of drugs on amines in the CNS. Ann. Rev. Pharmacol. 11, 209-230.
71. Sutherland, E.W., Rall, T.W., 1960. The relation of adenosine - 3, 5 - phosphate to the action of catecholamines. In: Adrenergic Mechanisms. Ciba Foundation Symposium, Little Brown and Co., Boston, pp. 295-304.
72. Vetulani, J., and Sulser, F., 1975. Action of various antidepressant treatments reduces the reactivity of the noradrenergic cyclic AMP - generating system in limbic forebrain. Nature 257, 495-496.
73. Vetulani, J., Stawarz, R. J., Sulser, F., 1976. Adaptive mechanisms of the noradrenergic cyclic AMP system in the limbic forebrain of the rat: Adaptation to persistent changes in the availability of norepinephrine. J. Neurochem. 27, 661-666.
74. Vogt, M., 1954. The concentration of sympathin in diff e rent parts of the central nervous system under normal conditions and after the administration of drugs. J. Physiol. 123, 451-481.
75. Weiner, N., 1970. Regulation of norepinephrine biosynthesis. Ann. Rev. Pharmacol. 10, 273-290.
76. Wolfe, B.B., Harden, T.K., Sporn, J.R., Molinoff, P.B., 1978. Presynaptic modulation of β-adrenergic receptors in rat cerebral cortex after treatment with antidepressants. J. Pharmacol. Exp. Ther. 207, 446-457.
77. Wong, M., Kling, M.A., Munson, P.J., Listwak, S., Licinio, J., Prolo, P., 2000. Pronounced and sustained central hypernoradrenergic function in major depression with melancholic features: Relation to hypercortisolism and corticotropin - releasing hormone.Proc. Natl. Acad. Sci. USA 97, 325-330.
78. Yoshikawa, K., Sabol, S.L., 1986. Expression of the enkephalin precursor gene in C6 glioma cells: Regulation by β-adrenergic agonists and glucocorticoids. Molec. Brain Res. 16, 75 -83.

CHAPTER 4

SEROTONIN AND THE NEUROTRANSMITTER ERA
IN NEUROPSYCHOPHARMACOLOGY

David Grahame Grahame-Smith

INTRODUCTION

My entrance into this story occurred in 1961. I had just finished a senior intern job in general medicine and felt the need to pit myself against a serious problem of biomedical science. The Professor of Medicine at St Mary's Hospital, Paddington, London was W. Stanley Peart, a man with a deceptively understated way of asking the right questions. I asked his advice. "Well", he said, "there is on the ward a patient with something called the carcinoid syndrome caused by a tumour which makes a substance by the name of serotonin. It appears that no one really knows how it is made. Why don't you find out?"

That question led to a train of research that lasted my working life.

DISCOVERY

The scientific story of serotonin starts sometime in the mid 1880s with the realisation that as blood clots vasoconstricting material appears in the serum (Stevens and Lee, 1884). In the late 1940s Page and his group (Page, 1954), at the Cleveland clinic were interested in finding a circulating substance (eventually identified as angiotensin) involved in hypertension but their efforts were continually thwarted by this substance which appeared when blood clots. So they set about finding out what it was. They crystallised it from ox serum (Rapport et al., 1948) and Rapport (1997) showed that chemically it was probably 5-hydroxytryptamine. Hamlin and Fisher (1951) confirmed this by synthesising it. These bald facts disguise a scientific adventure full of human struggle, interesting personalities, messy tissue pharmacology, incredible kitchen biochemistry and persistent trial and error until this serum vasoconstricting substance was tamed and identified. (See Whitaker-Azmitia, 1991, for a fascinating history of these early days).

However at the same time as these studies were going on in the USA equally revealing studies were afoot in Italy, no less full of adventure and persistence. Vittorio Erspamer (1909-1999) was to my mind a consummate investigative biologist. In the 1930s he was interested in the pharmacology of naturally occurring substances particularly those associated with enterochromaffin cells in mammalian (rabbit) gut an interest which spread to many other species, e.g., molluscs and other marine creatures. He extracted a smooth muscle contractile substance from rabbit intestinal mucosa, which he named *enteramine* (Erspamer and Vialli, 1937). Erspamer and Asero (1952) then chose two species of marine animal for their definitive studies on the isolation and identification of enteramine. They removed 30 kilos of posterior salivary gland tissue from 30,000 octopuses (Octopus Vulgaris) and removed the skin from 1020 Sicilian amphibians (Discoglossus Pictus). From these tissues they extracted the picrate salt of enteramine and identified it as 5-hydroxytryptamine. When synthetic 5-hydroxytryptamine became available they confirmed that indeed enteramine was 5-hydroxytryptamine (Erspamer, 1986).

These two lines of work were carried out without the two groups of workers being aware of each other's interests and findings and to my mind the honours for the discovery of *serotonin-enteramine-5-hydroxytryptamine* should be shared equally.

So in the history of serotonin we now have a chemically identified substance, 5-hydroxytryptamine, and I shall now refer to it as 5-HT (Bacq, 1952).

5-HT IN BRAIN

The story of 5-HT as a central neurotransmitter begins with the discovery of 5-HT in brain tissue, a discovery shared by two groups, Twarog and Page (1953) in the USA and Amin, Crawford and Gaddum (1954) in Scotland. These were investigations in which brains of various species were dissected and regions homogenised and the homogenate extracted and 5-HT identified and measured, high concentrations being found in the hypothalamus, mesencephalon, area postrema, nuclei gracilis and cuneatus and the colliculi.

Our understanding of the distribution of 5-HT in the central nervous system (CNS) was immensely refined by the application of the histochemical fluorescence technique to identifying groups of 5-HT cell bodies in the raphé nuclei of the brain stem and mesencephalon and tracing the distribution of their axons to distant parts of the brain (Baumgarten and Grozdanovic, 1997; Dahlstrom and Fuxe, 1964). These techniques were further refined later by conjoining them with micro-lesions of pathways, neurotoxic methodology, and immunocytochemical techniques using 5-HT antibodies (Wang and Peroutka, 1988).

Altogether the milestone anatomical studies mapped out the 5-HT systems in brain and raised the question of what can be the neurophysiological functions of these widely dispersed neural networks.

Very recently interest has turned to the mechanisms of cortical feedback to the raphé (Robbins, 2005). For instance uncontrollable shock stress in rats that leads to evidence of anxiety, "depressive" behaviour and physical evidence of stress (gastric ulcer) causes changes in dorsal raphé nucleus (DRN) activity and 5-HT function through a glutaminergic feedback pathway from the prefrontal cortex to the DRN. There the descending pathway interacts with GABAergic neurones that exert an inhibitory influence on DRN 5-HT neuronal firing. It is proposed that changes in 5-HT input to the cortex alters processing in the forebrain regions and change perceptual, motor, memory and cognitive functions relevant to depression. These findings make the raphé nuclei 5-HT neurones a much more vital and reactive set of neurones than was previously envisaged.

BRAIN 5-HT SYNTHESIS

Where does the 5-HT in neurones comes from? Udenfriend et al. (1956) demonstrated the 5-hydroxylation of L-tryptophan in toad venom glands. Gal, Poczic and Marshall (1963) showed that intracerebral injection of ^{14}C- tryptophan resulted in the formation of ^{14}C-5-HT in the brains of rat and pigeon. Grahame-Smith (1964, 1967) and Lovenberg et al. (1967) demonstrated that brain tissue contained tryptophan-5-hydroxylase which hydroxylated tryptophan to 5-hydroxytrptophan which was then decarboxylated to 5-HT, the decarboxylation step in brain by aromatic aminoacid decarboxylase having been shown by Lovenberg et al. (1962). Grahame-Smith (1967) postulated that 5-HT was made in neurones wherever both tryptophan-5-hydroxylase and 5-hydroxytrytophan decarboxylase were present together and that this occurred not only in 5-HT neuronal cell bodies but also at the terminals, as shown by the ability of synaptosomes to synthesise 5-HT. It is interesting that subsequent investigation by *in situ hybridisation* has demonstrated that tryptophan-5-hydroxylase is made in the cell bodies of the 5-HT neurones in the raphé nuclei and presumably transported along the axon to the terminals. Recent molecular genetic studies have shown that there are two forms of tryptophan hydroxylase (TPH). TPH2 is responsible for 5-HT neuronal synthesis. Studies by Zhang et al. (2005) have shown a single nucleotide polymorphism in TPH2 with a greater incidence in patients with unipolar depression that produces a great decrease in 5-HT production when that gene is expressed in PC12 cells. If this can be confirmed it will be a great step forward in understanding the involvement of 5-HT in depressive illness.

RELEVANCE TO PLASMA TRYPTOPHAN

The Km of tryptophan 5-hydroxylase is such that the enzyme would not, under physiological circumstances be expected to be saturated with its substrate L-tryptophan. This led Fernstrom and Wurtman (1971) and Grahame-Smith (1971) to investigate the dependence, under physiological circumstances and during tryptophan loading, of brain 5-HT synthesis on blood and brain tryptophan concentrations. Alec Coppen

(Coppen et al., 1963) however, with great perspicacity, had already seen all through this and had given L-trytophan and a monoamine oxidase inhibitor to patients with depression and had shown improvement in their condition. This was really the first experimental evidence that 5-HT might be involved in depressive illness. Tryptophan transport across the blood brain barrier and the various membranes separating blood from the intraneuronal environment is still a point of interest as being a step prior to biosynthesis capable of gentle manipulation that can be used to probe the effects of altering 5-HT synthesis on physiological functions.

As far as I know there has not been much progress in understanding the fine relationships between the various functional pools of 5-HT. Consider: where is tryptophan-5-hydroxylase? It is a soluble enzyme but is it bound to some intracellular structure? How and where is the 5-hydroxytryptophan formed spatially decarboxylated? When the 5-HT is formed how is it protected from the mitochondrial based monoamine oxidase before it is taken up by its storage vesicles? How is the soluble concentration of 5-HT controlled and is it important functionally?

This is not nitpicking. Answers to these questions may reveal points at which the function of 5-HT can be pharmacologically manipulated.

5-HT UPTAKE

Like the catecholamines, 5-HT is taken up after release by a Na+ dependent carrier mediated "reuptake" mechanism that is thought to be crucial in the termination of its action (Axelrod, 2003). Humphrey and Toh (1954) showed that dog platelets absorbed 5-HT. Blackburn et al. (1967) demonstrated 5-HT uptake by rat brain in vitro and Iversen (1975) deals comprehensively with the general background of monoamine uptake.

Briley and Langer (1979) went one important step further than uptake and studied the binding of imipramine to the uptake sites membranes prepared from rat cerebral cortex. Lesion studies showed these sites to be associated with 5-HT terminals.

BRAIN 5-HT METABOLISM

The major route of 5-HT metabolism is through oxidative deamination. Monoamine oxidase (MAO) was discovered in liver by Hare in 1928 (Hare, 1928); Blaschko (1952) showed that 5-HT was oxidatively deaminated by guinea pig tissues and posterior salivary glands of octopus vulgaris and Udenfriend et al. (1956), that the final product of this was 5-hydroxyindolic acid (5-HIAA) with 5-hydroxyindole-acetaldehyde as an intermediate. There are two distinct mitochondrial monoamine oxidases. MAO-A preferentially metabolises 5-HT, though strangely enough, platelets, which accumulate large amounts of 5-HT have MAO-B as the major isoform.

In the pineal gland, 5-HT is the precursor of melatonin, (Weissbach, et al., 1960), a subject worthy of a history in its own right.

ANIMAL BEHAVIOURAL MODELS

In the 1970s and 1980s animal behaviours associated with changes in 5-HT function had their proponents and uses. First was the reserpinised mouse thought superficially to be perhaps a model for depression upon which proposed antidepressant treatments might be tested. It was used as a screening test in the early days of tricyclic antidepressant drug development.

Various animal tests have been developed in the hope that they would act as a model for depression and be used both to explore 5-HT functional abnormalities which might be endogenous to "depression" and also to be used to test potential treatments. None of them are without their problems and uncertainties but they do have a use in screening molecules with likely antidepressant properties and are widely used by the pharmaceutical industry.

Other animal behavioural states have been used to explore 5-HT functions and the functional results of drug treatments. The hyperactivity serotonin syndrome in rats was first described by Hess and Doepfner (1961) and was produced by a combination of tryptophan and the MAO inhibitors (MAOIs) iproniazid or nialamide.. They were unable to find a quantitative correlation between brain concentrations of 5-HT and the severity of the hyperactivity syndrome. Grahame-Smith (1971) explored this further using the accumulation of brain 5-HT after the administration of tryptophan and tranylcypromine as an index of 5-HT synthesis and this did seem to correlate with measured aspects of the hyperactivity syndrome and it seemed likely that the hyperactivity syndrome was due to consequent spill over of 5-HT onto its receptor sites (which and where being unknown at that time). It was found that the same hyperactivity syndrome was produced by 5-hydroxytryptophan (5-HTP) plus a MAOI, and direct 5-HT agonists such as 5-methoxy-N, N-dimethytryptamine (5MeODMT). Utilising this model and the 5-HT$_2$ mediated head twitch in the mouse the actions of many drugs and procedures on 5-HT function were investigated (Green and Grahame-Smith, 1976; Green and Heal, 1985).

RECEPTORS

Gaddum and Picarelli (1957) using guinea pig ileum preparations showed that there were at least two types of "tryptamine" receptor. M receptors blocked by morphine and D receptors blocked by dibenzyline (phenoxybenzamine). The M receptor is probably the 5-HT$_3$ receptor and the D receptor the 5-HT$_2$ receptor. Early attempts to define brain 5-HT receptors utilised H^3-5HT binding with d-LSD displacement and also direct H^3-LSD binding with equilibrium dialysis. Although these early attempts showed different types of binding not much progress was made until Bennett and Snyder (1976) utilised the rapid filtration technique with 5-HT and LSD binding. Peroutka and Snyder (1981) concluded, correctly, that at least two distinct 5-HT receptors exist in brain, 5-HT_1 and 5-HT_2. As binding studies became more sophisticated and new putative ligands became available so the number of specific 5-HT binding sites increased. Some of us were sceptical at the time that 5-HT, within our experience almost an orphan hormone, could grow up to become such a sophisticate, but our scepticism has been replaced by wonder as the techniques of molecular biology coupled with radioligand binding have revealed at least 13 different 5-HT receptors. They fall into 7 different groups: five 5-HT_1 types (all linked to inhibition of adenylate cyclase), three 5-HT_2 types, (all linked to activation of phospholipase C) one 5-HT_3 type, (the one 5-HT gated ion channel), two 5-HT_5 receptors (signal transduction unknown) and one each of 5HT_6 & 5-HT_7 (linked to activation of adenylate cyclase). This has become a very complex and fascinating field, far too big to be reviewed here but Peroutka and Howell (1994) on reviewing the molecular evolution of G-protein coupled receptors conclude that these receptors have probably evolved over 750 million years and go so far as to speculate that all biogenic amine receptors might be considered direct descendants of the primordial 5-HT receptor.

THE WIDESPREAD FUNCTIONAL INFLUENCE OF 5-HT

This vast array of 5-HT receptors have been shown to control specific functions, some of them postsynaptic, acting as signal receptors on other neurones, others are presynaptic, or cell body auto-receptors acting on various functions of the 5-HT neurone itself (as a form of physiological self-discipline).

Work in multiple disciplines has shown why 5-HT seems to be involved in so many brain functions and why so many drugs which affect 5-HT functions have therapeutic effects in mental illnesses, e.g., in anxiety, depression, obsessive compulsive disorder, psychoses, or other striking effects upon mental functioning in normal people, e.g., hallucinogens, ecstasy.

The raphé nuclei in the mid-brain contain groups of 5-HT cell bodies the axons of which radiate to and influence the function of many parts of the brain. The 5-HT which is released may act with close synaptic apposition, may be released to form a more diffuse "cloud", may be released at nerve terminals, from axonal varicosities and from the cell bodies themselves. Its actions are therefore likely to be of various types

Released 5-HT may be transported by vesicular release dependent membrane depolarisation or by the release of cytoplasmic pools. Released 5-HT will then act within either precise anatomical boundaries or more diffusely upon appropriately placed receptors, of which there are 14 different types, many with fundamentally different effector mechanisms and functional outcomes.

THE EVOLUTION OF IDEAS ABOUT BRAIN 5-HT FUNCTION

In 1954 Amin, Crawford and Gaddum (Amin et al., 1954) suggested that 5-HT might have a specialised role to play in the brain and Twarog (Twarog and Page, 1953) was clearly aware of this as one of her interests was neuromuscular transmission in the byssus retractor muscle of the edible mussel (Mytilus Edulis).

Woolley and Shaw (1954) in a fascinating speculative paper, leapt into the future using a medicinal chemistry approach. The structure of 5HT had just been described and they looked around for substances that had chemical resemblance. One they identified was lysergic acid diethylamide (LSD). Some of the psychopharmacological properties of LSD were already known because of the experiences of its discoverer, Albert Hofmann in 1943 who, after ingesting 0.25 mg wrote; "Last Friday, April 16th, I was forced to stop my laboratory work in the middle of the afternoon and to go home as I was overcome by a peculiar restlessness associated with mild dizziness. Having reached home, I lay down and sank into a kind of delirium which was not unpleasant and which was characterised by extreme activity of the imagination. As I lay in a dazed condition with my eyes closed (I experienced day light as disagreeably bright), there surged in upon me an uninterrupted stream of phantastic images of extraordinary vividness and accompanied by an intense, kaleidoscopic-like play of colours. The condition passed of after about two hours" (Krantz and Carr 1965). These effects were likened (probably improperly) to some of the manifestations of schizophrenia.

Woolley and Shaw's (1954) account and thinking are so interesting that I should like to quote from their paper, (remember that this was in 1954 when receptor theory was still a theory): "It is now being widely recognised that some drugs have their effects on living things to the fact that they are related in chemical structure to one or other of the hormones, vitamins or other essential cell constituents and that by virtue of this relationship they are able to block the specific action of the cell constituent ...... the combined evidence both biochemical and pharmacological seems to be sufficient to encourage pursuit of the working hypothesis that this hormone-like compound (5-HT) plays an important part in the functioning of the nervous system." In their paper Woolley and Shaw foreshadowed 5-HT as a "neurohormone" in brain, that there were brain 5-HT receptors, that drugs would affect 5-HT receptors in brain and that there was a psychopharmacological function for 5-HT in brain. All predictions were correct!

5-HT IN DEPRESSION

Brodie and Shore (1957) did an important experiment in rats, administering reserpine, showing depletion of brain 5-HT (and norepinephrine), a resultant depression of behaviour (so called reserpinisation) and drew the conclusion that 5-HT and norepinephrine were chemical mediators in the brain and because there was the clinical knowledge that some patients taking reserpine for the treatment of hypertension developed depression as an adverse reaction, they suggested that decreased function of 5-HT or norepinephrine might be involved in the causation of depression. So the hunt was on to find out whether 5-HT dysfunction occurred in depression. Alec Coppen et al. (1963) did an important landmark clinical study. They compared a MAOI (tranylcypromine) alone and tranylcypromine plus trypto-phan in the treatment of depressed patients and found that the addition of trypto-phan to tranylcypromine was much more efficacious than the MAOI alone. It was assumed that the combination produced an increased accumulation of brain 5-HT that was confirmed later in rats by Grahame-Smith (1971). There is evidence that tryptophan alone is effective in the treatment of depression but less so, than when given in combination with a MAOI. Ashcroft et al. (1966) published evidence of low 5-hydroxyindoles in the spinal cerebrospinal fluid (CSF) of depressed patients and many such studies have been subsequently done with varying results but low CSF 5-HIAA does seem to be a feature in patients attempting suicide, particularly violent suicide (Asberg, 1997).

Kuhn (1958) demonstrated the clinical efficacy of imipramine in depression before its action on monoamine uptake was known. Nevertheless its effects and the general understanding of the significance of the uptake process for the therapeutic actions of the tricyclic antidepressants was important for the development of the selective serotonin re-uptake inhibitors (SSRIs).

The imipramine binding studies previously mentioned, the advent of the SSRIs and developments in molecular genetics have resulted in the identification of a polymor-phism of the serotonin transport gene and studies trying to identify a polymorphism associated with depressive disorder are being undertaken (Masson et al., 1999).

CLINICAL EXPERIMENTAL STUDIES

There are many abnormalities in the biochemical pharmacology and the pharmaco-logical and physiological functions of 5-HTwhich have been demonstrated in clinical studies in depression (Mann 1999):

1. Circumstantial evidence for a role of 5-HT in depression (Garlow and Nemeroff, 2004).
2. Precursor availability. Depletion of tryptophan results in depressive relapse in patients treated with antidepressants.
3. 5-HT synthesis. P-chloro-phenylalanine (PCPA), a tryptophan hydroxylase inhibitor, causes depressive relapse in antidepressant treated patients .
4. 5-HT storage. Reserpine, which depletes 5HT, may cause depression.
5. 5-HT release. Lithium, which augments 5-HT release, augments antidepressant action.

6. 5-HT transport. Vmax of platelet 5-HT uptake diminished and Bmax of imipramine binding decreased in depressed patients

7. 5-HT metabolism. Low CSF 5-HIAA, particularly in patients prone to violent suicide.

8. 5-HT postsynaptic receptor sites. $5\text{-}HT_2$ receptor increased Bmax on platelets of depressed patients. Some $5\text{-}HT_2$ agonists are antidepressants.

Experience and hindsight have taught us how difficult these studies are. Patient numbers must be adequate and calculating the necessary numbers to validate the *Power* of such studies can be very difficult, a priori, when the extent of the differences between depressed and non-depressed subjects is unknown. Many studies have been done which turn out to have had inadequate *Power* to back up the conclusions drawn.

History has taught us how painstaking and patient we must be in undertaking clinical studies in depression. Diagnostic criteria, blinding procedures, measurements of severity, time sequences of changes, state or disease dependence, responses to treatment, care in the application of biochemical, pharmacological or physiological measurement, experimental techniques (validity, reproducibility) are absolutely critical. At the clinical level progress can be very slow and one must be patient. There is no substitute for the results of clinical studies for understanding the relevance of purported neurotransmitter abnormalities in depression.

A ROLE FOR 5-HT IN NEURONAL AND SYNAPTIC ADAPTIVE RESPONSES

In recent years attention has turned to the understanding of the long-term effects of antidepressant treatments and the role of 5-HT. Depressive illness has a long-term biology in an individual as witnessed by its natural history. Antidepressant drugs take some weeks to act and electroconvulsive therapy (ECT) generally requires the several spaced out ECT sessions.

In this context studies on animals (Grahame-Smith 1988), and humans (neuroendocrine studies) (Cowen 1998), initially focussed on long term up and downregulation of receptors and their function. Although changes were found they have not contributed much to the understanding of either the endogenous pathology of 5-HT in depression or to a clear explanation of how the drugs affecting 5-HT act to relieve depression.

The latest development in the 1990s concerns the involvement of 5-HT in the adaptive responses to antidepressant drugs and also to the involvement of 5-HT in neuronal plasticity, synaptic adaptive change, and their relation to the causation of depression. This work is fuelled by Kandel's Nobel Prize winning studies on learning processes in Aplysia (Kandel and Hawkins, 1992) in which neurotransmission by 5-HT plays a crucial role and by a gradual understanding that 5-HT through its various receptors subtypes produces long lasting adaptive responses in neural targets through slow second messenger systems involving gene activation and neurotrophic factor (e.g., BDNF) release which results in synaptic adaptive responses. These ideas are being actively pursued (Duman, 2004 a, b) and I have attempted to summarise my view of this approach (Grahame-Smith, 1998).

CONCLUSION

We have travelled a journey from a hormone seeking a function (1950s), to a respectable neurotransmitter 1950s and 60s, to a substance involved in depression (the monoamine hypothesis of depression), a flirtation with schizophrenia (running through the 50s to date, e.g.,. clozapine), and producing a billion dollar industry in SSRIs, with all its controversies. Yet there is still an uncertain basis for all the attention that has been paid to 5-HT, except for the pragmatic fact that drugs affecting its function have a therapeutic effect in mental illness and can also produce profound mental change. It is here that the practical physician in me riles against the neuroscientist in me. The former is prepared to accept a serendipitous therapeutic benefit on the basis of an unknown pharmacology, while the latter demands to know at the reductionist level precisely what is going on. Will the role of 5-HT in neuronal network plasticity and its role in depression be an answer to this?

It has been a great trip (shades of LSD) -a dream, but like many dreams I think that for me it will pass without a clear conclusion. I remember a conversation in the 1980s with Brian Farrell, a highly respected psychologist and philosopher in Oxford, when I was bemoaning the fact that however much I knew about the functions of 5-HT it was not going to explain depression. He comforted me by saying, "Remember, however much you know about the molecular and atomic structure of water it won't explain why it feels wet."

For excellent early reviews of many aspect of 5-HT see: The Pharmacology of Psychotomimetic and Psychotherapeutic Drugs: Proceedings of a Conference (St. Whitelock, 1957).

REFERENCES
1. Amin, A. H., Crawford, T. B., Gaddum, J. H., 1954. The distribution of substance P and 5-hydroxytryptamine in the central nervous system of the day. J. Physiol. 126, 596-618.
2. Asberg, M., 1997. Neurotransmitters and suicidal behaviour. Annals of the New York Acad. Sci. 836, 158-181.
3. Ashcroft, G. W., Crawford, T. B. B., Eccleston, D., Sharman, D. F., MacDougall, E. J., Stanton, J. B., Binns, J. K., 1966. 5-hydroxyindole compounds in the cerebrospinal fluid of patients with psychiatric or neurological diseases. Lancet 2, 1049.
4. Axelrod, J., 2003. Journey of a late blooming biochemical neuroscientist. J. Biol. Chem. 278, 1-13.
5. Bacq, Z. M., 1952. Les amines biologiquement interessantes derivées des acides aminées. In: Rapport au 2e Congrés Internat, de Biochimie, Paris, 1952 , pp 59-74.

6. Baumgarten, H.G., Grozdanovic, Z., 1997. Anatomy of central serotonergic projection systems. In: Baumharten, H., Göthert, M. (Eds.), Serotonergic Neurons & 5HT Receptors in the CNS. Handbook of Experimental Pharmacology. Volume 129. Springer, Berlin/London.

7. Bennett, J, P., Snyder, S. H., 1976. Serotonin & lysergic acid diethylamide binding to rat brain membranes: relationship to postsynaptic serotonin receptors. Mol. Pharmacol. 12, 373-389.

8. Blackburn, K. J., French, P. C., Merrills, R. J., 1967. 5-Hydroxytryptamine uptake by rat brain in vitro. Life Sci. 6, 1653.

9. Blaschko, H., 1952. Amine oxidase and amine metabolism. Pharmacological Reviews 4, 415-58.

10. Briley, M., Langer, S. Z., 1979. High affinity ³H–imipramine binding sites in rat cerebral cortex. Eur. J. Pharmac. 54, 307-308.

11. Brodie, B. B., Shore, P. A., 1957. A concept for the role of serotonin and norepinephrine as chemical mediators in the brain. Ann. New York Acad. Sci. 66, 631-642.

12. Coppen, A., Shaw, D. M., Farrell, J. P., 1963. Potentiation of the antidepressant effect of a monoamine oxidase inhibitor by tryptophan. Lancet i, 79-81.

13. Cowen, P. J., 1998. Pharmcological challenge tests and brain serotonin function in depression and during SSRI treatment. In: Briley, M., Montgomery, S. (Eds.), Antidepressant Therapy at the Dawn of the Third Millennium. Martin Dunitz Ltd., London, pp. 175-189.

14. Dahlstrom, A., Fuxe, K., 1964. Evidence for the existence of monoamine containing neurones in the CNS. I. Demonstration of monoamines in the cell bodies of brain stem neurones. Acta. Physiol. Scand. 62 (Suppl. 232), 1-55.

15. Duman, R. S., 2004a. Role of neurotrophic factors in the aetiology and treatment of mood disorders. Neuro Molecular Medicine 5, 11-25.

16. Duman, R. S., 2004b. The neurochemistry of depressive disorders: preclinical studies. In: Charney, D.S., Nestler, E.J. (Eds.), Neurobiology of Mental Illness 2nd edition. Oxford University Press, Oxford/New York, pp. 421-439.

17. Erspamer, V., 1986. Historical introduction: the Italian contribution to the discovery of 5-hydroxytryptamine (enteramine, serotonin). J. Hypertens. 4 (Suppl.1), 53-55.

18. Erspamer, V., Asero, B., 1952. Identification of enteramine; specific hormone of enterochromaffin cells as 5-hydroxytrptamine. Nature 169, 800-801.

19. Erspamer, V., Vialli, M., 1937. Ricerche sul secreto delle cellule enterocromaffini. Boll d. Soc. Med-chir. Pavia. 51, 357-363.

20. Fernstrom, J. D., Wurtman, R. J., 1971. Brain serotonin content: physiological dependence on plasma tryptophan levels. Science 173, 149-152.

21. Gaddum, J.H., Picarelli, Z. P., 1957. Two kinds of tryptamine receptor. Brit. J. Pharmacol. 12, 323-328.

22. Gal, E. M., Poczik, M., Marshall, F. D., Jr., 1963. Hydroxylation of tryptophan to 5-hydroytryptophan by brain tissue in vivo. Biochem. Bioshys. Res. Commun. 12, 39-43.

23. Garlow, S.J., Nemeroff, C. B., 2004. The neurochemistry of depressive disorders: clinical studies. In: Charney, D.S., Nestler, E.J. (Eds.), Neurobiology of Mental Illness 2nd edition. Oxford University Press, Oxford/New York, pp. 440-460.

24. Grahame-Smith, D. G., 1964. Tryptophan hydroxylation in brain. Biochem. Biophys. Res. Commun. 16, 586-592.

25. Grahame-Smith, D. G., 1967. The biosynthesis of 5-hydroxytryptamine in brain. Biochem. J. 105, 351-360.

26. Grahame-Smith, D. G., 1971. Studies in vivo on the relationship between brain tryptophan, brain 5-HT synthesis and hyperactivity in rats treated with a monoamine oxidase inhibitor and L-tryptophan, J. Neurochem. 18, 1053-1066.

27. Grahame-Smith, D. G., 1988. Neuropharmacological adaptive effects in the actions of antidepressant drugs, ECT and lithium. In: Briley, M., Fillion, G. (Eds.), New Concepts in Depression. Pierre Fabre Monograph Series Vol. 2. Macmillan Press, Basingstoke, pp. 1-14.

28. Grahame-Smith, D. G., 1998. Disorder of synaptic homeostasis as a cause of depression and a target for treatment. In: Briley, M., Montgomery, S. (Eds.), Antidepressant Therapy at the Dawn of the Third Millennium. Martin Dunitz Ltd., London, pp. 111-139.

29. Green, A. R., Grahame-Smith, D. G., 1976. Effects of drugs on the processes regulating the functional activity of brain 5 hydroxytryptamine. Nature 260, 487-491.
30. Green, A. R., Heal D. L., 1985. Effects of drugs on serotonin mediated behavioural models. In: Green, A.R. (Ed.), Neuropharmacology of Serotonin. Oxford University Press, Oxford/New York, pp. 326-365.
31. Hamlin, K. E., Fischer, F. E., 1951. The synthesis of 5-hydoxytryptamine. J. Amer. Chem. Soc. 73, 5007.
32. Hare, M. L. C., 1928. Tyramine oxidase. 1. A new enzyme system in liver. Biochem. J. 22, 968.
33. Hess, S. M., Doepfner, W., 1961. Behavioural effects and brain amine content in rats. Arch. Int. Pharmacodyn. Therap. 134, 89-90.
34. Humphrey, J. H., Toh, C. C., 1954. Absorption of serotonin (5-hydroxytryptamine) and histamine by dog platelets. J. Physiol. 124, 300-304.
35. Iversen, L. L., 1975. Uptake processes for biogenic amines. In: Iversen, L.L, Iversen, S.D., Snyder, S.H. (Eds.), Handbook of Psychopharmacology. Vol.3. Plenum Press, New York, pp. 381-442.
36. Kandel, E. R., Hawkins, R. D., 1992. The biological basis of learning and individuality. Sci. Am. 267, 53-60.
37. Krantz, J. C. Jr., Carr, C. J., 1965. The Pharmacologic Principles of Medical Practice . The Williams and Wilkins Co., Baltimore, pp. 1-491.
38. Kuhn, R., 1958. The treatment of depressive states with G22355 (imipramine hydrochloride). Am. J. Psychiatry 115, 459-464.
39. Lovenberg, W., Jequier, E., Sjoerdsma, A., 1967. Tryptophan hydroxylation: measurement in pinal gland, brain stem and carcinoid tumour. Science 155, 217-219.
40. Lovenberg, W., Weissbach, H., Undenfriend S., 1962. Aromatic L-amino acid decarboxylase. J. Biol. Chem. 237, 89-93.
41. Mann, J. J., 1999. Role of the Serotonergic System in the pathogenesis of major depression and suicidal behaviour. Neuropsychopharmacology 21, 995-1055.
42. Masson, J., Sagne, C., Hamon, M., El-Mestikawy, S., 1999. Neurotransmitter transporters in the CNS. Pharmacol. Reviews 51, 439-464.
43. Page, I. H., 1954. Serotonin (5-hydroxytryptamine). Physiol. Rev. 34, 563-588.
44. Peroutka, S. J., Howell, T. A., 1994. The molecular evolution of G protein coupled receptors: focus on 5-hydroxytryptamine receptors. Neuropharmacology 33, 319-324.
45. Peroutka, S. J., Snyder, S. H., 1981. Two distinct serotonin receptors: regional variations in receptor binding in mammalian brain. Brain Research 208, 339-347.
46. Rapport, M. M., 1997. The discovery of serotonin. Perspectives in Biol. and Med. 40, 260-273.
47. Rapport, M. M., Green, A. A., Page, I. H., 1948. Crystalline serotonin. Science 108, 329-330.
48. Robbins, T. W., 2005. Controlling stress: how the brain protects itself from depression. Nature Neuroscience. 8, 261-262.
49. Stevens, L. T., Lee, F. S., 1884. Action of intermittent pressure and of defibrinated blood upon blood vessels of frog and terrapin. John Hopkins Biol. Studies 3, 99.
50. St. Whitelock, O. (Ed.), 1957. The Pharmacology of Psychotomimetic and Psychotherapeutic Drugs: Proceedings of a Conference. Annals New York Academy of Sciences 66, 417-870.
51. Twarog, B. M., Page, I. H., 1953. Serotonin content of some mammalian tissues and urine and a method for its determination. Am. J. Physiol. 175, 157-161.
52. Udenfriend, S., Titus, E., Weissbach, H., Peterson, R. E., 1956. Biogenesis and metabolism of 5-hydroxyindole compounds. J. Biol. Chem. 219, 335-344.
53. Wang, S. S., Peroutka, S. J., 1988. In: Saunders-Bush, E. (Ed.), The Serotonin Receptors. Humana Press, Clifton N. J., pp. 3 –15.
54. Weissbach, H., Redfield, B. G., Axelrod, J., 1960. Biosynthesis of melatonin: Enzymatic conversion of serotonin to N-acetylserotonin. Biochem. Biophys. Acta 43, 352-353.
55. Whitaker-Azmitia, P.M., 1991. The discovery of serotonin and its role in neuroscience. Neuropsychopharmacology 21, 25-75.

56. Woolley, D. W., Shaw, E., 1954. Some neurophysiological aspects of serotonin. Brit. Med. J. 4880, 122-126.
57. Zhang, X., Gainetdivinov, R. R., Beaulieu, J. M., Sotnikova, T. D., Burch, L. H., Williams, R. B., Schwartz, D. A., Krishnan, K. R., Caron, M. G., 2005. Loss-of-function mutation in tryptophan hydroxylase-2 identified in unipolar major depression. Neuron 45, 11-16.

CHAPTER 5

DOPAMINE AND DOPAMINE RECEPTORS

Philip Seeman

The history of dopamine and dopamine receptors is intertwined with the history of psychosis and antipsychotics. The research path of this field started with the development of antihistamines after the 2nd world war, especially with H. Laborit using these compounds to enhance analgesia in surgery and obstetrics (Lacomme et al., 1952). In patients receiving one of these medications, Laborit (in Lacomme et al., 1952) noticed a "euphoric quietude"; the patients were "calm and somnolent, with a relaxed and detached expression." Compound 4560, now known as chlorpromazine, emerged as the most potent of the Rhone Poulenc compounds synthesized in the series.

Chlorpromazine was tested by many French physicians for various medical illnesses. Although Sigwald and Bouttier (1953) were the first to use it as the sole medication for a psychotic patient, their work was not reported until 1953. The 1952 report by Delay et al. (1952) showed that within three days (Agid et al., 2003; Kapur et al., 2005) chlorpromazine alleviated hallucinations and stopped internal "voices" in 8 patients, a dramatic finding.

With the antipsychotic action of chlorpromazine capturing the attention of the psychiatric community, the specific target of action for chlorpromazine became a goal for the basic science community. The working assumption then, as now, was that the discovery of such a target might open the pathway to uncovering the biochemical cause of psychosis and possibly schizophrenia.

MEMBRANE STABILIZATION BY ANTIPSYCHOTICS

As a graduate student at Rockefeller University in New York in 1961, I became especially interested in the mechanism of action of chlorpromazine. If the target sites for antipsychotics could be found, then perhaps these sites were overactive in psychosis or schizophrenia. In the 1960s, no one agreed on what schizophrenia was. Inclusion criteria varied so much that it was impossible to decide which patients to study, let alone what to study. But everyone agreed that chlorpromazine and the many other new antipsychotic drugs alleviated the symptoms of schizophrenia, however defined.

Where in the brain does one start to look for the antipsychotic target?

With the advent of the electron microscope, the 1960s was an active decade of discovery of sub-cellular particles and cell membranes. It seemed reasonable to me, therefore, to start by examining the actions of antipsychotics on cell membranes. In particular, did antipsychotics readily locate to cell surfaces and cell membranes and thereby alter membrane structure and function?

To see if antipsychotics could enter membranes and be membrane-active, I first started with an artificial lipid film floating on water, and measured the film pressure with a piece of aluminum hanging into the bath (Wilhelmy method; Wilhelmy, 1863). When I added an antipsychotic to the water below the film, the film pressure immediately dropped. This indicated that the antipsychotic molecules had entered into the single layer of lipid molecules floating on the water surface, expanding the intermolecular spaces between the lipid molecules.

To my surprise, however, when I omitted the lipid molecules, the addition of the antipsychotic still caused a drop in the surface pressure of the water surface. In other words, I had inadvertently discovered that antipsychotics were surface active (Seeman and Bialy, 1963). While the surface-active potencies showed an excellent correlation with clinical antipsychotic potencies, the antipsychotic concentrations were all in the micromolar range, a concentration later found to be far in excess of that which was clinically effective.

I then extended the finding to show that the same thing occurred in human red blood cell membranes. That is, antipsychotics readily expanded red blood cell membranes by ~0.1-1% and, in doing so, exerted an anti-hemolytic action by allowing the cells to become somewhat larger and stabilized before hemolysis occurred (Seeman, 1966a,b, 1972; Seeman and Weinstein, 1966).

This membrane stabilization by antipsychotics was also associated with electrical stabilization of the membrane. That is, it soon became clear that the antipsychotics were potent anesthetics, blocking nerve impulses at antipsychotic concentrations of between 20 nM and 1,000 nM (Figure 1, top correlation line) (Seeman, 1972; Seeman and Lee, 1975; Seeman et al., 1974a.b), concentrations still in excess of those clinically found in the spinal fluid of treated patients.

THERAPEUTIC CONCENTRATION OF ANTIPSYCHOTICS

Although a variety of cellular and sub-cellular membrane-stabilizing actions occurre d with antipsychotics (Seeman, 1972), the antipsychotic concentrations were generally between 20 nM and 100 nM at their lowest. The actual therapeutic molarities were never obvious until the data on haloperidol were analyzed. For example, because only 8% of haloperidol was free and not bound to plasma proteins (Forsman and Öhman, 1977), the active free concentration of haloperidol in patients would be ~1-2 nM (Seeman, 1992, 1995; Zingales, 1971). Based on the standard pharmacological principle that the non-protonated form of tertiary amines readily permeate cell membranes (Seeman, 1966a), this concentration in the aqueous phase in the plasma is expected to be identical to the aqueous concentration of haloperidol in the spinal fluid.

Figure 1. All antipsychotic drugs inhibit the binding of [³H]haloperidol to dopamine-D₂ receptors (in calf striatal homogenate) in direct relation to the clinical antipsychotic potencies (lower line) (adapted from Seeman et al., 1975a,b, 1976). The upper line indicates that antipsychotics also block the stimulated release of [³H]dopamine (from rat striatal slices) at concentrations which correlate with their clinical potencies (adapted from Seeman and Lee, 1975); however, the antipsychotic concentrations required for this presynaptic action are much higher than those that inhibit [³H]haloperidol binding to the dopamine-D₂ receptors (lower line) or those which are found in the spinal fluid of patients being treated with antipsychotics (Seeman,1992).

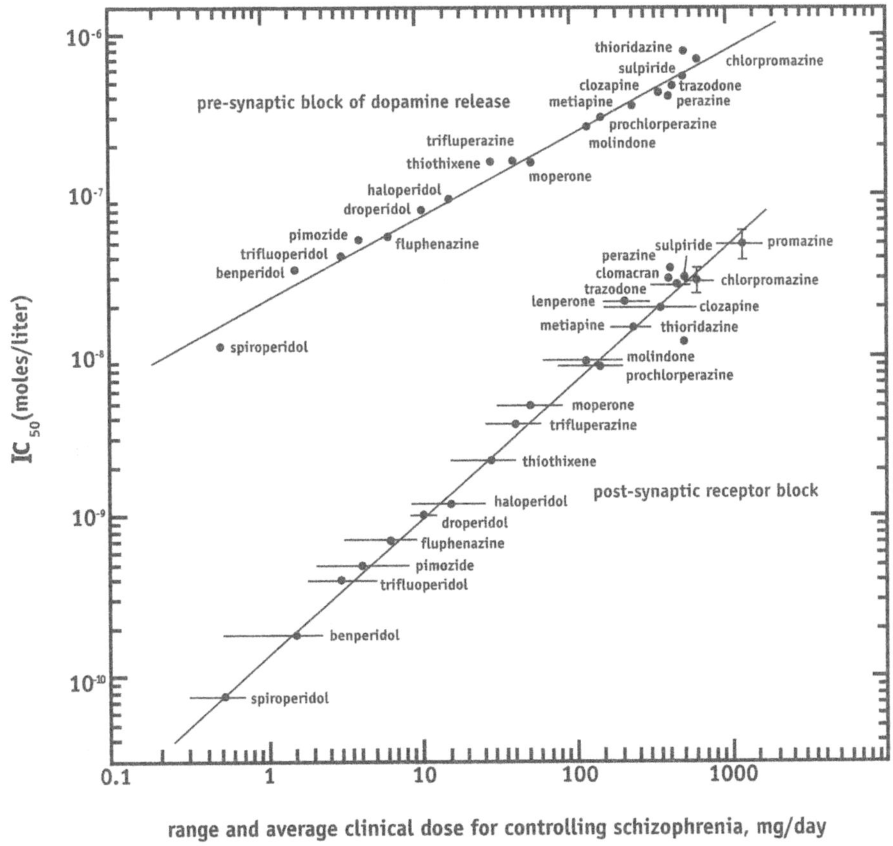

range and average clinical dose for controlling schizophrenia, mg/day

DISCOVERY OF THE ANTIPSYCHOTIC DOPAMINE RECEPTOR

The latter calculations were crucial for the discovery of the antipsychotic dopamine receptor (Seeman et al., 1974a, 1975a, b). That is, in order to detect or label a receptor with an affinity of ~1 nM for radioactive haloperidol, the specific activity of [³H]haloperidol would have to be at least 10 Ci/mmole. However, the [³H]haloperidol samples from Janssen Pharmaceutica (Belgium) kindly provided by Dr. J.J.P. Heykants in 1971 and by Dr. Jo Brugmans in 1972 only had a specific activity of 32-71 milliCi/mmole, too low to detect specific binding for a site with an expected dissociation constant of ~1 nM. I also asked New England Nuclear Corporation. (Boston, Massachusetts) to tritiate haloperidol, but the specific activity was only ~100 milliCi/mmole.

Finally, Dr. Paul A.J. Janssen and Dr. J. Heykants asked Mr. M. Winand at the National Institut Voor Radio-Elementen in Fleurus, Belgium (I.R.E. Belgique) to custom synthesize [³H]haloperidol for us. I.R.E. Belgique soon thereafter provided us with relatively high specific activity [³H]haloperidol (10.5 Ci/mmole) by June 1974. This [³H]haloperidol readily allowed us to detect the specific binding of [³H]haloperidol to brain striatal tissue, and our laboratory submitted an abstract describing this to the Society for Neuroscience before the annual May 1975 deadline (Seeman et al., 1975a). This report listed the following important IC₅₀% values to inhibit the binding of [³H]haloperidol: 2 nM for haloperidol, 20 nM for chlorpromazine, 3 nM for (+)butaclamol, and 10,000 nM for (-)butaclamol. The stereo-selective action of butaclamol and the good correlation between the IC₅₀% values and the clinical doses indicated that we had successfully identified the antipsychotic receptor. Moreover, of all the endogenous compounds tested, dopamine was the most potent in inhibiting the binding of [³H]haloperidol, thus indicating that the antipsychotic receptor was a dopamine receptor. The data of Seeman et al. (1975a) were confirmed by more extensive publications (Seeman et al., 1975b, 1976), showing a clear correlation between the clinical potencies and the antipsychotic dissociation constants (see figure 1, bottom correlation line).

At the CINP meeting held in Paris in July 1974, during the evening courtyard reception at the City Hall of Paris, I rushed up to Dr. Paul Janssen and showed him the chart correlating the average clinical antipsychotic doses with the *in vitro* antipsychotic potencies. He laughed and said that averaging the clinical doses for each antipsychotic was like averaging all the religions of the world. Nevertheless, the correlation remains a cornerstone of the dopamine hypothesis of schizophrenia, still the major contender for an explanatory theory of schizophrenia causation.

NOMENCLATURE OF DOPAMINE RECEPTORS

The receptor labeled by [³H]haloperidol was later termed the dopamine₂ (D₂) receptor (Kebabian and Calne, 1979). It is important to note that the data for the binding of [³H]haloperidol identifying the antipsychotic receptor (Seeman et al., 1975a,b) was very different from the pattern of [³H]dopamine binding described by Burt et al. (1976) and Snyder et al. (1975). For example, the binding of [³H]haloperidol was inhibited by ~10,000 nM dopamine, while that of [³H]dopamine was inhibited by ~7 nM dopamine. For several years, this latter [³H]dopamine binding site was termed the "dopamine3 (D3) site" (Seeman, 1980, 1982), a term which is not to be confused with the discovery of the dopamine₃ (D₃) receptor (Sokoloff et al., 1990). As summarized in table 1, there are now five different dopamine receptors that have now been cloned.

Table 1: Key findings related to dopamine and dopamine receptors

YEAR	FINDING	REFERENCE
1952	Analgesia and "euphoric quietude" with RP 4560 (chlorpromazine)	Laborit (in Lacomme et al.)
1952-53	Chlorpromazine has effective antipsychotic action	Delay et al.; Sigwald, Bouttier
1957-8	Dopamine found in brain tissue	Montagu; Carlsson et al.
1960	Very low amount of dopamine in Parkinson's diseased brain	Ehringer, Hornykiewicz
1963	Two antipsychotics increase normetanephrine and methoxytyramine	Carlsson, Lindqvist
1964	Three antipsychotics increase homovanillic acid (HVA) and dihydroxyphenylacetic acid (DOPAC); elimination delayed?	Andén et al.
1965	Dopamine can excite or inhibit neurones	Bloom et al.
1966	Dopamine hypothesis of schizophrenia outlined	van Rossum
1971	Dopamine stimulates adenylate cyclase	Kebabian, Greengard
1971	Haloperidol measured in patient's plasma (see 1977 below)	Zingales et al.
1974a	2.5 nM haloperidol blocks [^{3}H]dopamine receptors	Seeman et al.
1974	Haloperidol blocks excitation in *Helix*	Struyker Boudier et al.
1974	Fluphenazine blocks dopamine inhibition in *Aplysia*	Heiss, Hoyer
1975a,b	[^{3}H]haloperidol labels dopamine receptors	Seeman et al.
1975b	Antipsychotic doses correlate with block of dopamine receptors	Seeman et al.
1976	Sulpiride resolves two dopamine sites; no effect on adenylate cyclase	Roufogalis et al.
1976	Two dopamine receptors proposed: inhibitory and excitatory	Cools, van Rossum
1977	Dopamine stimulates adenylate cyclase in parathyroid	Brown et al.
1977	92% of plasma haloperidol bound, indicating 2 nM free in water	Forsman & Ohman
1978	Two dopamine receptors; coupled & uncoupled to adenylate cyclase	Spano et al.; Garau et al.
1978	Pre-synaptic action of apomorphine reduces release of dopamine	Starke et al.
1978	Elevated D_2 in post-mortem schizophrenia brain	Lee et al.
1979	Names of D_1 and D_2 used	Kebabian, Calne
1979	Dopamine inhibits adenylate cyclase in ant. pituitary	De Camili et al.
1983	Identical antipsychotic Ki values at striatum and limbic D_2 receptors	Seeman, Ulpian
1984	Kd values of D_2 ligands depend on final tissue concentration	Seeman et al.
1984	$D2^{High}$ and $D2_{Low}$ affinity states of D_2 receptors	Wreggett, Seeman
1985	$D2^{High}$ is functional state of D_2	George et al.
1986	[^{11}C]methylspiperone shows elevated D_2 in living schizophrenia patients	Wong et al.
1986	Labelling of D_2 receptors in living humans by positron tomography	Farde et al.
1988	Antipsychotics occupy 60-80% of D_2 in living schizophrenia patients	Farde et al.
1988-89	Cloning of the rat $D2_{Short}$ and $D2_{Long}$ receptors	Bunzow et al.; Giros et al.
1989	Cloning of the human $D2_{Short}$ and $D2_{Long}$ receptors	Grandy et al.
1989	90% of D_2 receptors are in $D2^{High}$ state in brain slices	Richfield et al.
1989	Endogenous dopamine lowers [^{3}H]raclopride binding; relevant to PET	Seeman et al.
1990-91	Dopamine D_1 and D_5 receptors cloned	Sunahara et al.

1990	Dopamine D_3 receptor cloned	Sokoloff et al.
1991	Dopamine D_4 receptor cloned	Van Tol et al.
1992	Block of D_2 >80% by antipsychotics associated with Parkinsonism	Farde et al
1992	Synaptic dopamine at rest is ~2 nM; ~100-200 nM during nerve impulses	Kawagoe et al.
1995	Drug Ki depends on fat solubilily of ligand	Seeman, Van Tol
1996	Amphetamine-induced release of dopamine is higher in schizophrenia	Laruelle et al.
1996	Glycine at position 194 in D_4 markedly reduces dopamine potency	Liu et al.
1998	$D2_{short}$ receptors located mostly in nigral neurones	Khan et al.
1999	Therapeutic doses of typical or atypical antipsychotics block 60-80% D_2	Kapur et al.
1999	Isoleucine at position 154 in D_2 causes myoclonus dystonia	Klein et al.
1999	Rapid release of clozapine and quetiapine from D_2 receptors	Seeman et al.
2000	New $D2_{longer}$ receptor	Seeman et al.
2003	Antipsychotics occupy more D_2 in limbic areas than striatum in patients	Bressan et al.
2005	Dopamine supersensitivily correlates with elevaled D^{High} states	Seeman et al.
2005	Dopamine receptor contribution to action of phencyclidine (PCP), lysergic acid diethylamide (LSD) and ketamine	Seeman et al.
2005	Higher D_2 density in healthy identical twins of schizophrenia patients	Hirvonen et al.
2005	Labeling of brain $D2^{High}$ receptors by $[^{11}C](+)$PHNO	Wilson et al.

At the same 1974 CINP meeting where I showed the correlation chart to Dr. Janssen, I happened to meet Dr. Sol Snyder in the lobby of the convention hotel and told him that I had custom prepared [³H]haloperidol and that it was now available. The pattern of [³H]haloperidol binding later published by Snyder et al. (1975) and by Burt et al. (1976) agreed with my findings. The paper by Snyder et al. (1975) in Psychopharmacology Communications kindly cited my Proceedings of the National Academy of Sciences paper of November, 1975, describing the [³H]haloperidol-labelled antipsychotic receptor (Seeman et al., 1975b), and the publication of Burt et al. (1976) kindly acknowledged the receipt of the drug samples of (+)- and (-)-butaclamol from our laboratory so that they could demonstrate stereo-selective binding of [³H]haloperidol.

DISCOVERY OF DOPAMINE AND ANTIPSYCHOTIC–ACCELERATED TURNOVER OF DOPAMINE

As listed in table 1, Montagu (1957) in Weil-Malherbe's laboratory (Weil-Malherbe and Bone, 1957, 1958), and Carlsson et al. (1958) discovered dopamine in brain tissue. This finding soon became clinically relevant with the dramatic finding by Ehringer and Hornykiewicz (1960) that the content of dopamine was extremely low in the post-mortem brains of patients who died with Parkinson's disease.

These findings naturally stimulated brain research on dopamine. Carlsson and Lindqvist (1963) soon reported that chlorpromazine and haloperidol increased the production of normetanephrine and methoxytyramine, metabolites of epinephrine and dopamine, respectively. To explain the increased production of these metabolites, these authors suggested that "the most likely [mechanism] appears to be that chlorpromazine and haloperidol block monoaminergic receptors in brain; as is well known, they block the effects of accumulated 5-hydroxytryptamine..."

In other words, these authors proposed that antipsychotics might block all three types of receptors for noradrenaline, dopamine and serotonin, but they did not identify which receptor was selectively blocked or how to identify or test any of these receptors directly *in vitro*. The paper by Carlsson and Lindqvist (1963) is often mistakenly cited as discovering the principle that antipsychotic drugs selectively block dopamine receptors. Even the students of the Carlsson laboratory, Andén et al. (1964), limited their speculation to proposing that "chlorpromazine and haloperidol delays the elimination of the (metabolites)...", a hypothesis no longer held. Moreover, as late as seven years later, although Andén et al. (1970) reported that antipsychotics increased the turnover of both dopamine and noradrenaline, they could not show that the antipsychotics were selective in blocking dopamine; for example, chlorpromazine enhanced the turnover of noradrenaline and dopamine equally. Therefore, it remained for in vitro radio-receptor assays to detect the dopamine receptor directly and to demonstrate antipsychotic selectivity for the dopamine receptor.

In fact, when the antipsychotic dopamine receptor was discovered (Seeman, 1975a,b), there was a peak surge in the rate of citations of the paper by Carlsson and Lindqvist (1963), a peak stimulated by the actual discovery of the dopamine receptor method, as shown in figure 2. This figure also shows that there was approximately a twelve-year interval between the onset of dopamine research and the research on dopamine receptors, indicating that the two fields were stimulated by separate developments.

THE DOPAMINE HYPOTHESIS OF SCHIZOPHRENIA AND DOPAMINE RECEPTORS IN HUMAN BRAIN

The paper by Carlsson and Lindqvist (1963) is often mistakenly cited as the origin of the dopamine hypothesis of schizophrenia. The dopamine hypothesis of schizophrenia was first outlined by Van Rossum (1967) (Baumeister and Francis, 2002), as follows:

"The hypothesis that neuroleptic drugs may act by blocking dopamine receptors in the brain has been substantiated by preliminary experiments with a few selective and potent neuroleptic drugs. There is an urgent need for a simple isolated tissue that selectively responds to dopamine so that less specific neuroleptic drugs can also be studied and the hypothesis further tested ...... When the hypothesis of dopamine

Figure 2. Top: Annual number of publications on "dopamine" and on "dopaminereceptors", as listed by PubMed online. Dopamine was found in brain tissue by Montagu (1957) in Weil-Malherbe's Laboratory (Weil-Malherbe and Bone, 1957, 1958) and by Carlsson (1958). There is approximately a twelve year interval between the two sets of publications, suggesting that the two onsets of publications were stimulated by separate other publications. Bottom: Annual rate of citations (Web of Science, Thomson Scientific, Philadelphia, Pennsylvania) of the article by Carlsson and Lindqvist (1963), describing the increased production of normetanephrine and methoxytyramine by chlorpromazine or haloperidol. The citation rate of this 1963 article peaked in 1975 when the dopamine receptors were discovered (Seeman et al., 1974a, 1975a, b).

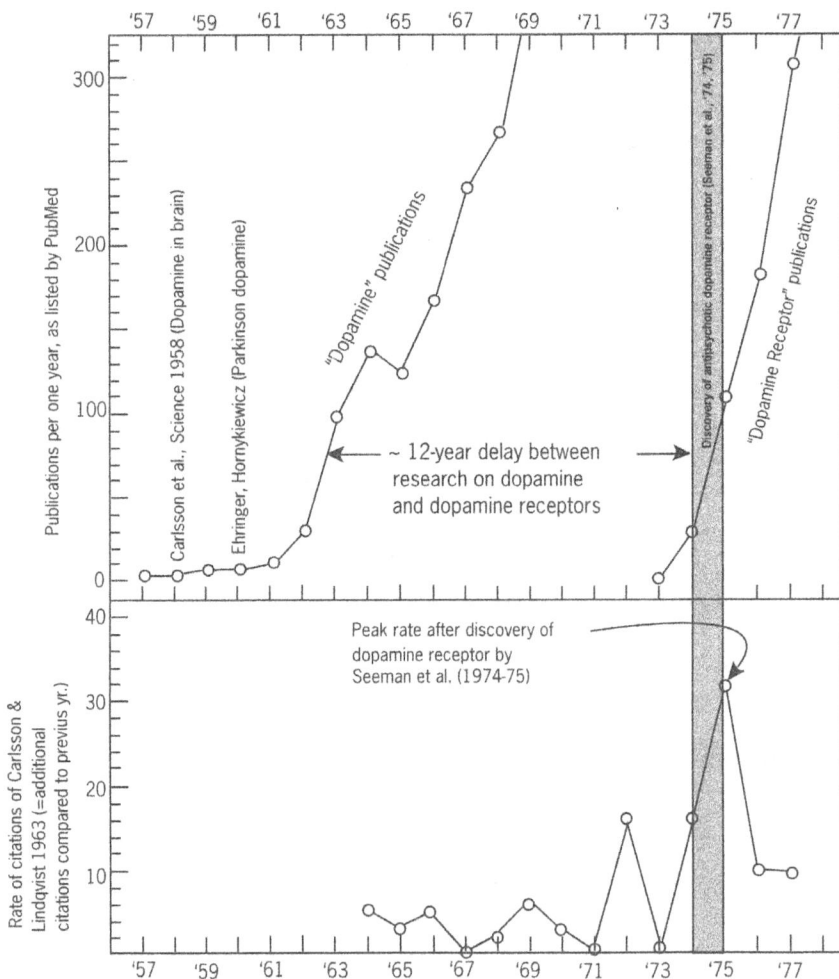

blockade by neuroleptic agents can be further substantiated it may have fargoing consequences for the pathophysiology of schizophrenia. Over-stimulation of dopamine receptors could then be part of the etiology."

With the discovery of the antipsychotic dopamine receptor *in vitro*, it became possible to measure the densities and properties of these receptors not only directly in animal brain tissues, but also in the post-mortem human brain and, at a later time, in living humans by means of positron emission tomography. Many, but not all, of these findings directly or indirectly support the dopamine hypothesis of schizophrenia.

KEY FINDINGS RELATED TO DOPAMINE RECEPTORS

Many of the significant advances in dopamine receptors and the dopamine hypothesis of psychosis or schizophrenia are listed in table 1. Between 1976 and 1979, it became clear that there were two main groups of dopamine receptors, D1 and D2 (Cools and Van Rossum, 1976; Garau et al., 1978; Kebabian and Calne, 1979; Spano et al., 1978). The D1-like group of receptors were associated with dopamine-stimulated cyclase (Brown et al., 1977; Kebabian and Greengard, 1971), but were not selectively labeled by [^{3}H]haloperidol. The antipsychotic potencies at these D1 receptors did not correlate with clinical antipsychotic potency (Seeman, 1980). The D1 receptors now consist of the cloned D_1 and D_5 receptors (Sunahara et al., 1990, 1991).

The D2-like receptors did not stimulate adenylate cyclase and are now known to inhibit adenylate cyclase (De Camilli et al., 1979; Garau et al., 1978; Meunier and Labrie, 1982; Onali et al., 1985; Roufogalis et al., 1976; Spano et al., 1978). The D2-like group now includes the cloned D2$_{Short}$ (Bunzow et al., 1988; Grandy et al., 1989), D2$_{Long}$ (Giros et al., 1989), D2$_{Longer}$ (Seeman et al., 2000), D_3 (Sokoloff et al., 1990) and D_4 dopamine receptors (Van Tol et al., 1991).

Moreover, each of these receptors has a state of high affinity and a state of low affinity for dopamine, with D2^{High} being the functional state in the anterior pituitary (George et al., 1985), in nigral dopamine terminals (presynaptic receptors, Starke et al., 1978) and presumably in the nervous system itself. Although this latter point has not been unequivocably established, Richfield et al. (1986) have found that 90% of the D_2 receptors in brain slices are in the D2^{High} state. The D2^{High} state can be quickly converted into the D2$_{Low}$ state by guanine nucleotide (Wreggett and Seeman, 1984).

The differences in findings on dopamine receptors between laboratories are explained by technically different methods and ligands. For example, the dissociation constant of a ligand at the D_2 receptor can vary enormously, depending on the final concentration of the tissue (Seeman et al., 1984a). Moreover, fat-soluble ligands, such as [^{125}I]iodosulpride, [^{3}H]nemonapride, and [^{3}H]spiperone, invariably yield higher dissociation constants than less fat-soluble ligands (such as [^{3}H]raclopride) for competing drugs (Seeman, 2002; Seeman and Van Tol, 1995). This technical effect also occurs with postiron emission tomography ligands (Hagberg et al., 1998).

Although the density of D_2 receptors in post-mortem human schizophrenia tissues is elevated (Lee et al., 1978; Lee and Seeman, 1980; Seeman, 1980, 1987; Seeman et al., 1984b), some of this elevation may have resulted from the antipsychotic administered during the lifetime of the patient. An example of this elevation is shown in figure 3, where it may be seen that the post-mortem tissues from half of the patients who died with schizophrenia revealed elevated densities of [^{3}H]spiperone-labeled D_2 receptors in the caudate-putamen tissue. The other half of the post-mortem schizophrenia tissues were normal in D_2 density even though most of the patients were known to have been also treated with antipsychotics during their lifetime.

It is often surprising to encounter people who are resistant to such advances in science. For example, I vividly recall one British psychiatrist standing up and shouting at me from the audience: "Post-mortem dopamine receptors? Do you actually expect me to believe that these dead receptors come to life and bind your radioactive material?" I answered that the same type of question was raised a century ago when people seriously questioned whether ferments could be isolated and still have activity, but that we can now buy crystallized enzymes for a few dollars and that these ferments are fully active.

Although the density of D_2 receptors labeled by [^{11}C]methylspiperone is elevated in drug-naive schizophrenia patients (Wong et al., 1986), [^{11}C]raclopride does not show this (Farde et al., 1986, and subsequent work). The recent work by Hirvonen et al. (2005) shows that the D_2 density is elevated in healthy identical co-twins of patients who have schizophrenia. This finding suggests that while the elevation of D_2 receptors might be necessary for psychosis, it is not a sufficient condition to cause disease.

Current active areas of research on the dopamine hypothesis of schizophrenia are: 1. Dopamine D_2 receptor occupancy by antipsychotics (Bressan et al., 2003; Farde et al. 1988, 1992), inquiring whether the contribution of serotonin-2 block assists in alleviating psychosis and affecting D_2 occupancy (Kapur et al., 1999; Knable et al., 1997; Nyberg and Farde, 1997), and whether the antipsychotic occupancy is higher or not in limbic regions (Bressan et al., 2003; Kapur and Seeman, 2001; Seeman, 2002; Seeman and Tallerico, 1999; Talvik et al., 2001). These problems relate to the question of the mechanism of action for atypical antipsychotics which elicit less Parkinsonism than the traditional antipsychotics such as chlorpromazine and haloperidol. The work from our laboratory shows that a significant feature of the atypical action of clozapine and quetiapine is that these compounds dissociate rapidly from the D_2 receptor (Seeman, 2002). 2. The molecular basis of dopamine super-sensitivity by monitoring the $D2_{High}$ state (Seeman et al., 1993, 2003, 2005a,b; Wilson et al., 2005); and 3. The use of amphetamine-induced release of endogenous dopamine as a possible marker of psychosis (Laruelle et al., 1996; Seeman, 2004; Seeman et al., 1989a).

The vision, the objective, and the questions still remain. What is the molecular pathway for antipsychotic action? Are any of these steps specifically altered in schizophrenia? At present, the most promising direction in this field is to examine the molecular basis of dopamine supersensitivity (Seeman et al., 2005b), because up to 70% of patients are supersensitive to either methylphenidate or amphetamine

Figure 3. Elevation of D_2 receptors in post-mortem caudate-putamen tissues from patients who had died with schizophrenia. Each box indicates the D_2 density measured by saturation analysis with [^{3}H]spiperone (Scatchard method for Bmax; centrifugation method)(adapted from Seeman et al., 1984b, 1987, 1989b). The D_2 densities in the post-mortem striata from schizophrenia patients exhibit a bimodal pattern, with half the values being two or three times the normal density. Most of the schizophrenia patients had been treated with antipsychotics during their lifetime. Although the Alzheimer patient tissues also revealed a small elevation of D_2 densities, the magnitude and pattern were different than that for schizophrenia.

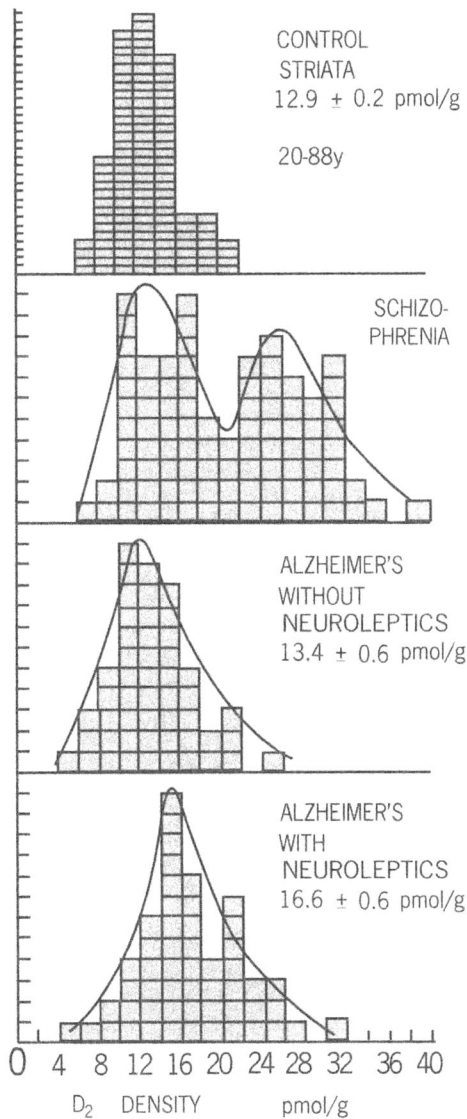

CONTROL STRIATA 12.9 ± 0.2 pmol/g 20-88y

SCHIZO-PHRENIA

ALZHEIMER'S WITHOUT NEUROLEPTICS 13.4 ± 0.6 pmol/g

ALZHEIMER'S WITH NEUROLEPTICS 16.6 ± 0.6 pmol/g

D_2 DENSITY pmol/g

at doses which do not affect control humans. Moreover, a wide variety of brain alterations (lesions, drug treatment, receptor knockouts) all lead to the final common *target* of elevated proportions of D_2 receptors in the $D2^{High}$ state. Therefore, the molecular control of the high-affinity state of D_2 is emerging as a central problem in this field. At present, there is uncertainty as to whether this high-affinity state of D_2 is controlled through Go or one of the Gi proteins, because this varies from cell to cell.

It is currently proposed that there are multiple pathways in the various types of psychosis that all converge to elevate the $D2^{High}$ state in specific brain regions and that this elevation elicits psychosis (Seeman et al., 2005a). This proposition is supported by the dopamine supersensitivity that is a common feature of schizophrenia and that also occurs in many types of genetically-altered, drug-altered, and lesion-altered animals. Dopamine supersensitivity, in turn, correlates with $D2^{High}$ states. The finding that all antipsychotics, traditional and recent ones, act on D_2 receptors further supports the proposition.

Altogether, the dawn of the neurotransmitter era has proven to be an exciting chapter in neuropsychopharmacology. The art of psychiatry is becoming a science. It has been a privilege to participate in these developments. I thank my fellow students for making it possible.

REFERENCES

1. Agid, O., Kapur, S., Arenovich, T., Zipursky, R.B., 2003. Delayed-onset hypothesis of antipsychotic action: a hypothesis tested and rejected. Arch. Gen. Psychiatry 60, 1228-1235.
2. Andén, N.-E., Roos, B.-E., Werdinius, B., 1964. Effects of chlorpromazine, haloperidol and reserpine on the levels of phenolic acids in rabbit corpus striatum. Life Sci. 3, 149-158.
3. Andén, N.-E., Butcher, S.G., Corrodi, H., Fuxe, K., Ungerstedt, U., 1970. Receptor activity and turnover of dopamine and noradrenaline after neuroleptics. Eur. J. Pharmacol. 11, 303-314.
4. Baumeister, A.A., Francis, J.L., 2002. Historical development of the dopamine Van Tol hypothesis of schizophrenia. J. History Neurosci. 11, 265-277.
5. Bloom, F.E., Costa, E., Salmoiraghi, G.C., 1965. Anesthesia and the responsiveness of individual neurons of the caudate nucleus of the cat to acetylcholine, norepinephrine and dopamine administered by microelectrophoresis. J. Pharmacol. Exp. Ther. 150, 244-252.
6. Bressan, R.A., Erlandsson, K., Jones, H.M., Mulligan, R., Flanagan, R.J., Ell, P.J., Pilowsky, L.S., 2003. Is regionally selective D_2/D_3 dopamine occupancy sufficient for atypical antipsychotic effect? An in vivo quantitative [$_{123}$I]epidepride SPEC study of amisulpride-treated patients. Am. J. Psychiatry 160, 1413-1420.
7. Brown, E.M., Carroll, R.J., Aurbach, G.D., 1977. Dopaminergic stimulation of cyclic AMP accumulation and parathyroid hormone release from dispersed bovine parathyroid cells. Proc. Natl. Acad. Sci. USA. 74, 4210-4213.
8. Bunzow, J.R., Van Tol, H.H., Grandy, D.K., Albert, P., Salon, J., Christie, M., Machida, C.A., Neve, K.A., Civelli, O., 1988. Cloning and expression of a rat D_2 dopamine receptor cDNA. Nature 336, 783-787.
9. Burt, D.R., Creese, I., Snyder, S.H., 1976. Properties of [₃H]haloperidol and [₃H]dopamine binding associated with dopamine receptors in calf brain membranes. Mol. Pharmacol. 12, 800-812.

10. Carlsson, A., Lindqvist, M., 1963. Effect of chlorpromazine or haloperidol on formation of 3-methoxytyramine and normetanephrine in mouse brain. Acta Pharmacol. Toxicol. (Copenh.) 20,140-144.
11. Carlsson, A., Lindqvist, M., Magnusson, T., Waldeck, B., 1958. On the presence of 3-hydroxytyramine in brain. Science 127, 471.
12. Cools, A.R., Van Rossum, J.M., 1976. Excitation-mediating and inhibition-mediating dopamine-receptors: a new concept towards a better understanding of electrophysiological, biochemical, pharmacological, functional and clinical data. Psychopharmacologia 45, 243-254.
13. De Camilli, P., Macconi, D., Spada, A., 1979. Dopamine inhibits adenylate cyclase in human prolactin-secreting pituitary adenomas. Nature 278, 252-254.
14. Delay, J., Deniker, P., Harl, J.-M., 1952. Traitement des états d'excitation et d'agitation par une méthode médicamenteuse dérivée de l'hibernithérapie. [Therapeutic method derived from hiberno-therapy in excitation and agitation states.] Ann. Méd-Psychol. (Paris) 110, 267-273.
15. Ehringer, H., Hornykiewicz, O., 1960. Distribution of noradrenaline and dopamine (3-hydroxytyramine) in the human brain and their behavior in diseases of the extrapyramidal system. Klin. Wochenschr. 38, 1236-1239.
16. Farde, L., Hall, H., Ehrin, E., Sedvall, G., 1986. Quantitative analysis of D_2 dopamine receptor binding in the living human brain by PET. Science 231, 258-261.
17. Farde, L., Wiesel, F.-A., Halldin, C., Sedvall, G., 1988. Central D_2-dopamine receptor occupancy in schizophrenic patients treated with antipsychotic drugs. Arch. Gen. Psychiatry 45, 71-76.
18. Farde, L., Nordstrom, A.L., Wiesel, F.A., Pauli, S., Halldin, C., Sedvall, G., 1992. Positron emission tomographic analysis of central D_1 and D_2 dopamine receptor occupancy in patients treated with classical neuroleptics and clozapine. Relation to extrapyramidal side effects. Arch. Gen. Psychiatry 49, 538-544.
19. Forsman, A., Öhman, R., 1977. Studies on serum protein binding of haloperidol. Curr. Ther. Res. Clin. Exp. 21, 245-255.
20. Garau, L., Govoni, S., Stefanini, E., Trabucchi, M., Spano, P.F., 1978. Dopamine receptors: pharmacological and anatomical evidences indicate that two distinct dopamine receptor populations are present in rat striatum. Life Sci. 23, 1745-1750.
21. George SR, Watanabe M, Di Paolo T, Falardeau P, Labrie F, Seeman P., 1985. The functional state of the dopamine receptor in the anterior pituitary is in the high affinity form. Endocrinology 117, 690-697.
22. Giros, B., Sokoloff, P., Martres, M.P., Riou, J.F., Emorine, L.J., Schwartz, J.C., 1989. Alternative splicing directs the expression of two D_2 dopamine receptor isoforms. Nature 342, 923-926.
23. Grandy, D.K., Marchionni, M.A., Makam, H., Stofko, R.E., Alfano, M., Frothingham, L., Fischer, J.B., Burke-Howie, K.J., Bunzow, J.R., Server, A.C., Civelli, O.,1989. Cloning of the cDNA and gene for a human D_2 dopamine receptor. Proc. Natl. Acad. Sci. USA 86, 9762-9766.
24. Hagberg, G., Gefvert, O., Bergström, M., Wieselgren, I.-M., Lindstrom, L., Wiesel, F.-A., Langström, B., 1998. N-[¹¹C]methylspiperone PET, in contrast to [¹¹C]raclopride, fails to detect D_2 receptor occupancy by an atypical neuroleptic. Psychiatry Res. 82, 147-160.
25. Heiss WD, Hoyer J., 1974. Dopamine receptor blockade by neuroleptic drugs in *Aplysia* neurones. Experientia 30, 1318-1320.
26. Hirvonen, J., van Erp, T.G., Huttunen, J., Aalto, S., Nagren, K., Huttunen, M., Lonnqvist, J., Kaprio, J., Hietala, J., Cannon, T.D., 2005. Increased caudate dopamine D_2 receptor availability as a genetic marker for schizophrenia. Arch. Gen. Psychiatry 62, 371-378.
27. Kapur, S., Seeman, P., 2001. Does fast dissociation from the dopamine D2 receptor explain the action of atypical antipsychotics? - A new hypothesis. Am. J. Psychiat. 158, 360-369.
28. Kapur, S., Zipursky, R.B., Remington, G., 1999. Clinical and theoretical implications of 5-HT₂ and D_2 receptor occupancy of clozapine, risperidone, and olanzapine in schizophrenia. Am. J. Psychiatry 156, 286-293.
29. Kapur, S., Arenovich, T., Agid, O., Zipursky, R., Lindborg, S., Jones, B., 2005. Evidence for onset of antipsychotic effects within the first 24 hours of treatment. Am. J. Psychiatry 162, 939-946.

30. Kawagoe, K.T., Garris, P.A., Wiedemann, D.J., Wightman, R.M., 1992. Regulation of transient dopamine concentration gradients in the microenvironment surrounding nerve terminals in the rat striatum. Neuroscience 51, 55-64.

31. Kebabian, J.W., Calne, D.B., 1979. Multiple receptors for dopamine. Nature 277, 93-96.

32. Kebabian, J.W., Greengard, P., 1971. Dopamine-sensitive adenyl cyclase: possible role in - synaptic transmission. Science 174, 1346-1349.

33. Khan, Z.U., Mrzljak, L., Gutierrez, A., de la Calle, A., Goldman-Rakic, P.S., 1998. Prominence of the dopamine D2$_{short}$ isoform in dopaminergic pathways. Proc. Natl. Acad. Sci. USA. 95, 7731-7736.

34. Klein, C., Brin, M.F., Kramer, P., Sena-Esteves, M., de Leon, D., Doheny, D., Bressman, S., Fahn, S., Breakefield, X.O., Ozelius, L.J., 1999. Association of a missense change in the D$_2$ dopamine receptor with myoclonus dystonia. Proc. Natl. Acad. Sci. USA. 96, 5173-5176.

35. Knable, M.B., Heinz, A., Raedler, T., Weinberger, D.R., 1997. Extrapyramidal side effects with risperidone and haloperidol at comparable D2 receptor occupancy levels. Psychiatry Res. 75, 91-101.

36. Lacomme, M., Laborit, H., Le Lorier, G., Pommier, M., 1952. Obstetric analgesia potentiated by associated intravenous dolosal with RP 4560. Bull. Féd. Soc. Gynecol. Obstet. Lang. Fr. 4, 558-562.

37. Laruelle, M., Abi-Dargham, A., van Dyck, C.H., Gil, R., D'Souza, C.D., Erdos, J., McCance, E., Rosenblatt, W., Fingado, C., Zoghbi, S.S., Baldwin, R.M., Seibyl, J.P., Krystal, J.H., Charney, D.S., Innis, R.B., 1996. Single photon emission computerized tomography imaging of amphetamine-induced dopamine release in drug-free schizophrenic subjects. Proc. Natl. Acad. Sci. USA. 93, 9235-9240.

38. Lee, T., Seeman, P., 1980. Elevation of brain neuroleptic/dopamine receptors in schizophrenia. Amer. J. Psychiat. 137, 191-197.

39. Lee, T., Seeman, P., Tourtellotte, W.W., Farley, I.J., Hornykiewicz, O., 1978. Binding of ^{3}H-neuroleptics and ^{3}H-apomorphine in schizophrenic brains. Nature 274, 897-900.

40. Liu, I.S.C., Seeman, P., Sanyal, S., Ulpian, C., Rodgers-Johnson, P.E.B., Serjeant, G.R., Van Tol, H.H.M., 1996. The dopamine D$_4$ receptor variant in Africans, D4$_{Valine194Glycine}$, is insensitive to dopamine and clozapine. Report of a homozygous individual. Amer. J. Med. Gen. 61, 277-282.

41. Meunier, H., Labrie, F., 1982. The dopamine receptor in the intermediate lobe of the rat pituitary gland is negatively coupled to adenylate cyclase. Life Sci. 30, 963-968.

42. Montagu, K.A., 1957. Catechol compounds in rat tissues and in brains of different animals. Nature 180, 244-245.

43. Nyberg, S, Farde, L., 1997. The relevance of serotonergic mechanisms in the treatment of schizophrenia has not been confirmed. J. Psychopharmacol. 11, 13-14.

44. Onali, P., Olianas, M.C., Gessa, G.L., 1985. Characterization of dopamine receptors mediating inhibition of adenylate cyclase activity in rat striatum. Mol. Pharmacol. 28, 138-145.

45. Richfield, E.K., Young, A.B., Penney, J.B., 1986. Properties of D$_2$ dopamine receptor autoradiography: high percentage of high-affinity agonist sites and increased nucleotide sensitivity in tissue sections. Brain Res. 383, 121-128.

46. Roufogalis BD, Thornton M, Wade DN., 1976. Specificity of the dopamine sensitive adenylate cyclase for antipsychotic antagonists. Life Sci. 19, 927-934.

47. Seeman, P., 1966a. Erythrocyte membrane stabilization by local anesthetics and tranquilizers. Biochem. Pharmacol. 15, 1753-1766.

48. Seeman, P., 1966b. Membrane stabilization by drugs: Tranquilizers, steroids and anesthetics. Int. Rev. Neurobiol. 9, 145-221.

49. Seeman, P., 1972. The membrane actions of anesthetics and tranquilizers. Pharmacol. Rev. 24, 583-655.

50. Seeman, P., 1980. Brain dopamine receptors. Pharmacol. Rev. 32, 229-313.

51. Seeman, P., 1982. Nomenclature of central and peripheral dopaminergic sites and receptors. Biochem. Pharmacol. 31, 2563-2568.

52. Seeman, P., 1987. Dopamine receptors and the dopamine hypothesis of schizophrenia. Synapse 1, 133-152.

53. Seeman, P., 1992. Dopamine receptor sequences. Therapeutic levels of neuroleptics occupy D_2, clozapine occupies D_4. Neuropsychopharmacology 7, 261-284.

54. Seeman, P., 1995. Therapeutic receptor-blocking concentrations of neuroleptics. Int. Clin. Psychopharmacol. 10 (Suppl. 3), 5-13.

55. Seeman, P., 2002. Atypical antipsychotics: Mechanism of action. Can. J. Psychiat. 47, 27-38.

56. Seeman, P., 2004. Comment: Diverse psychotomimetics act through a common signaling pathway. Science 305, 180.

57. Seeman, P., Bialy, H.S., 1963. The surface activity of tranquilizers. Biochem. Pharmacol. 12, 1181-1191.

58. Seeman, P., Lee, T., 1975. Antipsychotic drugs: Direct correlation between clinical potency and presynaptic action on dopamine neurones. Science 188, 1217-1219.

59. Seeman, P., Tallerico, T., 1999. Rapid release of antipsychotic drugs from dopamine D_2 receptors: An explanation for low receptor occupancy and early clinical relapse upon drug withdrawal of clozapine or quetiapine. Amer. J. Psychiat. 156, 876-884.

60. Seeman, P. Ulpian, C., 1983. Neuroleptics have identical potencies in human brain limbic and putamen regions. Europ. J. Pharmacol. 94, 145-148.

61. Seeman, P., Van Tol, H.H.M., 1995. Deriving the therapeutic concentrations for clozapine and haloperidol: The apparent dissociation constant of a neuroleptic at the dopamine D_2 or D_4 receptor varies with the affinity of the competing radioligand. Eur. J. Pharmacol. – Mol. Pharmacol. 291, 59-66.

62. Seeman, P., Weinstein, J., 1966. Erythrocyte membrane stabilization by tranquilizers and anti-histamines. Biochem. Pharmacol. 15, 1737-1752.

63. Seeman, P., Wong, M., Lee, T., 1974a. Dopamine receptor-block and nigral fiber impulse-blockade by major tranquilizers. Fed. Proc. 33, 246.

64. Seeman, P., Staiman, A., Chau-Wong, M., 1974b. The nerve impulse-blocking actions of tranquilizers, and the binding of neuroleptics to synaptosome membranes. J. Pharmacol. Exp. Ther. 190, 123-130.

65. Seeman, P., Wong,M., Tedesco, J., 1975a. Tranquilizer receptors in rat striatum. Soc. Neurosci. Abstr. 1, 405.

66. Seeman, P., Chau-Wong, M., Tedesco, J, Wong, K., 1975b. Brain receptors for antipsychotic drugs and dopamine: direct binding assays. Proc. Natl. Acad. Sci. USA. 72, 4376-4380.

67. Seeman, P., Lee, T., Chau-Wong, M., Wong, K., 1976. Antipsychotic drug doses and neuroleptic/dopamine receptors. Nature (Lond.) 261, 717-719.

68. Seeman, P., Ulpian, C., Wreggett, K.A., Wells, J., 1984a. Dopamine receptor parameters detected by ^{3}H-spiperone depend on tissue concentration: analysis and examples. J. Neurochem. 43, 221-235.

69. Seeman, P., Ulpian, C., Bergeron, C., Riederer, P., Jellinger, K., Gabriel, E., Reynolds, G.P., Tourtellotte, W.W., 1984b. Bimodal distribution of dopamine receptor densities in brains of schizophrenics. Science 225, 728-731.

70. Seeman, P., Guan, H.-C., Niznik, H.B., 1989a. Endogenous dopamine lowers the dopamine D2 receptor density as measured by [^{3}H]raclopride: Implications for positron emission tomography of the human brain. Synapse 3, 96-97.

71. Seeman, P., Niznik, H.B., Guan, H.-C., Booth, G., Ulpian, C., 1989b. Link between D_1 and D_2 dopamine receptors is reduced in schizophrenia and Huntington diseased brain. Proc. Nat. Acad. Sci., USA. 86, 10156-10160.

72. Seeman, P., Ulpian, C., Larsen, R.D., Anderson, P.S., 1993. Dopamine receptors labelled by PHNO. Synapse 14, 254-262.

73. Seeman, P. Nam, D., Ulpian, C., Liu, I.S.C., Tallerico, T., 2000. A new dopamine receptor, $D2_{longer}$, with a unique TG splice site, in human brain. Mol. Brain Res. 76, 132-141.

74. Seeman, P., Tallerico, T., Ko, F., 2003. Dopamine displaces [^{3}H]domperidone from high-affinity sites of the dopamine D2 receptor, but not [^{3}H]raclopride or [^{3}H]spiperone in isotonic medium: Implications for human positron emission tomography. Synapse 49, 209-215.

75. Seeman, P., Weinshenker, D., Quirion, R., Srivastava, L., Bhardwaj, S.K., Grandy, D.K., Premont, R., Sotnikova, T., Boksa, P., El-Ghundi, M., O'Dowd, B.F., George, S.R., Perreault, M.L., Mannisto, P.T., Robinson, S., Palmiter, R.D., Tallerico, T., 2005a. Dopamine supersen-

sitivity correlates with D2^{High} states, implying many paths to psychosis. Proc. Nat. Acad. Sci. USA. 102, 3513-3518.

76. Seeman, P., Ko, F., Tallerico, T., 2005b. Dopamine receptor contribution to the action of PCP. LSD, and ketamine psychotomimetics. Mol. Psychiatry (online April 26, 2005).

77. Sigwald, J., Bouttier, D., 1953. 3-Chloro-10-(3'-dimethylaminopropyl)-phenothiazine hydrochloride in current neuro-psychiatry. Ann. Méd. Interne (Paris) 54, 150-182.

78. Snyder, S.H., Creese, I., Burt, D.R., 1975. The brain's dopamine receptor: labeling with [^{3}H]dopamine and [^{3}H]haloperidol. Psychopharmacol. Commun. 1, 663-673.

79. Sokoloff, P., Giros, B., Martres, M.P., Bouthenet, M.L., Schwartz, J.C., 1990. Molecular cloning and characterization of a novel dopamine receptor (D$_3$) as a target for neuroleptics. Nature 347, 146-151.

80. Spano, P.F., Govoni, S., Trabucchi, M., 1978. Studies on the pharmacological properties of dopamine receptors in various areas of the central nervous system. Adv. Biochem. Psychopharmacol. 19, 155-165.

81. Starke, K., Reimann, W., Zumstein, A., Hertting, G., 1978. Effect of dopamine receptor agonists and antagonists on release of dopamine in the rabbit caudate nucleus in vitro. Naunyn Schmiedebergs Arch. Pharmacol. 305, 27-36.

82. Struyker Boudier, H.A.J., Gielen, W., Cools, A.R., van Rossum, J.M., 1974. Pharmacological analysis of dopamine-induced inhibition and excitation of neurones of the snail *Helix Aspersa*. Arch. Int. Pharmacodyn. Ther. 209, 324-331.

83. Sunahara, R.K., Niznik, H.B., Weiner, D.M., Stormann, T.M., Brann, M.R., Kennedy, J.L., Gelernter, J.E., Rozmahel, R., Yang, Y., Israel, Y., Seeman, P., O'Dowd, B.F., 1990. Human dopamine D$_1$ receptor encoded by an intronless gene on chromosome 5. Nature 347, 80-83.

84. Sunahara, R.K., Guan, H.-C., O'Dowd, B., Seeman, P., Laurier, L.G., Ng, G., George, S., Torc, J., Van Tol, H.H.M., Niznik, H.B., 1991. Cloning of the gene for a human dopamine D5 receptor with higher affinity for dopamine than D$_1$. Nature 350, 614-619.

85. Talvik, M., Nordström, A.L., Nyberg, S., Olsson, H., Halldin, C., Farde, L., 2001. No support for regional selectivity in clozapine-treated patients: a PET study with [^{11}C]raclopride and [^{11}C]FLB 457. Am. J. Psychiatry 158, 926-930.

86. Van Rossum, J.M., 1967. The significance of dopamine-receptor blockade for the action of neuroleptic drugs. In: Brill, H., Cole, J.O., Deniker, P., Hippius, H., Bradley, P.B. (Eds.), Neuro-Psycho-Pharmacology, Proceedings of the Fifth International Congress of the Collegium Internationale Neuro-Psycho-pharmacologicum, March 1966, Excerpta Medica Foundation, Amsterdam, pp. 321-329.

87. Van Tol, H.H.M., Bunzow, J.R., Guan, H.-C., Sunahara, R.K., Seeman, P., Niznik, H.B., Civelli, O., 1991. Cloning of the gene for a human dopamine D$_4$ receptor with high affinity for the antipsychotic clozapine. Nature 350, 610-614.

88. Weil-Malherbe, H., Bone, A.D., 1957. Intracellular distribution of catecholamines in the brain. Nature 180, 1050-1051.

89. Weil-Malherbe, H., Bone, A.D., 1958. Effect of reserpine on the intracellular distribution of catecholamines in the brain stem of the rabbit. Nature 181, 1474-1475.

90. Wilhelmy, L., 1863. Ann. Physik., Lpz. 119, 177.

91. Wilson, A.A., McCormick, P., Kapur, S., Willeit, M., Garcia, A., Hussey, D., Houle, S., Seeman, P., Ginovart, N., 2005. Radiosynthesis and evaluation of [^{11}C]-(+)-PHNO as a potential radiotracer for in vivo imaging of the dopamine D2 high affinity state with positron emission tomography (PET). J. Med. Chem. 48, 4153-4160.

92. Wong, D.F., Wagner, H.N. Jr., Tune, L.E., Dannals, R.F., Pearlson, G.D., Links, J.M., Tamminga, C.A., Broussolle, E.P., Ravert, H.T., Wilson, A.A., Toung, T., Malat, J., Williams, J.A., O'Tuama, L.A., Snyder, S.H., Kuhar, M.J., Gjedde, A., 1986. Positron emission tomography reveals elevated D$_2$ dopamine receptors in drug-naive schizophrenics. Science 234, 1558-1563.

93. Wreggett, K.A., Seeman, P., 1984. Agonist high- and low-affinity states of the D2 dopamine receptor in calf brain: partial conversion by guanine nucleotide. Mol. Pharmacol. 25, 10-17.

94. Zingales, I.A., 1971. A gas chromatographic method for the determination of haloperidol in human plasma. J. Chromatogr. 54, 15-24.

PART THREE

PHARMACOLOGICAL ACTIONS

AND CLINICAL EFFECTS

LEVODOPA AND THE EMERGENCE OF BRAIN NEUROTRANSMITTER REPLACEMENT IN NEUROPSYCHOPHARMACOLOGY

Oleh Hornykiewicz

The year 1956, which witnessed the founding of the Collegium Internationale Neuro-Psychopharmacologicum (CINP), also proved to be decisive for the direction that my own research has since taken. Although our first clinical trials with levodopa (3,4-dihydroxy-phenylalanine, L-dopa) in Parkinson's disease (PD) patients did not start before 1961, my first experience with levodopa as a pharmacological agent dates back to 1956, the year in which I had joined (from Vienna's Pharmacological Institute) Hermann Blaschko's laboratory in the department of pharmacology of Oxford University.

DOPAMINE AND LEVODOPA IN 1956: A GOOD STARTER (FOR ME)

It was also in 1956, that Blaschko postulated, for the first time, that dopamine (DA), the decarboxylation product of levodopa in the body (Holtz et al., 1938), must have "*some regulatory functions of its own, which are not yet known*" (Blaschko, 1957). Until then, DA had been regarded as being a mere intermediate in the formation of noradrenaline (NA) and adrenaline (Blaschko, 1939; Holtz, 1939). Now Blaschko asked me to test his idea experimentally. To do this, I chose to examine the action of DA on the blood pressure of the guinea pig. In this species, DA has an action opposite to that of NA and adrenaline: instead of raising the blood pressure, as the latter do, DA lowers it. In my study, I included iproniazid, the first in vivo effective inhibitor of the DA degrading enzyme monoamine oxidase (MAO). The results of my study were clear: Iproniazid, instead of abolishing the fall in blood pressure, as expected on the basis of earlier explanations (Holtz and Credner, 1942), actually potentiated DA's effect, proving that the fall in blood pressure was due to DA itself. I also examined levodopa, which behaved exactly like DA, and whose DA-like effect was also potentiated by inhibition of MAO. The results of my study, which I had finished by early summer of 1957, convinced me that DA was a biologically active substance in its own right, different from the other two catecholamines NA and adrenaline.

DA OCCURS IN THE BRAIN AND IS ACTED UPON BY LEVODOPA, RESERPINE AND MAO INHIBITORS

In August 1957, Kathleen Montagu from Hans Weil-Malherbe's Runwell laboratory in Wickford, London, reported on the presence of DA (and L-dopa) in the brain of several species, including the human brain (Montagu, 1957). In November 1957, Weil-Malherbe confirmed and extended this discovery (Weil-Malherbe and Bone, 1957). At the same time, between September and December 1957, three levodopa studies appeared in print. First, Peter Holtz, in Germany, observed, for the first time, that levodopa caused "central excitation", especially in MAO inhibitor (MAOI) pre-treated animals, and also prevented hexobarbital anesthesia (Holtz et al., 1957); Arvid Carlsson, in Sweden, reported that levodopa, in addition to causing central excitation, abolished the "tranquillizing" effect of reserpine (Carlsson et al., 1957); and Alfred Pletscher, in Switzerland, found that levodopa increased brain catecholamine levels, especially after MAO inhibition (Pletscher, 1957). Finally, early in 1958, both Carlsson (in "Science", February 28) and Weil-Malherbe (in "Nature", May 24) reported that reserpine depleted the brain of DA and levodopa restored the DA to normal (or above-normal) levels (Carlsson et al., 1958; Weil-Malherbe and Bone, 1958).

For the historical record it should be noted that of the three research groups involved in this cluster of closely related levodopa studies, only Holtz concluded that levodopa's central excitatory effect must be due to the "*hydroxytyramine [DA] formed from dopa in the brain*" (Holtz et al., 1957). While Pletscher (1957) stated that "*the composition of the catecholamines following treatment with DOPA has not yet been examined*", Carlsson confined himself to "*the assumption*" that the effect of levodopa "*was due to an amine formed from it*" (Carlsson et al., 1957).

While these papers were published, my 1957 Oxford study, which had convinced me of DA's biological importance, appeared in print (Hornykiewicz, 1958). Aware of the reports about brain DA, I started – now back in Vienna's Institute of Pharmacology – in the summer of 1958, a study (in the rat) with several centrally acting substances, including the parkinsonism-inducing chlorpromazine and bulbocapnine, as well as cocaine and MAOIs. I found that from the various substances employed only MAOIs affected (increased) the levels of brain DA (Holzer and Hornykiewicz, 1959). While I was conducting my research one more paper was published on brain DA. It was the most exciting report, authored by the Swedish investigators, Åke Bertler and Evald Rosengren (Bertler and Rosengren, 1959a).

DA'S STRIATAL LOCALISATION HINTS AT ITS FUNCTION IN THE BRAIN

In 1954, Marthe Vogt, in Edinburgh, had published her landmark study on NA's regional distribution in the dog brain, and inferred, from the amine's uneven distribution pattern, NA's possible role in brain function (Vogt, 1954). Following this pattern, Bertler and Rosengren examined, also in the dog, DA's regional brain distribution and found the bulk of the amine in the corpus striatum, i.e. caudate and putamen (Bertler and Rosengren, 1959a). Isamu Sano in Japan published similar findings in the human brain (Sano et al., 1959). In their January 1959 report, Bertler and Rosengren (1959a) concluded that their *"results favour the assumption that dopamine is connected with the function of the corpus striatum and thus with the control of movement"*; and Sano considered *"dopamine to function in the extrapyra - midal system which regulates the central motoric function"*. Bertler and Rosengren (1959a), when referring to the DA depleting action of reserpine, were quick to point out the possible involvement of striatal DA in the reserpine-induced parkinsonism; however, neither they nor Sano drew attention to, or hinted at, the possibility of striatal DA being involved in human basal ganglia disease.

CONNECTING STRIATAL DA TO PD, AND THE MANY PROBLEMS OF THE RESERPINE MODEL

The possibility of a connection between basal ganglia DA and reserpine-induced parkinson-like conditions, prompted me to move from animal studies to the human brain and its diseases in my reserach. I was already familiar with basal ganglia disease from my first postdoctoral work in the early 1950s, when I had studied ceruloplasmin's polyphenol oxidase activity in the blood serum of patients with Wilson's disease; and I had already done work on peripheral DA in Oxford and on brain DA in Vienna. Thus, the idea of connecting the observations in laboratory animals with human basal ganglia disorders, specifically PD, came quite naturally to me.

Although reserpine was an invaluable pharmacological tool, the drug, in addition to DA depleted also NA and serotonin in the brain, so that the relative contribution of these changes to reserpine's central action remained obscure. Starting in about 1956, fierce battles were fought about the central action of reserpine between the proponents of serotonin (Brodie) and the proponents of NA (Carlsson) in the two laboratories. Since those debates did not at all concern themselves with reserpine's well-known and well-defined extrapyramidal effects (Bein, 1956) - revolving, instead, around the drug's "sedative" or "tranquillizing" actions, considered to be, rightly or wrongly, the animal behavioural correlate of reserpine's antipsychotic action in humans - they generated more heat than light in this difficult field of research. This being so, I thought it best to avoid the reserpine model and look directly into the PD brain, and determine whether there was a change in DA or not.

STRIATAL DA DEFICIENCY IN THE PD BRAIN – BUT NOT IN EVERYONE'S MIND

Immediately after the Bertler and Rosengren report was published in January 1959, I started, together with my postdoctoral collaborator Herbert Ehringer, a study on DA in postmortem brains of patients with PD and other basal ganglia disorders. Five months later, in June 1959 – the same time when Carlsson's contribution to a symposium was published (Carlsson, 1959) that is often quoted as containing the concept that DA plays a role in human PD – we already had analysed two PD brains, clearly observing the typical striatal DA deficiency. Our study, which we had finished in late spring of 1960, included brains of 17 adult controls, 2 brains of Huntington's disease, 6 brains of patients with extrapyramidal disorders of unknown etiology, and 6 PD brains, as well as 2 neonate brains and one infant brain. Of the 14 cases with basal ganglia disease, only the 6 PD cases had a severe loss of DA in the caudate and putamen (Ehringer and Hornykiewicz, 1960). We concluded that our observations "*could be regarded as com - parable in significance to the histological changes in substantia nigra*" so that "*a partic - ularly great importance would have to be attributed to dopamine's role in the pathophys - iology and symptomatology of idiopathic Parkinson's disease*". This discovery was pub- lished in December 1960. Ever since, it has proved to be a solid, rational basis for all the research that followed into the mechanisms, the causes, and new treatments, of PD.

It is interesting to note that what appeared to me so logical, and indeed necessary, i.e. the move from reserpine/DA/levodopa research in animals to the PD brain, had not occurred to any of the authors of the respective animal studies. Thus, there is no hint to be found in any of these reports (Bertler and Rosengren, 1959a; Carlsson, 1959; Carlsson et al., 1958; Weil-Malherbe and Bone, 1958) – in none of the publications prior to our December 1960 DA/PD paper – that such a study should be done. Even more surprising is that, when Bertler and Rosengren (1959b) – Carlsson's graduate students at that time – published a study that included analysis of DA in normal human brain (published in the fall of 1959), they did not think that it would be impor- tant to study the PD brain, or at least mention that possibility. The first suggestion that it would be desirable to analyse PD brains, was made nearly two years later, in a "Science" article by André Barbeau, Gerard Murphy and Theodore Sourkes in Montreal, reporting on low urinary DA in PD patients (Barbeau et al., 1961). Published on May 26, 1961, their suggestion was published six months after our study in Vienna had appeared in print.

LEVODOPA FOR THE PD PATIENT – BASIC RESEARCH PUT TO GOOD USE

With the results of our study in PD brain in my hands, I did not need much help to take the step from human brain homogenates to DA replacement (Hornykiewicz,

2002). DA's precursor, levodopa, was a logical (pro)-drug of choice. I had already noted, in my 1957 Oxford study, levodopa's DA-like biological effects and the potentation of these effects by MAO inhibition. In November 1960, I asked the clinical neurologist Walther Birkmayer to conduct a clinical trial with intravenously administered levodopa in patients with PD. I gave him my total supply of levodopa, about 2 grams, donated to me earlier by F.Hoffmann-LaRoche's Medical Director Alfred Pletscher, a pioneer and supporter of brain monoamine research. The intravenous route offered the most economical procedure. To make treatment even more economical I suggested pre-treatment with MAOI.

In July 1961, after many reminders, Birkmayer finally administered 50 to 150 mg. of levodopa intravenously to several patients who were pre-treated with MAOI. The effect was spectacular. Our first report, published in November 1961, reads as follows: "*The effect of a single i.v. administration of L-dopa was, in short, a complete abolition or substantial relief of akinesia. Bed-ridden patients who were unable to sit up; patients who could not stand up when seated; and patients who when standing could not start walking, performed after L-dopa all these activities with ease. They walked around with normal associated movements and they even could run and jump. The voiceless, aphonic speech, blurred by pallilalia and unclear articulation, became forceful and clear as in a normal person. For short periods of time the patients were able to perform motor activities which could not be prompted to any comparable degree by any other known drug*" (Birkmayer and Hornykiewicz, 1961).

At the same time, and independent from us, Ted Sourkes in Montreal suggested to André Barbeau a clinical trial with oral levodopa. In their report, published in 1962, they wrote: "*In all cases with Parkinson's disease L-dopa ameliorated the rigidity, espe - cially when combined with an inhibitor of monoamine oxidase*" (Barbeau et al., 1962).

It took six more years, before levodopa found its way into clinical practice. In 1967, George Cotzias in New York – aware of our prior levodopa studies in PD patients (Cotzias et al., 1964) – published the findings of a study in which they administered D, L-dopa in gradually increasing oral doses (3 to 16 grams/day) chronically (Cotzias et al., 1967). In this way, a strong and sustained effect was obtained, that was suitable for continuous treatment – a regimen that in principle is still used today. Two years later, a double blind, placebo-controlled study, conducted by Melvin Yahr, showed that levodopa was superior to any other known antiparkinson drug (Yahr et al., 1969). A further important advance at the time was the development of so-called "peripheral dopa decarboxylase inhibitors", which are used today generally as adjuvants in levodopa treatment (Pletscher, 1994).

In the years between 1961 and 1967, several confirmatory, but also a few negative reports were published on the use of levodopa in the treatment of PD. The negative findings were mostly due to diagnostic problems, uncritical patient selection, and unsuitable trial conditions. One such negative report was Isamu Sano's, who, after finding, in the summer of 1959, low DA in a single PD brain, injected 2 patients with 200 mg of levodopa intravenously. He did not evaluate the effect of the substance clinically. Instead, he kept the patients on the examination table, because he was "*more interested in* [the patients'] *subjective complaints* " than in the effect of the drug on PD (Letter of I. Sano to O.Hornykiewicz, dated March 20, 1962). In a lecture (in Japanese), delivered in 1960, Sano concluded that "*treatment with dopa has no ther-apeutic value*" (Sano, 2000).

THE NEW AND UNEXPECTED, ESPECIALLY WHEN SUCCESSFUL, PROVOKES OPPOSITION

Despite of the unprecedented success of levodopa, there were doubts expressed about its "miraculous" effect in patients. Some of the doubts questioned the rationale on which the drug's use was based. Some neurologists suggested that intravenous injections have a placebo effect. Such a suggestion was possible only by dismissing our 1962 report, in which we had shown the ineffectiveness of intravenously inject-ed compounds related to levodopa, such as D-dopa, 3-O-methyldopa, DA, and D,L-dops, in the treatment of PD. It was only levodopa that produced in the same patients on each occasion when given, a strong, reproducible therapeutic anti-akinesia effect (Birkmayer and Hornykiewicz, 1962).

More damaging than these doubts were statements by prominent neuroscientists. Some of the adherents of the old reserpine-NA story claimed that "*the actions* [on motor behaviour] *of DOPA and DOPS* [the direct precursor of NA] *were similar*", and insisted that "*dopamine can activate not only its own receptors* [in the brain], *but also those of noradrenaline, and vice versa*" (Carlsson, 1964, 1965), whereas others declared that "*the effect of L-dopa was too complex to permit a conclusion about dis-turbances of the dopamine system in Parkinson's disease*" and concluded that "*with the facts so far available, it is not possible to say what functions dopamine has in the central nervous system*" (Bertler and Rosengren, 1966). There were also those who simply decided that levodopa was "*the right therapy for the wrong reason*" (Ward, 1970; Jasper, 1970). Furthermore, there was, also a suspicion expressed that "*since L-dopa floods the brain with dopamine, to relate its* [antiparkinson] *effects to the natural function of dopamine neurons may be erroneous*" (Vogt, 1973). Statements like these not only diminished the status of levodopa as a specific DA replacing agent, but also put in doubt the whole concept of DA replacement therapy of PD, without which the striatal DA deficit would have to be looked upon as one of the several unspecific bio-chemical accompaniments of the neurodegenerative process as such.

None of the criticisms withstood the test of time. Guy Everett in Chicago convinc-ingly demonstrated DA's principal role in the reserpine-induced motor disturbance, disproving the claims made for the involvement of brain NA (or DOPS) (Everett, 1970). In 1975, Ken Lloyd, in Toronto, conducted a study in PD brains, in which he showed directly that levodopa treated patients had more DA in their corpus striatum than untreated patients, with the highest DA levels measured shortly after the last pre-mortem dose of levodopa (Lloyd et al., 1975). In 1974, the first study about the antiparkinson effect of bromocriptine, a direct DA receptor agonist, was published by Donald Calne in London, indicating that the drug had qualitatively the same antiparkinson action as levodopa (Calne et al., 1974). The latter two studies provided the definitive proof of the DA replenishing action of levodopa in PD.

A NEW (DA FIBRE) CONNECTION IN THE BRAIN

The question why the morphologically intact striatum in PD had such a severe loss of DA, had direct bearing on the specificity of our biochemical findings in PD. In 1938, Rolf Hassler, in Germany, had established that in PD, the loss of the substantia nigra melanin-containing compacta neurons was the most specific morphological change (Hassler, 1938). Taking up that lead, I started in 1962 a study of the substantia nigra in PD, and discovered markedly reduced DA in this nucleus, similar to the DA loss in the striatum. I concluded that the *"cell loss in the substantia nigra [in PD] could well be the cause of the DA deficit in the striatum"* (Hornykiewicz, 1963). I still like to think of this study as the true beginning of the discovery of the nigrostriatal DA pathway. In the spring of 1963, I sent reprints of my paper to Ted Sourkes and Louis Poirier in Montreal, and to Annica Dahlström and Kjell Fuxe in Stockholm, knowing that both groups were interested in this question. And indeed, soon afterwards both groups were able to present experimental evidence for the existence of this DA pathway in the rat by DA histofluorescence (Dahlström and Fuxe, 1964), and in the primate (rhesus monkey) by means of electrolytic midbrain lesions (Poirier and Sourkes, 1965). Both groups graciously acknowledged my substantia nigra work in the PD brain.

However, not all neuroanatomists were convinced of the existence of this pathway. For many years it was controversial and debated especially between Louis Poirier in Montreal and Malcolm Carpenter in New York. I was also drawn into the controversy. Although Hassler was in favour of substantia nigra's involvement in PD, he rejected the idea of a nigrostriatal fibre connection. When I sent him reprints of my work, he wrote back: *"Your interpretation of your observations does not agree with many known facts, this being so, because you accept the American opinion about the direction of the nigrostriatal connection. I believe that all your observations can be equally well, or even better, explained by the striatonigral direction"* (of the DA pathway) (Letter of R. Hassler to O.Hornykiewicz, dated February 9, 1967). An influential opponent of the connection between substantia nigra and PD was Derek Denny-Brown in Boston, the "father" of modern American neurology. In 1962 he stated, in a monograph on basal ganglia and movement disorders, that *"we have presented reasons against the common assumption that lesions of the substantia nigra are responsible for Parkinson's disease"* (Denny-Brown, 1962). I cannot forget a meeting in New York in the early 1970s, when, after my lecture, Denny-Brown got quickly up from his seat and declared that he had

seen autopsied brains of non-parkinsonian patients with completely depigmented substantia nigra, asking how I would explain that. Not knowing him at that time, I rather
nonchalantly retorted that I would be only too happy if he could *"kindly send me such
brains for biochemical analyses"*. Judging from the expression on Denny-Brown's face,
I could clearly see that he was not pleased with my answer.

A POSTSCRIPT

Besides being of obvious consequence for the diseased patient, the work on DA and
levodopa in PD has been of considerable conceptual significance. The demonstration
that neurotransmitter replacement in a degenerative brain disease was possible, held
out prospects for discovery of similar treatments of other neurodegenerative diseases,
e.g., Alzheimer's disease, in which, as recently commented by Hardy and Langston
(2004), *"the current cholinergic therapy is the intellectual heir of dopamine replace -
ment therapy for Parkinson's disease"*.

REFERENCES
1. Barbeau, A., Murphy, G.F., Sourkes, T.L., 1961. Excretion of dopamine in diseases of basal
   ganglia. Science 133, 1706-1707.
2. Barbeau, A., Sourkes, T.L., Murphy, G.F., 1962. Les catécholamines dans la maladie de
   Parkinson: In: deAjuriaguerra, J. (Ed), Monoamines et système nerveux centrale. Georg,
   Genève and Masson, Paris, pp 247-262.
3. Bein, H.J., 1956. The pharmacology of Rauwolfia. Pharmacol. Rev. 8, 435-483.
4. Bertler, Å., Rosengren, E., 1959a. Occurrence and distribution of dopamine in brain and
   other tissues. Experientia 15, 10-11.
5. Bertler, Å., Rosengren, E., 1959b. On the distribution in brain monoamines and of enzymes
   responsible for their formation. Experientia 15, 382-383.
6. Bertler, Å., Rosengren, E.,. 1966. Possible role of brain dopamine. Pharmacol. Rev. 18, 769-773.
7. Birkmayer, W., Hornykiewicz, O., 1961. Der L-Dioxyphenylalanin (DOPA)-Effekt bei der
   Parkinson-Akinese. Wien. Klin. Wschr. 73, 787-788.
8. Birkmayer, W., Hornykiewicz, O., 1962. Der L-Dioxyphenylalanin (DOPA)-Effekt beim
   Parkinson-Syndrom des Menschen: zur Pathogenese und Behandlung der Parkinson-
   Akinese. Arch. Psychiat. Nervenkr. 203, 560-574.
9. Blaschko, H., 1939. The specific action of L-dopa decarboxylase. J. Physiol. 96, 50.
10. Blaschko, H., 1957. Metabolism and storage of biogenic amines. Experientia 13, 9-12.
11. Calne, D.B., Teychenne, P.F., Claveria, L.E., Eastman, R., Greenacre, J.K., Petrie, A., 1974.
    Bromocriptine in parkinsonism. Brit. Med. J. 4, 442-444.
12. Carlsson, A., 1959. The occurrence, distribution and physiological role of catecholamines
    in the nervous system. Pharmacol. Rev. 11, 490-493.
13. Carlsson, A., 1964. Functional significance of drug-induced changes in brain monoamine
    levels. In: Himwich, H.E., Himwich, W.A. (Eds.), Progr. Brain Res. 8: Biogenic Amines.
    Elsevier, Amsterdam, pp 9- 27.
14. Carlsson, A., 1965. Drugs which block the storage of 5-hydroxytryptamine and related
    amines. In. Eichler, O., Farah, A. (Eds.), 5-Hydroxytryptamine and Related
    Indolealkylamines. Handbook of Experimental Pharmacology, Vol.19. Springer, Berlin/
    Heidelberg/ New York, pp. 529-592.

15. Carlsson, A., Lindqvist, M., Magnusson, T., 1957. 3,4-Dihydroxyphenylalanine and 5-hydroxytryptophan as reserpine antagonists. Nature 180, 1200.

16. Carlsson, A., Lindqvist, M., Magnusson, T., Waldeck, B., 1958. On the presence of 3-hydroxy-tyramine in brain. Science 127, 471.

17. Cotzias, G.C., Papavasiliou, P.S., Van Woert, M.H., Sakamoto, A., 1964. Melanogenesis and extrapyramidal diseases. Fed. Proc. 23, 713-718.

18. Cotzias, G.C., Van Woert, M.H., Schiffer, I.M., 1967. Aromatic amino acids and modification of Parkinsonism. New Engl. J. Med. 276, 374-379.

19. Dahlström, A., Fuxe, K., 1964. Evidence for the existence of monoamine-containing neurons in the central nervous system. I. Demonstration of monoamines in the cell bodies of brain stem neurons. Acta Physiol. Scand. 62 (Suppl . 232).

20. Denny-Brown, D, 1962. The Basal Ganglia and Their Relation to Disorders of Movement, Oxford University Press, Oxford.

21. Ehringer, H., Hornykiewicz, O., 1960. Verteilung von Noradrenalin und Dopamin (3-Hydroxy-tyramin) im Gehirn des Menschen und ihr Verhalten bei Erkrankungen des extrapyramidalen Systems. Klin. Wschr. 38, 1236-1239.

22. Everett, G.M., 1970. Evidence for dopamine as a central modulator: neurological and behavioral implications. In: Barbeau, A., McDowell, R.H. (Eds.), L-Dopa and Parkinsonism, F.A. Davis, Philadelphia, pp. 364-368.

23. Hardy, J., Langston, W.J., 2004. How many pathways are there to nigral death? Ann. Neurol. 56: 316-318.

24. Hassler, R., 1938. Zur Pathologie der Paralysis agitans und des postenzephalitischen Parkinsonismus. J. Psychol. Neurol. 48, 387-476.

25. Holtz, P., 1939. Dopadecarboxylase. Naturwissenschaften 27, 724-725.

26. Holtz, P., Credner, K., 1942. Die enzymatische Entstehung von Oxytyramin im Organismus und die physiologische Bedeutung der Dopadecarboxylase. Naunyn-Schmiedeberg's Arch. Exp. Path. Pharmakol. 200, 256-288.

27. Holtz, P., Heise, R., Lüdtke, L., 1938. Fermentativer Abbau von L-Dioxyphenylalanin (Dopa) durch Niere. Naunyn-Schmiedeberg's Arch. Exp. Path. Pharmakol. 191, 87-118.

28. Holtz, P., Balzer, H., Westermann, E., Wezler, E., 1957. Beeinflussung der Evipannarkose durch Reserpin, Iproniazid und biogene Amine. Naunyn-Schmiedeberg's Arch. Exp. Path. Pharmakol. 231, 333-348.

29. Holzer, G., Hornykiewicz, O., 1959. Über den Dopamin-(Hydroxytyramin-) Stoffwechsel im Gehirn der Ratte. Naunyn Schmiedeberg's Arch. Exp. Path. Pharmakol. 237, 27-33.

30. Hornykiewicz, O., 1958. The action of dopamine on the arterial blood pressure of the guinea pig. Brit. J. Pharmacol. 13, 91-94.

31. Hornykiewicz, O., 1963. Die topische Lokalisation und das Verhalten von Noradrenalin und Dopamin (3-Hydroxytyramin) in the Substantia nigra des normalen und Parkinsonkranken Menschen. Wien. Klin. Wschr. 75, 309-312.

32. Hornykiewicz, O., 2002. Dopamine miracle: from brain homogenate to dopamine replacement. Movement Disord. 17, 501-508.

33. Jasper, H.H., 1970. Neurophysiological mechanisms in parkinsonism. In: Barbeau, A., McDowell, F.H. (Eds.), L-Dopa and Parkinsonism, FA Davis, Philadelphia, pp 408-411.

34. Lloyd, K.G., Davidson, L., Hornykiewicz, O., 1975. The neurochemistry of Parkinson's disease: effect of L-dopa therapy. J. Pharmacol. Exp. Ther. 195, 453-464.

35. Montagu, K.A., 1957. Catechol compounds in rat tissues and in brains of different animals. Nature 180, 244-245.

36. Pletscher, A., 1957. Wirkung von Isopropyl-isonicotinsäurehydrazid auf den Stoffwechsel von Catecholaminen und 5-Hydroxytryptamin im Gehirn. Schweiz. Med. Wschr. 87, 1532-1534.

37. Pletscher, A., 1994. From levodopa to Madopar In: Poewe, W., Lees, A.J. (Eds.), 20 Years of Madopar – New Avenues, Editiones Roche, Basel, pp. 43-51.

38. Poirier, L.J., Sourkes, T.L., 1965. Influence of the substantia nigra on the catecholamine content of the striatum. Brain 88, 181-192.

39. Sano, I., 2000. Biochemistry of the extrapyramidal system. Parkinsonism Relat. Disord. 6, 3-6.

40. Sano, I., Gamo, T., Kakimoto, Y., Taniguch,i K., Takesada, M., Nishinuma, K., 1959. Distribution of catechol compounds in human brain. Biochim. Biophys. Acta 32, 586-587.
41. Vogt, M., 1954. The concentration of sympathin in different parts of the central nervous system under normal conditions and after the administration of drugs. J. Physiol. 123, 451-481.
42. Vogt, M., 1973. Functional aspects of the role of catecholamines in the central nervous system. Brit. Med. Bul.l 29, 168-172.
43. Ward, A.A., 1970. Physiological implications in the dyskinesias. In: Barbeau, A,, McDowell, F.H. (Eds.) L-Dopa and Parkinsonism, F.A. Davis, Philadelphia, pp 151-159.
44. Weil-Malherbe, H., Bone, A.D., 1957. Intracellular distribution of catecholamines in the brain. Nature 180, 1050-1051.
45. Weil-Malherbe, H., Bone, A.D., 1958. Effect of reserpine on the intracellular distribution of catecholamines in the brain stem of the rabbit. Nature 181, 1474-1475.
46. Yahr, M.D., Duvoisin, R.C., Schear, M.J., Barrett, R.E., Hoehn, M.M., 1969. Treatment of parkinsonism with levodopa. Arch. Neurol. 21, 343-354.

CHAPTER 7

MONOAMINE OXIDASES, THEIR INHIBITORS AND THE OPENING OF THE NEUROTRANSMITTER ERA IN NEUROPSYCHOPHARMACOLOGY

Moussa B. H. Youdim

INTRODUCTION

In 1928 Mary Hare-Bernheim described tyramine oxidase, an enzyme that was able to metabolize tyramine (Bernheim, 1931), and in 1933 Herman Blaschko demonstrated that tyramine oxidase, noradrenaline oxidase and aliphatic oxidase were the same enzyme that was capable of metabolizung primary, secondary and tertiary amines (Blaschko, 1952). The name mitochondrial monoamine oxidase (MAO) was given to this enzyme by Albert Zeller to differentiate it from diamine oxidase (DAO) that was known to deaminate mono and diamines (see Zeller, 1979). Iproniazid was the first MAO inhibitor (MAOI) that was discovered by Zeller (1963) and introduced into clinical use as an antidepressant (Bailey et al., 1959; Saunders et al., 1959). Iproniazid together with reserpine opened up the neurotransmitter era in neuropsychopharmcology. Although in the late 1950s and 1960s, iproniazid and other MAOIs were shown to possess antidepressant activity, their clinical usefulness was seriously limited because of liver toxicity and by what was to become known as the "cheese reaction," manifest in hypertension and cerebral hemorrhage with fatality in some patients. The "cheese reaction" was the consequence of tyramine formation from tyrosine present in many fermented foodstuffs, including cheese, wine, that was not deaminated by MAO in the intestine and in the liver of patients treated with MAOIs. The side effects of MAOIs, together with the hasty 1965 Medical Research Council (MRC) report in the United Kingdom on the lack of antidepressant activity of these drugs virtually halted interest in the enzyme, and the development of other MAOIs as antidepressants. Although the problem of hepatotoxicity was resolved with the development of non-hydrazine derived drugs such as tranylcypromine and pargyline, the cheese reaction remained the major reason for the fall from favor of these effective antidepressants. Tyramine and other indirectly acting sympathomimetic amines are present in food and beverages and metabolized by MAO to inactive substances. If peripheral, including liver and intestinal MAO is inhibited these amines can gain access to the circulatory system and cause a significant release of noradrenaline from sympathetic neurons (Figure 1). The consequence of the released noradrenaline can be a severe hypertensive reaction and sometimes death. The advent of tricyclic amine uptake inhibitors replaced MAOIs as first line antidepressants. Nevertheless MAOIs have remained in use in the treatment of depression with some dietary restriction to prevent such side effects.

Interest in the neuropharmacology and biochemistry of the enzyme received a great impetus from its purification from outer mitochondrial membrane and its identification as a flavoprotein, where the flavin is covalently and irreversibly bound to the enzyme in propargyl possessing inhibitors, such as pargyline, L-deprenyl and clorgyiline (Edmondson et al., 2004; Tipton et al., 2004; Youdim et al., 1988, 2005).

REVIVAL OF MAO INHIBITORS AS PSYCHOTROPIC DRUGS

The idea that MAO was not a single enzyme but existed in several forms, was first reported by Gorkin (1966) working in Moscow. From what we established about the physicochemical properties of the enzyme it was apparent that at least two forms were present in the liver and brain of rats having different heat stability, optimal pH, and inhibitory specificity and sensitivity (Youdim and Sourkes, 1965). These findings were strengthened by the observation of Johnson (1968) that the propargyl containing irreversible inhibitor, clorgyline, could differentiate between two forms Type A and Type B of MAO in brain and most of the tissues of animals. MAO-A form was inhibited selectively by clorgyline (see figure 1) and was responsible for the oxidative deamination of noradrenaline and serotonin. By contrast, MAO-B was resistant to inhibition by clorgyline and preferentially metabolized benzylamine, and phenylethylamine, as later on shown by Neff and his colleagues (Yang and Neff, 1973). Tyramine and dopamine were metabolized equally well by both forms of the enzyme (O'Carroll et al., 1983). Clorgyline was shown to have antidepressant effects in a series of double blind clinical trials (Wheatley, 1970). Although the cheese reaction that was consistently observed with clorgyline and other irreversible MAO-A inhibitors, led to the abandonment of the use of these drugs as antidepressants (Youdim et al., 1988), research with these irreversible MAOIs continued and contributed to progress in neuropharmacology.

L-Deprenyl (selegiline) (see figure 1) was developed originally from L-methamphetamine as a psychic energizer to be used as an antidepressant. It was the first MAOI that was shown to be devoid of the "cheese reaction" (Knoll and Magyar, 1972). Selegiline had no antidepressant action. At its selective dosage it inhibited the oxidation of phenylethylamine and benzylamine, but not of serotonin and noradrenaline. Its lack of tyramine potentiation was rather puzzling. Knoll and Magyar (1972) attributed it to an inherent pharmacological activity of the drug. However, Finberg and colleagues (Finberg and Tenne, 1982; Finberg et al., 1981) showed that at higher doses L-deprenyl inhibited MAO-A that led to the potentiation of the sympathomimetic action of tyramine in vivo. These studies indicated that other MAO-B inhibitors would also lack tyramine potentiation at their selec-

Figure 1. Structures of earlier classical, propargylamine possessing, reversible, and novel brain selective MAO inhibitors

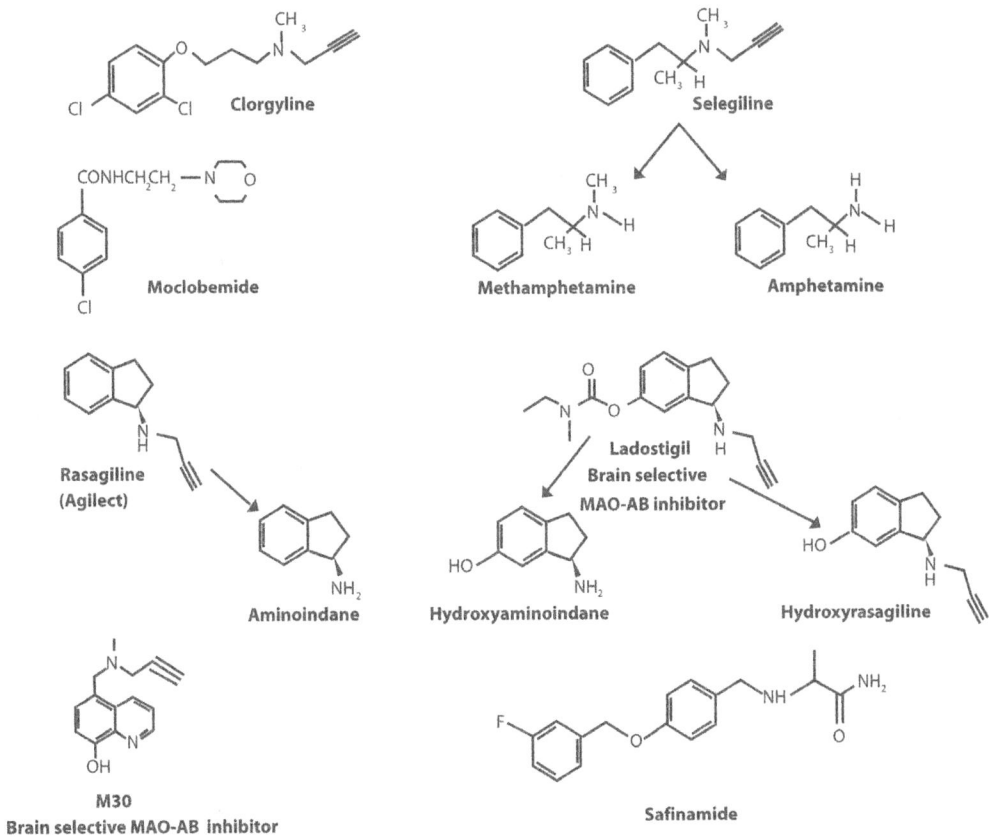

tive dosage, because MAO-A is present only in the peripheral adrenergic neurons. Confirmation that other MAO-B inhibitors also lack tyramine potentiation at their selective dosage came from AGN 1135 (N-propargyl-1-aminoindan), the second propargylamine possessing irreversible selective MAO-B inhibitor, that was later to be known as rasagiline (see figure 1) (Feinberg and Youdim, 2002; Feinberg et al., 1981; Youdim et al., 2001a).

SELECTIVE MONOAMINE OXIDASE B INHIBITORS AS ANTI-PARKINSON DRUGS

L-DEPRENYL (SELEGILINE)

Reports of the presence of both MAO-A and MAO-B enzymes in human brain and the predominance of MAO-B activity (80%) in the basal ganglia as compared to other brain regions (Collins et al., 1970; O'Carroll et al., 1983) led to the suggestion that selective inhibitors could be developed that would be effective in treating depression and neurological disorders without the occasional dangerous side effects inherent in older MAOIs (Youdim et al., 1972). MAO-B accounts for about 80% of total MAO activity in human basal ganglia. It is mainly localized in the glia cells, astrocytes and in a few specific neuronal cells, e.g., raphé nuclei. MAO-A is present in the extraneuronal compartment (glia cells and astrocytes) and within the dopaminergic, serotonergic and noradrenergic nerve terminals, where it is involved in the intraneuronal metabolism of these amines, maintaining their cytoplasmic concentrations low (Youdim et al., 1988).

The lack of cheese reaction with L-deprenyl and the experimental finding that dopamine but not noradrenaline and serotonin was a substrate for MAO-B (Green and Youdim, 1975; Green et al., 1977), was the basis of the use of L-deprenyl in Parkinson's disease (PD) (Birkmayer et al., 1975, 1977). Peter Riederer was looking for a MAOI, free from the cheese reaction, to use it as an adjunct in PD patients already treated with L-dopa, and the obvious choice was L-deprenyl because human brain basal ganglia contains predominantly MAO–B (Collins et al., 1970; Youdim et al., 1972). The first clinical trial in patients treated with L-dopa was successful and unlike in the earlier 1961 studies of Birkmayer carried out in 1961 (Birkmayer and Hornykiewicz, 1961) none of the patients showed a cheese reaction. (Birkmayer et al., 1975). Several other clinical trials followed in which L-deprenyl was added to L-dopa and L-deprenyl became an accepted part of therapy for PD in Europe, although patients in the United States had to wait for another 15 years before the Food and Drug Administartion (FDA) licensed the drug and gave it a new name in the process, selegiline. By now selegiline is used as monotherapy in the treatment PD and has been shown to postpone the need for levodopa in early PD. It is also useful in the management of end-of-dose akinesia in the fully developed disease (Birkmayer et al., 1975, 1977; Group, 1989, 1993; Lees et al., 1977).

REVIVAL OF MAO INHIBITORS AS ANTIPARKINSON AND ANTI-DEPRESSANT DRUGS

RASAGILINE (AZILECT, AGILECT)

The antiparkinson action of L-deprenyl was responsible for the resurgence of interest in developing selective MAO-A and MAO-B inhibitors as antidepressant and antiparkinson drugs, which are devoid of the cheese reaction. The first of these drugs was AGN 1135 (Finberg et al., 1981; Kalir et al., 1981), a restricted analogue of L-deprenyl . Its optical R-isomer, rasagiline (Azilect, Agilect, N-propargyl-1-[R]-aminoindan) was developed as an antiparkinson drug (Blandini, 2005; Rascol, 2005; Youdim et al., 2001a,b, 2005). It is a potent selective irreversible MAO-B inhibitor, with 10 to 20 times greater potency than L-deprenyl in vivo (Finberg and Youdim, 2002; Youdim et al., 2001a). Unlike L-deprenyl , rasagiline has no sympathomimetic activity (Finberg et al., 1999) because instead of metabolising to L-methamphetamine it metabolises to aminoindan. Consequently, rasagiline does not possess the L–methamphetamine dependent cardiovasclaur effects seen with L-deprenyl (Finberg and Youdim, 2002). Furthermore, unlike L-methamphetamine, aminoindan has neuroprotective activity in vitro and in vivo (Youdim et al., 2005). Controlled studies have recently shown that rasagiline is effective both as monotherapy and as adjuvant to L-dopa in early and late parkinsonian subjects. The drug has been approved for clinical use in Europe, Israel and USA. Recently clnical studies have indicated that it may possess disease-modifying activity in PD subjects.

The first selective reversible MAO-A inhibitor (RIMA) antidepressant was moclobemide (Cesura and Pletscher, 1992; Da Prada et al., 1983, 1988 ; Haefley et al., 1992) (see figure 1). The idea being that drugs such as RIMAs, even at extremely high dosages can be displaced by tyramine from the active site of the MAO-A enzyme thereby enabling this amine and other amines to be metabolized and preventing their access into the circulation (Figure 2). Since tyramine does not cross the blood brain barrier and therefore is not able to displace the inhibitor from its active site on the enzyme, brain MAO-A will continue to be inhibited, noradrenaline and serotonin levels increased and antidepressant effects achieved with RIMAs (Haefely et al., 1992). Other RIMAs with antidepressant activity, similar to moclobemide, include befloxatone and toloxetone. Reversible MAO-B inhibitors such lazabemide, milacemide and safinamide (see figure 1) were shown to possess antiparkinson activity without inducing "cheese reaction." These drugs do not have an inhibitory action on MAO-A, the predominant enzyme in the gastrointestinal tract, portal system and adrenergic neurons. However, none of these drugs, except moclobemide, is in clinical use so far.

REVERSIBLE MAO-A INHIBITORS AND PARKINSON'S DISEASE

In brains of PD patients after two weeks or four years of L-selegiline treatment, a highly significant (>3000%) increase in phenylethylamine and moderate (40-70%) increase in dopamine levels were found in the substantia nigra, caudate nucleus, putamen and globus pallidus, without any changes in the concentrations of serotonin, noradrenaline or their metabolites (Riederer and Youdim, 1986; Riederer et

Figure 2. Mechanism of action of RIMAs. Interaction of RIMA with the flavin containing active site substrate recognition sites and its displacement by a substrate (tyramine) can result in the metabolism of tyramine before reaching the circulation and peripheral adrenergic neurons. RIMA is also metabolized. Since tyramine cannot cross the blood-brain-barrier, it does not have the opportunity of displacing the inhibitor from the enzyme in the brain, thus MAO will continue to be inhibited resulting in raised brain levels of serotonin and noradrenaline.

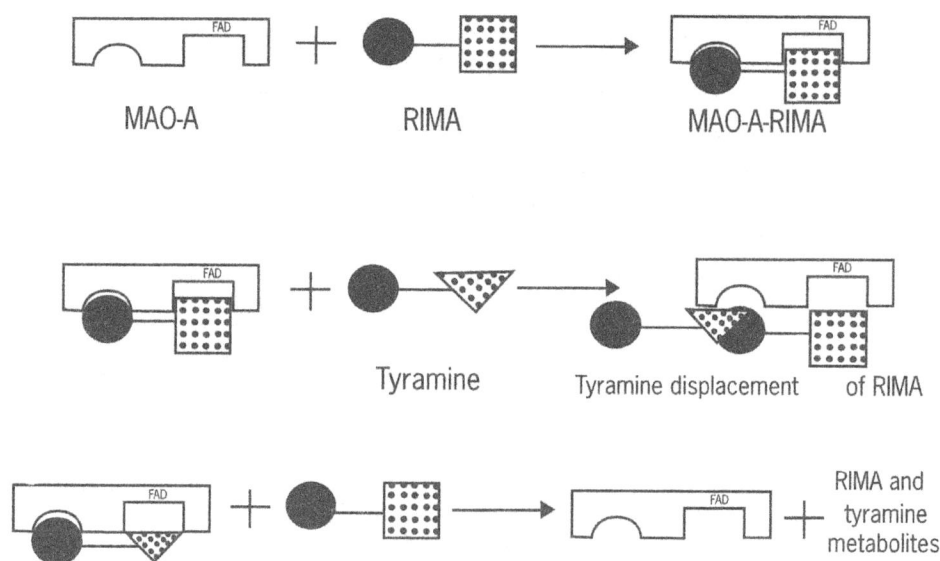

al., 1987). By contrast, clorgyline, a selective MAO-A inhibitor, significantly increased both noradrenaline and serotonin levels but produced only a small rise in dopamine levels in human basal ganglia (Youdim and Riederer, 1993). In spite of the fact that dopamine is equally well metabolized by MAO-A and MAO-B in human and rat striatum little attention was paid to MAO-A inhibition in PD (O'Carrdl et al., 1983). Thus, the contribution of MAO-A to dopamine metabolism in the parkinsonian striatum was not known, since L-selegiline produced less elevation of dopamine than of phenylethylamine in PD brains (Riederer and Youdim, 1986). These data and those of Green and Youdim (1975) and Green et al. (1977) on rat brains clearly indicate that when one form of MAO is selectively inhibited, the other can metabolize dopamine equally well. Thus, the level of this amine will not change appreciably in the striatum (Green et al., 1977; Youdim and Riederer, 1993) (Figure 3). To determine the role of MAO-A inhibition on dopamine metabolism and its potential clinical effect in PD, we compared the effects of the RIMA, moclobemide on motor performance to the standard therapy with levodopa and dopaminergic agonists in idiopathic PD (Sieradzan et al., 1995). Moclobemide was chosen since in subjects with major depression, moclobemide was found to improve vigilance, psychomotor speed and longterm memory (Allain et al., 1993; Fairweather et al., 1993; Kerr et al., 1992) Moclobemide also improves memory and choice reaction time in elderly subjects (Amrein et al., 1999; Wesnes et al., 1989). Moclobemide is safe, devoid of major side effects and does not produce hypertensive reactions when tyramine is ingested (Bieck et al., 1993; Da Prada et al., 1988; Haefely et al., 1992; Korn et al., 1987). It is also well tolerated by PD patients when administered with levodopa and benserazide (Sieradzan et al., 1995). The good tolerance of moclobemide in standard therapy suggests that moclobemide and other MAO-A inhibitors (lacking the cheese reaction) may be particularly useful antidepressants in patients with PD (Sieradzan et al., 1995). The shortening of the latency and prolongation of the duration of the motor response in moclobemide treated patients to a single levodopa challenge may be explained by the known effects of moclobemide on the metabolism of exogenous levodopa and its oxidative deamination by MAO-A. Moclobemide treatment seems to provide a mild symptomatic benefit in PD (Ruggieri et al., 1996; Sieradzan et al., 1995; Sternic et al., 1998). In particular motor disturbances improve during moclobemide treatment. These findings suggest that bradykinesia may be more amenable to moclobemide treatment than the other disabilities in PD. In the absence of depression moclobemide does not significantly influence cognitive function in PD patients. But moclobemide influences cognitive function in PD patients with depression (Jansen Steur and Ballering, 1999). Numerous studies in rodents have shown that inhibition of MAO-A with either reversible (moclobemide) or irreversible (clorgyline) inhibitors increases brain noradrenaline and serotonin levels but has little effect on dopamine levels. Nevertheless, using striatal microdialysis in rats it was shown that moclobemide and clorgyline significantly increased dopamine release (Colzi et al., 1992). This indicates that intraneuronal MAO-A inhibition does indeed affect dopamine metabolism. The increased release of dopamine during MAO-A inhibition may account for the prolonged duration of the motor response to a single L-dopa challenge in PD patients. The relatively mild symptomatic effect of moclobemide in PD patients may be associated with the pharmacokinetics of the drug. Since moclobemide is a reversible inhibitor it could be displaced from its binding site on MAO-A (Colzi et al., 1992; Sieradzan et al., 1995). This would lead to a reduction in dopamine accumulation and release. Thus, special attention needs to be paid to the ratio of daily dosage of moclobemide to that of L-dopa for a more effective action of moclobemide on dopamine metabolism in PD.

NOVEL IRREVERSIBLE BRAIN-SELECTIVE MAO-A AND MAO-B INHIBITOR ANTIDEPRESSANTS

The relatively mild response observed with either selegiline or moclobemide in monotherapy or as adjuvant to L-dopa in PD, indicates that with the inhibition of one enzyme is insufficient to obtain full functional activity of dopamine. This is attributed to the findings that when one form of the enzyme is inhibited in the basal ganglia, dopamine formed from L-dopa either extraneuronally or neuronally by the remaining dopamine neurons can be metabolized by the other form of MAO (Green et al., 1977) (see figure 3). Thus, there is a need for the development of either a non selective reversible MAO-AB inhibitor or an irreversible inhibitor that is brain-selective to help us to understand the contribution of MAO-A and MAO-B inhibition to serotonin or dopamine metabolism in depressive illness and PD respectively. Such a drug could then also serve as an antidepressant, and for the treatment of PD and Alzheimer's disease (AD) with depressive symptoms.

Figure 3. Pathway of dopamine synthesis and metabolism by MAO-A and B and sites of action of selective and non selective MAO inhibitors. TH (tyrosine hydroxylase); DDC (dopa decarboxylase); DT (dopamine transporter); D_1 and D_2 dopamine receptors; SV (synaptic vesicles); AR (amine reuptake).

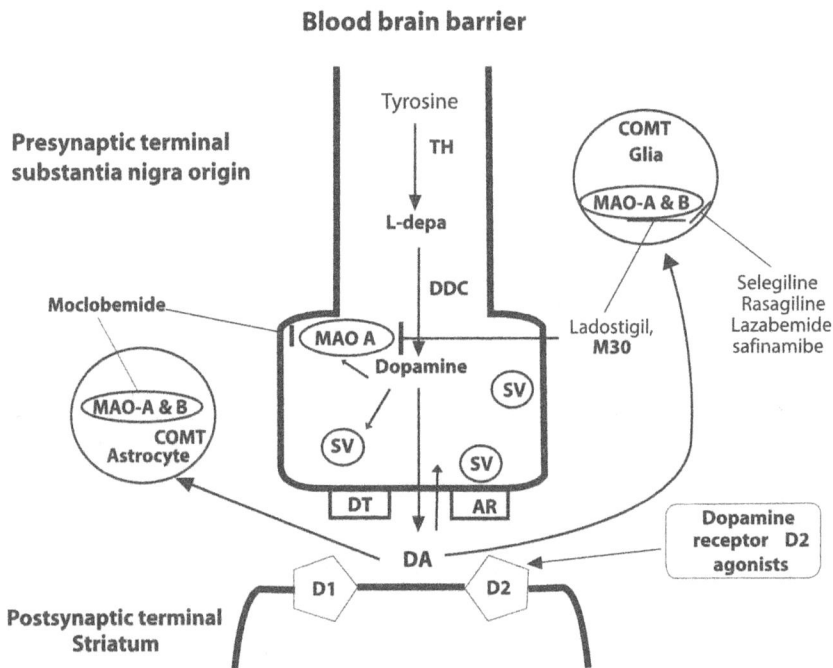

LADOSTIGIL

Recently several novel third generation novel brain selective MAO-AB inhibitors have been developed which do not produce a "cheese reaction" with high doses of tyramine.. Included among them are ladostigil (TV 3326). (Weinstock et al., 2000a; Sterling et al., 2002; Youdim and Buccafusco, 2005) and M30 [5-(N-methyl-N-propargylaminomethyl)-8-hydroxyqinoline] (Gal et al., 2005; Zheng et al., 2005) (see figure 3). Ladostigil is a carbamate derivative [N-propargyl-(3R)-aminoindan-5-yl-ethyl methyl carbamate, hemitartrate] of rasagiline (Weinstock et al., 2000a). It is a potential treatment for AD and dementia with Lewy bodies (Weinstock et al., 2000b) or Parkinsonism with dementia by increasing cortical cholinergic transmission and nigrostriatal dopamine levels since in addition to the cholinergic deficit, a significant proportion of AD patients also have a slowing of motor activity and extrapyramidal dysfunction resembling that seen in PD (Honig and Mayeux, 2001; Tsolaki et al., 2001). Depressive symptoms occur in a large proportion of subjects with AD, Lewy Body disease (DLB) (Newman, 1999) and with PD (Tandberg et al., 1996), and this may be related to degeneration of noradrenaline and serotonin neurones innervating the limbic system (Palmer et al., 1988). MAO inhibition should preserve the levels of these amines in AD and PD patients and reduce depressive symptoms. Although rasagiline is a selective inhibitor of MAO-B the introduction of the carbamate moiety into the 6 position of the aminoindan resulted in a marked reduction in MAO-B inhibitory activity and loss of MAO-B selectivity. However, after chronic oral administration to rats the drug showed brain-selective inhibition of both MAO-A and MAO-B, with increases in dopamine, noradrenaline and serotonin levels. There was little if any inhibition of these enzymes in the intestine and liver (Weinstock et al., 2000a). This was probably due to the formation of a 6-hydroxy derivative of rasagiline, which is a potent non-selective inhibitor of MAO. M 30 (Zheng et al., 2005; Gal et al., 2005), the other substance in this group is a potent inhibitor of the MAO-A and the MAO-B enzymes in vitro and in vivo, with selectivity for the brain enzymes. It is similar to ladostigil in that it lacks inhibition of the enzymes in liver and small intestine.

CHEESE REACTION

The finding that ladostigil causes little or no MAO-A inhibition in the intestine suggests that patients receiving the drug should develop a much smaller increase in blood pressure on ingestion of tyamine-containing foods or beverages than those treated with other irreversible, non-selective MAOIs, like iproniazid and tranylcypromine. This was confirmed in conscious rabbits in which it was shown that chronic oral administration of ladostigil (26 mg/kg) for 2 weeks, in a dosage that inhibited brain MAO-A and MAO-B by more than 90%, increased the pressor response to oral and intravenous tyramine to the same extent as seen with the RIMA inhibitor, moclobemide. This was in marked contrast to the effect of the non-selective inhibitor of MAO, tranylcypromine, which inhibited brain MAO to a similar extent but increased the pressor response to oral tyramine 20-fold since it also inhibited MAO-A in the intestine by more than 80% (Weinstock et al., 2002a).

ANTIDEPRESSANT ACTIVITY OF LADOSTIGIL

The finding that ladostigil inhibits brain MAO-A and MAO-B, indicates that ladostigil should show antidepressant activity, like tranylcypromine, phenelzine and clorgyline. This was demonstrated by findings with the forced swim, or "Porsolt test" which is used for the screening in rats for potential antidepressants (Porsolt et al., 1977). Daily oral administration of ladostigil, (26 mg/kg/day) for two weeks, which inhibited brain MAO-A and MAO-B by more than 65%, produced a similar alteration in rat behaviour to that seen after chronic treatment with amitriptyline (10 mg/kg/day) or moclobemide (20 mg/kg/day). The antidepressant effect of TV-3326 was associated with a twofold increase in the brain levels of serotonin (Weinstock et al., 2002b).

M 30

M30 (see figure 3) is a propargylamine derivative with pharmacological properties similar to VK-28 {5-[4-(2-hydroxyethyl) piperazine-1-ylmethyl]-quinoline-8-ol}, an iron chelator that permeates the brain. It has a similar profile of tissue MAO–A and MAO-B inhibition to ladostigil in that it is selective for brain MAO-A and MAO-B inhibition with little affinity for the enzymes in liver and small intestine. It is expected to have a similar profile to ladostigil with regards to cheese reaction and antidepressant activity. Both inhibitors have neuroprotective properties similar to rasagiline (Figure 4) and anti Parkinson activity in the current N-methyl-4-phenyl-1236-tetrahydropyridine (MPTP)-induced mice model of PD (Gal et al., 2005; Sagi et al., 2003). M 30 raises the brain levels of dopamine, noradrenaline and serotonin in striatum, hippocampus, raphe nucleus and hypothalamus. The mechanism by which ladostigil and M 30 have selectivity for brain MAOs is not known but may be related to their metabolism by cytochrome P450. Elucidation of this mechanism may help to design other brain selective MAOIs.

Figure 4. Molecular mechanism of the neuroprotective-neurorescue activities of propargy-lamine possessing MAOIs. The propargylaines prevent the collapse of mitochondrial membrane potential in response to a neurotoxin. The result is up regulation of the anti-apoptotic Bcl-2 family proteins, while down regulating the pro-apoptotic genes. This results in the activation of cell survival protein kinase C (PKC)α and ε and their translocation to the membrane. Inhibitors of PKC and ERK prevent the neuroprotective effects of these

MAOIs. Furthermore these inhibitors activate the TRKB pathway of PKC which may explain their ability to induce mRNA and proteins of the glial neurotrophic factor (GDNF) and brain derived neurotrophic factor (BDNF) which may contribute to their neurorescue activity (Youdim and Buccafusco, 2005; Youdim et al., 2005). Aβ (Aβ amyloid); sAPPα (soluble amyloid precursor protein α); Bad, Bax, pro-apoptotic proteins; Bcl-2 and Bcl-Xl; anti-apoptotic proteins; APP (amyloid precursor protein).

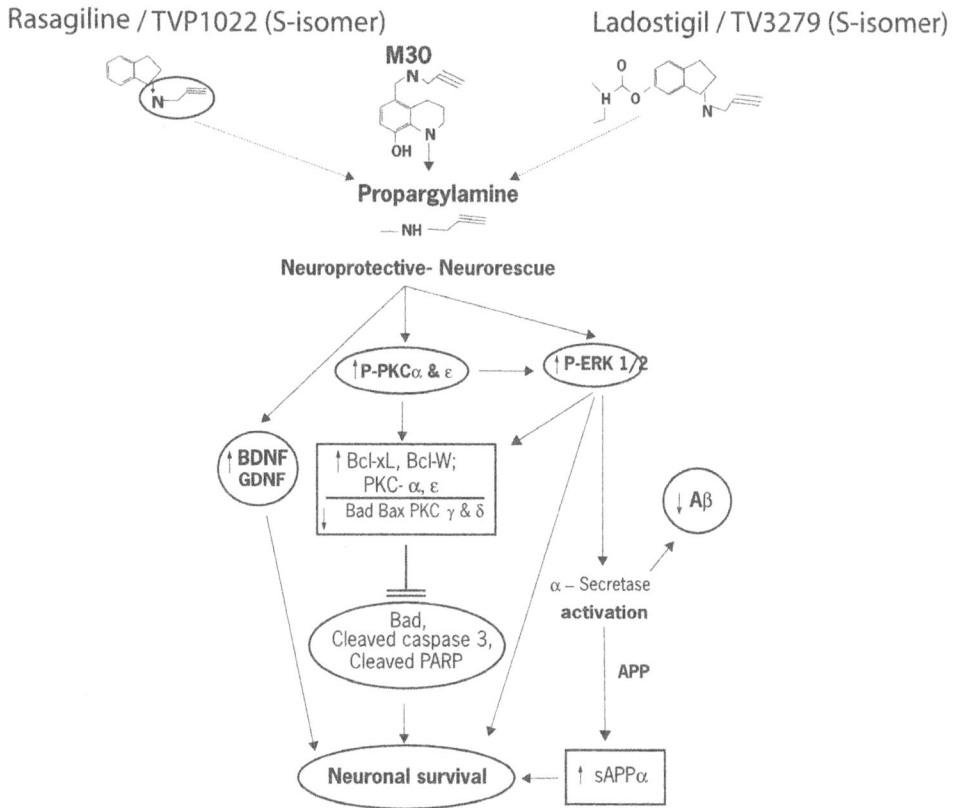

Increases of MAO activity and dysregulation of brain iron which occurs in ageing PD and AD are thought to contribute to the neurodegenerative porsess. This is thought to results from the interaction of hydrogen peroxide produced by MAO and other oxidative processes and its interaction with iron to induce oxidative stress, a consequence of Fenton reaction, dependent oxygen radical formation (Zecca et al., 2004). Thus MAO inhibitors and iron chelators may be neuroprotective in both disorders (Gal et al., 2005). In AD interactions of iron with holo-APP may contribute to the Alzheimer's amyloid pathology. Thus, metal chelation could be a therapeutic strategy for AD pathogenesis. Alternatively, a complementary approach would be to target the stimulation of APP to induce non-amyloidogenic processing in releasing sAPPα and the consequent reduction of Aβ production. It has been demonstrated that propargylamines, including the propargylamine rasagiline and ladostigil enhance secretion of sAPPα via PKC and mitogen activated protein (MAP) kinases signaling cascades. Therefore we designed a non-toxic, lipophilic brain-permeable multifunctional drug, M 30, that contains the pharamcophore of the iron chelator, VK 28 plus the propargyl moiety of rasagiline, as a potential therapeutic agent for AD. M 30 markedly reduces the levels of cellular APP, β-C-terminal fragment (β-CTF) and the levels of the amyloidogenic Aβ peptide in the medium, in SH-SY5Y (human dopaminergic neuroblastoma) cells and CHO cells stably transfected with the APP "Swedish" mutation. In addition, the levels of the non- amyloidogenic soluble APPα and α- CTF in medium and cell lysate were respectively increased. M 30 decreased apoptosis of SH-SY5Y cells in a neuro rescue, serum deprivation model, via multiple protection mechanisms. This resulted from reduction of the pro-apoptotic proteins, Bad, Bax; and Ser139 phosphorylated H2A.X; induction of Bcl-2 (see figure 4, as shown for other propargylamines) and inhibition of the cleavage and activation of caspase-3. M-30 promoted morphological changes, resulting in axonal growth-associated protein-43 (GAP-43) implicating neuronal differentiation. Thus, the multifunctional drug, M 30 possessing both MAO inhibitory and iron chelating activity has the ability to limit holo-APP expression and Aβ secretion and stimulate the non-amyloidogenic processing of APP, making it a highly potential drug for treatment of not only PD but also of AD (Youdim and Buccafesco, 2005).

NEUROPROTECTION AND NEURORESCUE ACTIVITIES OF PROPARGYLAMINE POSSESSING MAO INHBITORS

NEUROPROTECTION

By 1980 L-deprenyl plus L-dopa was well established as therapy in PD and our group had accumulated data from a 6-year study of this treatment. Our preliminary analysis of clinical response and survival of the PD patients indicated that those receiving L-deprenyl plus L- dopa had a better survival rate than those treated with L-dopa alone. The results suggested that L-deprenyl was slowing the rate of degeneration in dopaminergic neurons, an effect referred to as neuro-protection (Birkmayer et al., 1985). No such effect had been observed or discussed previously, with any other treatment for PD. In 1983 MPTP was shown to be selectively toxic to the dopaminergic neurones in the substantia nigra in animals and to cause PD-like syndrome in humans (Langston and Irwin, 1986) This compound had been inadvertently synthesized by a drug addict as an impurity in his preparation of meperidine and after using it, he had developed PD like symptoms while still in his twenties. However this neurotoxin could now be used to induce PD-like neurodegeneration in animal models and has proved to be most valuable in studies of the development of this disease. Heikkila et al. (1984) had found that pretreatment with non-selective MAOIs (iproniazid or tranylcypromine) protected the nigrostriatal neurons in mice against the damage caused by MPTP. With the selective inhibitors, it was soon clear that L-deprenyl, and not clorgyline, was protective and that the neurotoxin was being metabolized selectively by MAO-B to the active toxin MPP+ (dihydropyridine ion) (Chiba et al., 1984). Similar results were obtained with another selective MOA-B inhibitor, AGN 1135 ((Heikkila et al., 1985) and its substrate, pheylethylamine (Melamed and Youdim, 1985). The neuroprotective effect of phenylethylamine was attributed to its occupancy at the active site of MAO-B and thus competing with MPTP, which is also a selective substrate of MAO-B (Chiba et al., 1984; Yang and Neff, 1973) and thus preventing the depletion of striatal dopamine. This combination of an agent inducing PD-like neurodegeneration and a means to prevent it in animal models raised hopes that a similar cause and prevention might be found in humans. Regrettably, no MPTP like neurotoxin has been identified either as an endogenous factor or in the environment and, although we have a possible mechanism, we still have not established the cause of PD.

Nevertheless, these studies with MPTP and L-deprenyl, rasagiline and other MAO-B inhibitors have contributed greatly to the concept of neuroprotection not only in PD but other neurodegenerative diseases. An analogy may be made with rheumatic disease. Here ibuprofen and similar anti-inflammatory agents alleviate the pain, edema, stiffness and other consequences of the disease without affecting its progression. Disease modifying agents such as corticosteroids, methotrexate or leflunomide actually modify the underlying disease process and are meant to slow the progression of the disease. Neuroprotective agents would prevent the progression of PD and perhaps other neurodegenerative diseases, not just control the symptoms of neuronal loss. Such agents might also counteract the effect of exposure to the causative agent(s) when they are finally identified, slowing or even preventing critical damage to the neurones. Nevertheless L-deprenyl, rasagiline and a number of other propargylamines not being MAOIs have been shown to possess neuroprotective activity in several neuronal cell cultures and animal models in vivo (Foley et al., 2000; Youdim et al., 2005).

NEURORESCUE

Tatton and co-workers (Ansari et al., 1993) showed that L-deprenyl was able to prevent degeneration of neurons when administered after neurotoxin or physical insult. He (Tatton and Greenwood, 1991) proposed that the phenomenon should more appropriately regarded as being one of "neurorescue", in which L-deprenyl somehow prevents the death and degeneration of neurons after damage that would otherwise be considered lethal. Indeed, such protective effects with L-deprenyl has also been shown with primary cultures of non-neuronal cells and tissue explants from radiation damage by a process that involves BCl-2 elevation (Seymour et al., 2003).

The mechanisms involved do not appear to involve inhibition of MAO-B, since the doses of L-deprenyl, and rasagiline required are lower than those necessary to inhibit the enzyme and not all selective MAO-B inhibitors appear to be effective in this respect. Furthermore, L-deprenyl and rasagiline are effective in protecting serum-deprived partially differentiated PC-12 (pheochromocytoma) and human SHSY-5Y cells, which possess only MAO-A activity (Youdim et al., 1986). L-Deprenyl and rasagiline have some intrinsic antiapoptotic property that is unrelated to MAO-B inhibition, since the S-optical isomer of rasagiline, TVP 1022 not being an MAO inhibitor has similar neuroprotective activity to the latter MAOIs (Youdim et al., 2001b). Some other propoargylamine-containing MAO-B inhibitors, including aliphatic propargylamines (Berry and Boulton, 2002; Youdim et al., 2005a) and PF 9601N (Cuttillas et al., 2002) and, in some but not all, systems, the MAO-A inhibitor clorgyline exhibit similar activity. *In vivo* studies with a number of propoargylamine-containing MAO-B inhibitors have confirmed their neuroprotective activity in several animal models (Youdim and Weinstock, 2002; Youdim et al., 2005). Neuroprotection/neurorescue was associated with protein synthesis resulting in induction of, *inter alia*, Bcl-2 and superoxide dismutase (SOD), which can be prevented by the protein-synthesis inhibitors, such as cycloheximide and actinomysin D.

Structure-activity studies with derivatives and metabolites of deprenyl and rasagiline indicate that the neuroprotection and neurorescue by these inhibitors resides in their propargyl moiety. The propargylamine derivative CGP 3466 (N-dimethyl-N-propargyl-10-aminomeyhyl-dibenzo [b,f] oxepin) is as effective as L-deprenyl as a neuroprotectant, although it does not inhibit MAO (Kragten et al., 1998). More recently, propargylamine, which is a poor inhibitor of MAO-A and MAO-B, has been shown to be neuroprotective and possess neurorescue activity, with similar potencies to that of L-deprenyl and rasagiline (Bar Am et al., 2005). Furthermore TVP 1022, the *S*-isomer of rasagiline, which is a poor inhibitor of MAO-B (Youdim et al., 2001a), has similar neuroprotective activity to that of rasagiline (Youdim et al., 2001b) .

The propargylamine-derived neuroprotective agents are generally anti-apoptotic. They include prevention of mitochondrial swelling, permeability-transition pore opening and cytochrome-c release, associated with preservation of the mitochondrial membrane potential and permeability-transition pore function (Akao et al., 2002; Berry and Boulton, 2002). The ubiquitin-proteasome system and caspase-3 activation are also inhibited. The effects on gene expression have shown that L-deprenyl, rasagiline and ladostigil up regulate the anti-apoptotic (Bcl-2, Bcl-xl and Bcl-w) and suppress the pro-apoptotic (Bad, Bax) members of the Bcl-2 family (see figure 4). This process has been shown to be associated with PKC-dependent-MAP-kinase pathway, resulting from activation of PKCα and ε and their translocation. This results in down regulation of death-initiating PKCδ and γ as consequence of the induction of ERK1/2 phosphorylatio (see figure 4). This property of rasagiline and presumably L-deprenyl may be associated with their ability to induce mRNAs of glia derived neuro t rophic factor (GNF), brain derived neuro t rophic factor (BDNF) and nerve growth factor (NGF) and their proteins in cultu red astrocytes and SHSY-5Y cells. Inhibition of PKC by GF109293X/Calphostin C and ERK1/2 by PD98059/UO126 reduces the neuroprotective-neurorescue activity and the e ffects on the Bcl-2 family proteins (Bar Am et al., 2004). Furthemo re, they prevent PKC-dependent MAPkinase induced release of neuroprotective-neurotrophic sAPPα and holo-APP in vivo as induced by rasagiline and its derivatives (Youdim and Buccafesco, 2005; Youdim et al., 2005) (see figure 4). These processes are directly dependent on the propargyl moiety of propargylamine derived MAOIs, since propargy-lamine has similar potency effects (Weinreb et al., 2004). It has been suggested that a key event in these processes is the specific binding of propargylamines to glyceralde-hyde-3-phosphate dehydrogenase, which has been shown to be an important mediator of neuronal apoptosis (Akao et al., 2002; Maruyama et al., 2001; Tatton et al., 2003).

CONCLUSION

It is 60 years since MAOIs were among the first antidepressants to be discovered and used as such. Now they might have therapeutic value in several major neurodegen-erative conditions because monoamine oxidase plays a role in oxidative stress induced neurodegeneration. But many claims and some counter-claims have been made about the physiological importance of these enzymes and the potential of their inhibitors. These have been evaluated in the light of what we know, and still have to learn, of the structure, function and genetics of the MAOIs and how to employ the disparate actions of their inhibitors in the clinic.

Studies have established that inhibition of MAO-A with selective irreversible and reversible inhbitors increase serotonin and noradrenaline in various brain regions with little change in dopamine metabolism and clinical studies have shown them to possess antidepressant activities. In contrast non-selective MAOIs, which inhibit both enzyme forms, increase brain levels of all three neurotransmitters. Furthermore, it is apparent that non-selective MAOIs or a combination of MAO-A and MAO-B inhibitors is more effective in increasing brain serotonin and noradrenaline, than the selective MAO-A inhibitors. Nevertheless, selective MAO-A inhibitors have consistently been shown to have antidepressant and anti-Parkinson activity. However the antiparkinson activity of reversible MAOIs have not been fully appreciated. Although it was believed that dopamine can be metabolized by MAO-B in the presence of MAO-A inhibition a significant increase in intraneuronal dopamine was found by microdialysis in rats treated with clorgyline or moclobemide (Colzi et al., 1992). This indicates that intra-neuronal MAO-A does indeed affect dopamine metabolism, even though this is less than that is obtained with non-selective MAOIs. The increased release of dopamine obtained with moclobemide in the rat studies may well account for the prolonged duration of motor response in a single-dose levodopa challenge observed in Parkinsonian subjects (Sieradzan et al., 1995). Since the first generation of non-selective (iproniazid, tranylcypromine, phenelzine) MAOIs were shown to produce "cheese reaction" as a consequence of systemic MAO inhibition, it has not been possible to compare the clinical response of Parkinsonian patients to these drugs, with that of selective, reversible MAO-A or irreversible MAO-B inhibitors in controlled studies. Availability of the novel brain selective MAO-AB inhibitor devoid of cheese reaction, such as ladostigil and M 30, may eventually answer the question whether such drugs would be more effective or not. We learned from the pharmacology and mechanism of neuroprotective/neurorescue activities of these novel third generation of non-selective MAO-AB inhibitors, as compared to selective MAO-A or MAO-B inhibitors, in animal studies and neuronal cell cultures, is that they might be more effective as antidepressants and antiparkinson drugs. And in PD and AD they may possess disease modifying activities more effective than that reported for rasagiline recently (Parkinson Study Group, 2004, 2005; Rascol et al., 2005).

REFERENCES

1. Akao, Y., Maruyama, W., Shimizu, S., Yi, H., Nakagawa, Y., Shamoto-Nagai, M., Youdim, M.B., Tsujimoto, Y., Naoi, M., 2002. Mitochondrial permeability transition mediates apoptosis induced by N-methyl(R)salsolinol, an endogenous neurotoxin, and is inhibited by Bcl-2 and Rasagiline, N-Propargyl-1(R)-aminoindan. J. Neurochem. 82, 913-23.

2. Allain, H., Lieury, A, Brunet-Bourgin, F., Mirabaud, C., Trebon, P., Le Coz, F., Gandon, J.M.,.1993. Antidepressants and cognition: comparative effects of moclobemide, viloxazine and maprotiline. Psychopharmacology (Berl). 106 (Suppl), S56-S61.

3. Amrein, R., Martin, J. R., Cameron, A., 1999. Moclobemide in patients with dementia and depression. Adv. Neurol. 80, 509-519.

4. Ansari, K. S., Yu, P. H., Kruck, T. P., Tatton, W. G., 1993. Rescue of axotomized immature rat facial motoneurons by R(-)-deprenyl: stereospecificity and independence from monoamine oxidase inhibition. J. Neurosci. 13, 4042-4053.

5. Bailey, S.D., Bucci, L., Gosline, E., Kline, N.S., Park, I.H., Rochlin, D., Saunders, J.C., Vaisberg, M., 1959. Comparison of iproniazid with other amine oxidase inhibitors, including W-1544, JB-516, RO 4-1018, and RO 5-0700. Ann. N. Y. Acad. Sci. 80, 652-668.

6. Bar-Am, O., Yogev-Falach, M., Amit, T., Sagi, I., Youdim, M. B. H., 2004. Regulation of protein kinase C by the anti-Parkinson drug, MAO-B inhibitor, rasagiline and its derivatives, J. Neurochem. 89, 1119-1125.

7. Bar Am, O., Weinreb, O., Amit, T., Youdim, M. B. H., 2005. Neurorescue activity of N-propargylamine associated with regulation of BCL-2 family proteins, neurotrophic factors and amyloid precursor protein (APP) processing. FASEB J. 19, 1899-1901.

8. Bernheim, N.L.C., 1931. Tyramine oxidation II. The course of oxidation. J.Biol.Chem. 155, 299-309.

9. Berry, M. D., Boulton, A.A., 2002. Aliphatic propargylamines as symptomatic and neuroprotective treatments for neurodegenerative diseases. Neurotoxicol. Teratolog. 24, 667-673.

10. Bieck, P. R., Antonin, K H, Schmidt, E., 1993. Clinical pharmacology of reversible monoamine oxidase-A inhibitors. Clin. Neuropharmacol. 16 (Suppl 2), S34-S41.

11. Birkmayer, W, Hornykiewicz, O., 1961. The L-3,4-dioxyphenylalanine (DOPA)-effect in Parkinson-akinesia. Wien. Klin. Wochenschr. 73, 787-788.

12. Birkmayer, W., Riederer, P., Youdim, M. H. G. H., Linuaer, W., 1975. The potentiation of the anti-akinetic effect after L-dopa treatment by an inhibitor of MAO-B, deprenyl. J. Neural. Transm. 36, 303-326.

13. Birkmayer, W., Riederer, P., Youdim, M.B.H., Ambrozi, A., 1977. Implications of combined treatment with Madopar and L-deprenyl in Parkinson's disease. A long-term study. Lancet 1(8009), 439-443.

14. Birkmayer, W., Knoll, J., Riederer, P., Youdim, M. B., Hars, V., Marton, J., 1985. Increased life expectancy resulting from addition of L-deprenyl to Madopar treatment in Parkinson's disease: a longterm study. J. Neural. Transm. 64. 113-127.

15. Blandini, F., 2005. Neuroprotection by rasagiline: a new therapeutic approach to Parkinson's disease? CNS Drug Rev. 11, 183-194.

16. Blaschko, H., 1952. Amine oxidase and amine metabolism. Pharmacol.Rev. 4, 415-453.

17. Cesura, A. M., Pletscher, A., 1992. The new generation of monoamine oxidase inhibitors. Prog. Drug Res. 38, 171-297.

18. Chiba, K., Trevor, A., Castagnoli, N. Jr., 1984. Metabolism of the neurotoxic tertiary amine, MPTP, by brain monoamine oxidase. Biochem. Biophys. Res. Commun. 120, 574-578.

19. Collins, G. G., Sandler, M., Williams, A., Pare, C. M. B., Youdim, M B. H., 1970. Multiple forms of human brain mitochondrial monoamine oxidase. Nature 225, 817-820.

20. Colzi, A., d'Agostini, F., Cesura, A. M., Da Prada, M., 1992. Brain microdialysis in rats: a technique to reveal competition in vivo between endogenous dopamine and moclobemide, a RIMA antidepressant. Psychopharmacology (Berl) 106 (Suppl.), S17-S20.

21. Cuttillas, B., Ambrosio, S., Unzeta, M., 2002. Neuroprotective effect of the monoamine oxidase inhibitor PF 9601N [N-(2-propynyl)-2-(5-benzyloxy-indolyl) methylamine] on rat nigral neurons after 6-hydroxydopamine-striatal lesion. Neurosci. Lett. 329, 165-168.

22. Da Prada, M., Kettler, R., Keller, H. H., Haefely, W. E., 1983. Neurochemical effects in vitro and in vivo of the antidepressant Ro 11-1163, a specific and short-acting MAO-A inhibitor. Mod. Probl. Pharmacopsychiatry 19, 231-245.

23. Da Prada, M., Zurcher, G., Wuthrich, I., Haefely, W. E., 1988. On tyramine, food, beverages and the reversible MAO inhibitor moclobemide. J. Neural Transm. 26, 31-56.

24. Edmondson, D. E., Binda, C., Mattevi, A., 2004. The FAD binding sites of human monoamine oxidases A and B. Neurotoxicology 25, 63-72.

25. Fairweather, D. B., Kerr, J. S., Hindmarch, I., 1993. The effects of moclobemide on psychomotor performance and cognitive function. Int. Clin. Psychopharmacol. 8, 43-47.

26. Finberg, J. P., Tenne, M., 1982. Relationship between tyramine potentiation and selective inhibition of monoamine oxidase types A and B in the rat vas deferens. Br. J. Pharmacol. 77, 13-21.

27. Finberg, J., Youdim, M. B. H., 2002. Pharmacological properties of the anti-Parkinson drug rasagiline; modification of endogenous brain amines, reserpine reversal, serotonergic and dopaminergic behaviours. Neuropharmacology 43, 1110-1118.

28. Finberg, J. P., Tenne, M., Youdim, M. B. H., 1981. Tyramine antagonistic properties of AGN 1135, an irreversible inhibitor of monoamine oxidase type B. Br. J. Pharmacol. 7, 65-74.

29. Finberg, J. P., Lamensdorf, I., Weinstock, M., Schwartz, M., Youdim, M. B. H., 1999. Pharmacology of rasagiline (N-propargyl-1R-aminoindan). Adv. Neurol. 80, 495-499.

30. Foley, R., Gerlach, M., Youdim, M. B. H., Riederer, R., 2000. MAO-B inhbitors; Multiple roles in the therapy of neurodegenrative disorders. PARD 6, 25-47.

31. Gal, S., Zheng, H., Fridkin, M., Youdim, M. B. H., 2005. Novel multifunctional neuroprotective iron chelator-monoamine oxidase inhibitor drugs for neurodegenerative diseases. II; In vivo selective brain monoamine oxidase inhibition and prevention of MPTP induced striatal dopamine depletion. J. Neurochem. 95, 79-88.

32. Gorkin, V.Z., 1966. Monoamine oxidases. Pharmacol. Rev. 18, 115-20.

33. Green, A. R., Mitchell, B. D., Tordoff, A., Youdim, M. B. H., 1977. Evidence for dopamine deamination by both type A and type B monoamine oxidase in rat brain in vivo and for the degree of inhibition of enzyme necessary for increased functional activity of dopamine and 5-hydroxytryptamine. Br. J. Pharmacol. 60, 343-349.

34. Green, A. R., Youdim, M. B. H., 1975. Effects of monoamine oxidase inhibition by clorgyline, deprenil or tranylcypromine on 5-hydroxytryptamine concentrations in rat brain and hyperactivity following subsequent tryptophan administration. Br. J. Pharmacol. 55, 415-422.

35. Group, T. P. S., 1989. Effect of deprenyl on the progression of disability in early Parkinson's disease. N. Engl. J. Med. 321, 1364-1371.

36. Group, T. P. S., 1993. Effects of tocopherol and deprenyl on the progression of disability in early Parkinson's disease. N. Engl. J. Med. 328, 176-183.

37. Haefely, W., Burkard, W. P., Cesura, A. M., Kettler, R., Lorez, H. P., Martin, J. R, Richards, J. G., Scherschlicht, R., Da Prada, M., 1992. Biochemistry and pharmacology of moclobemide, a prototype RIMA. Psychopharmacology (Berl) 106 (Suppl), S6-S14.

38. Heikkila, R. E., Duvoisin, R. C., Finberg, J. P., Youdim, M.B., 1985. Prevention of MPTP-induced neurotoxicity by AGN-1133 and AGN-1135, selective inhibitors of monoamine oxidase-B. Eur. J. Pharmacol. 116, 313-317.

39. Heikkila, R. E., Manzino, L., Cabbat, F. S., Duvoisin, R. C., 1984. Protection against the dopaminergic neurotoxicity of 1-methyl-4-phenyl-1,2,5,6-tetrahydropyridine by monoamine oxidase inhibitors. Nature 311, 467-469.

40. Honig, L. S., Mayeux, R., 2001. Natural history of Alzheimer's disease. Aging (Milano) 13, 171-182.

41. Jansen Steur, E. N., Ballering, A. L., 1999. Combined and selective monoamine oxidase inhibition in the treatment of depression in Parkinson's disease. Adv. Neurol. 80: 505-508.

42. Johnson, J. P., 1968. Some observations upon a new inhibitor of monoamine oxidase in brain tissue. Biochem. Pharmacol. 1, 1285-1297.

43. Kalir, A., Sabbagh, A., Youdim, M. B. H., 1981. Selective acetylenic 'suicide' and reversible inhibitors of monoamine oxidase types A and B. Br. J. Pharmacol. 73, 55-64.

44. Kerr, J. S., Fairweather, D. B., Mahendran, R., Hindmarch, I., 1992. The effects of acute and repeated doses of moclobemide on psychomotor performance and cognitive function in healthy elderly volunteers. Human Psychopharmacol. Clin. Experi. 7, 273-279.

45. Knoll, J., Magyar, K., 1972. Some puzzling pharmacological effects of monoamine oxidase inhibitors. Adv. Biochem. Psychopharmacol. 5, 393-408.

46. Korn, A., Da Prada, M., Raffesberg, W., Allen, S., Gasic, S., 1987. Tyramine pressor effect in man: studies with moclobemide, a novel, reversible monoamine oxidase inhibitor J. Neural Transm. 26, 57-71.

47. Kragten, E., Lalande, I., Zimmermann, K., Roggo, S., Schindler, P., Muller, D., van Ostrum, J., Waldmeier, P., Furst, P., 1998. Glyceraldehyde-3-phosphate dehydrogenase, the putative target of the anti-apoptotic compounds CGP 3466 and R-(-)-deprenyl. J. Biol. Chem. 273, 5821-5828.

48. Langston, J.W., Irwin, I., 1986. MPTP: current concepts and controversies. Clin. Neuropharmacol. 9, 485-507.

49. Lees, A. J., Shaw, K., Stern, G., Sandler, M., Youdim, M. B. H., 1977. Deprenyl in Parkinson's disease. Lancet 2, 791-795.

50. Maruyama, W., Akao, Y., Youdim, M. B., Davis, B. A., Naoi, M., 2001. Transfection-enforced Bcl-2 overexpression and an anti-Parkinson drug, rasagiline, prevent nuclear accumulation of glyceraldehyde-3-phosphate dehydrogenase induced by an endogenous dopaminergic neurotoxin, N-methyl(R)salsolinol. J. Neurochem. 78, 727-735.

51. Melamed, E., Youdim, M. B., 1985. Prevention of dopaminergic toxicity of MPTP in mice by phenylethylamine, a specific substrate of type B monoamine oxidase. Br. J. Pharmacol. 86, 529-531.

52. Newman, S. C., 1999. The prevalence of depression in Alzheimer's disease and vascular dementia in a population sample. J. Affect. Disord. 52, 169-176.

53. O'Carroll, A. M., Fowler, C. J., Tipton, K. F., 1983. The deamination of dopamine by human brain monoamine oxidase. Specificity for the two enzyme forms in seven brain regions. Naunyn-Schmiedebergs Arch. Pharmacol. 322, 198-202.

54. Palmer, A. M., Stratmann, G. C., Procter, A. W., Bowen, D. M., 1988. Possible neurotransmitter basis of behavioral changes in Alzheimer's disease. Ann. Neurol. 23, 616-620.

55. Parkinson Study Group, 2004. A controlled, randomized, delayed-start study of rasagiline in early Parkinson disease. Arch. Neurol. 61, 561-566.

56. Parkinson Study Group, 2005. A randomized placebo-controlled trial of rasagiline in levodopa-treated patients with Parkinson disease and motor fluctuations: the PRESTO study. Arch. Neurd. 62, 241-248.

57. Porsolt, R.D., Bertin, A., Jalfre, M., 1977. Behavioral despair in mice: a primary screening test for antidepressants. Arch. Int. Pharmacodyn. Ther. 229, 327-336.

58. Rascol, O., 2005. Rasagiline in the pharmacotherapy of Parkinson's disease - a review. Expert Opin. Pharmacother. 6, 2061-2075.

59. Rascol, O., Brooks, D. J., Melamed, E., Oertel, W., Poewe, W., Stocchi, F., Tolosa, E., 2005. Rasagiline as an adjunct to levodopa in patients with Parkinson's disease and motor fluctuations. Lancet 365 (9463), 947-954.

60. Riederer, P., Youdim, M. B. H., 1986. Monoamine oxidase activity and monoamine metabolism in brains of parkinsonian patients treated with L-deprenyl. J. Neurochem. 46, 1359-1365.

61. Riederer, P., Konradi, C., Birkmayer, W., Youdim, M. B. H., 1987. Localization of MAO-A and MAO-B in human brain: a step in understanding the therapeutic action of L-deprenyl. Adv. Neurolog. 45, 111-118.

62. Ruggieri, S., Fabbrini, G., Bramante, L., DePandis, F., Stocchi, F., Barbanti, P., Vacca, L., Manfredi, M., 1996. An open study with reversible MAO-A inhibitors in complicated Parkinson's disease. Adv. Neurol. 69, 595-598.

63. Sagi, Y., Weinstock, M., Youdim, M. B. H., 2003. Attenuation of MPTP-induced dopaminergic neurotoxicity by TV 3326, a cholinesterase-monoamine oxidase inhibitor. J. Neurochem. 86, 290-297.

64. Saunders, J. C., Radinger, N., Rochlin, D., Kline, N. S., 1959. Treatment of depressed and regressed patients with iproniazid and reserpine. Dis. Nerv. Syst.. 20, 31-39.

65. Seymour, C. B., Mothersill, C., Mooney, R., Moriarty, M., Tipton, K. F., 2003. Monoamine oxidase inhibitors L-deprenyl and clorgyline protect nonmalignant human cells from ionising radiation and chemotherapy toxicity. Br. J. Can. 89, 1979-1986.

66. Sieradzan, K., Channon, S., Ramponi, C., Stern, G. M., Lees, A. J., Youdim, M. B., 1995. The therapeutic potential of moclobemide, a reversible selective monoamine oxidase A inhibitor in Parkinson's disease. J. Clin. Psychopharmacol. 154 (Suppl. 2), S51-S59.

67. Sterling, J., Herzig, Y., Goren, T., Finkelstein, N., Lerner, D., Goldenberg, W., Miskolczi, I., Molnar, S., Rantal, F., Tamas, T., Toth, G., Zagyva, A., Zekany, A., Finberg, J., Lavian, G., Gross, A., Friedman, R., Razin, M., Huang, W., Krais, B., Chorev, M., Youdim, M. B., Weinstock, M., 2002. Novel dual inhibitors of AChE and MAO derived from hydroxy aminoindan and phenethylamine as potential treatment for Alzheimer's disease. J. Med. Chem. 45, 5260-5279.

68. Sternic, N., Kacar, A., Filipovic, S., Svetel, M., Kostic, V. S., 1998. The therapeutic effect of moclobemide, a reversible selective monoamine oxidase A inhibitor, in Parkinson's disease. Clin. Neuropharmacol. 21, 93-96.

69. Tandberg, E., Larsen, J. P., Aarsland, D., Cummings, J. L., 1996. The occurrence of depression in Parkinson's disease. A community-based study. Arch. Neurol. 53, 175-179.

70. Tatton, W. G., Greenwood, C. E., 1991. Rescue of dying neurons: a new action for deprenyl in MPTP parkinsonism. J. Neurosci. Res. 30, 666-372.

71. Tatton, W., Chalmers-Redman, R. Tatton, N. 2003. Neuroprotection by deprenyl and other propargylamines: glyceraldehyde-3-phosphate dehydrogenase rather than monoamine oxidase B. J. Neural Transm. 110, 509-515.

72. Tipton, K. F., Boyce, S., O'Sullivan, J., Davey, G. P., Healy, J., 2004. Monoamine oxidases: certainties and uncertainties. Curr. Med. Chem. 11, 1965-1982.

73. Tsolaki, M., Kokarida, K., Iakovidou, V., Stilopoulos, E., Meimaris, J., Kazis, A., 2001. Extrapyramidal symptoms and signs in Alzheimer's disease: prevalence and correlation with the first symptom. Am. J. Alzheimers Dis. Other Demen. 16, 268-278.

74. Weinreb, O., Bar Am, O., Amit, T., Chillag-Talmor, O., Youdim, M. B. H., 2004. Neuroprotection via pro-survival protein kinase C isoforms associated with Bcl-2 family members. FASEB J, 18, 1471-1474.

75. Weinstock, M., Bejar, C., Wang, R. H., Poltyrev, T., Gross, A., Finberg, J. P., Youdim, M. B., 2000a. TV3326, a novel neuroprotective drug with cholinesterase and monoamine oxidase inhibitory activities for the treatment of Alzheimer's disease. J. Neural. Transm. (Suppl. 60), 157-169.

76. Weinstock, M., Goren, T., Youdim, M. B. H., 2000b. Development of a novel neuroprotective drug (TV 3326) for the treatment of Alzheimer's disease, with cholinesterase and monoamine oxidase inhibitory activities. Drug Develop. Res. 50, 216-222.

77. Weinstock, M., Gorodetsky, E., Wang, R. H., Gross, A., Weinreb, O., Youdim, M. B., 2002a. Limited potentiation of blood pressure response to oral tyramine by brain-selective

monoamine oxidase A-B inhibitor, TV-3326 in conscious rabbits. Neuropharmacology; 43, 999-1005.

78. Weinstock, M., Poltyrev, T., Weinreb, O., Youdim, M. B. H., 2002b. Effect of TV 3326, a novel monoamine-oxidase cholinesterase inhibitor, in rat models of anxiety and depression. Psychopharmacology (Berl) 160, 318-324.

79. Wesnes, K.A., Simpson, P.M., Christmas, L., Anand, R., McClelland, G.R., 1989. The effects of moclobemide on cognition. J. Neural Transm. 28 (Suppl.), 91-102.

80. Wheatley, D., 1970. Comparative trial of a new monoamine oxidase inhibitor in depression. J. Ppsychiat. 117, 573-576.

81. Yang, H. Y., Neff, N. H., 1973. β-Phenylethylamine: a specific substrate for type B monoamine oxidase of brain. J. Pharmacol. Exp. Ther. 187, 365-371.

82. Youdim, M. B. H., Buccafesco. J. J., 2005. Multi-functional Drugs for Various CNS Targets in the Treatment of Neurodegenerative Disorders. TIPS. 26, 27-35.

83. Youdim, M. B. H., Riederer, P., 1993. Dopamine metabolism and neurotransmission in primate brain in relationship to monoamine oxidase A and B inhibition. J. Neural. Transm. 91, 181-195.

84. Youdim, M. B. H., Sourkes, T.L., 1965. Effects of heat, pH and inhbitors on rat liver and brain monoamine oxidase. Can..J. Biochem. 43, 225-258.

85. Youdim, M. B. H., Weinstock, M., 2002. Molecular basis of neuroprotective activities of rasagiline and the anti alzheimer drug, TV 3326, {[N-propargyl-(3R)aminoindan-5-YL]-ethyl methyl carbamate}. Cell. Mol. Neurobiol. 21, 555-573.

86. Youdim, M. B. H., Collins, G. G., Sandler, M., Pare C. M. B., Bevan Jones, A., 1972. Human brain monoamine oxidase: multiple forms and selective inhibitors. Nature 236 (5344), 225-228.

87. Youdim, M. B. H., Heldman, E., Pollard, H. B., Fleming, P. McHugh, E., 1986. Contrasting monoamine oxidase activity and tyramine induced catecholamine release in PC12 and chromaffin cells. Neuroscience 19, 1311-1318.

88. Youdim, M. B. H., Finberg, J. P. M., Tipton, K. F., 1988. Monoamine oxidase. Catecholamine II. In: Trendelenburg, U., Weiner N (Eds.), Handbook of Experimental Pharmacology. Springer-Verlag, Berlin, pp. 127-199.

89. Youdim, M. B. H., Gross, A. Finberg, J. P. M., 2001a. Rasagiline [N-propargyl-1R(+)-aminoindant], A selective and potent inhibitor of mitochondrial monoamine oxidase B. Br. J. Pharmacol. 132, 500-506.

90. Youdim, M. B., Wadia, A., Tatton, W., Weinstock, M., 2001b. The antiparkinson drug rasagiline and its cholinesterase inhibitor derivatives exert neuroprotection unrelated to MAO inhibition in cell culture and in vivo. Ann. N. Y. Acad. Sci. 939, 450-458.

91. Youdim, M. B. H., Maruyama, W., Naoi, M., 2005. Neuropharmacological, neuroprotective and amyloid precursor processing properties of selective MAO-B inhibitor antiparkinsnian drug, rasagiline. Drugs of Today 41, 369-391.

92. Zecca, L., Youdim, M. B., Riederer, P., Connor, J. R., Crichton, R. R., 2004. Iron, brain ageing and neurodegenerative disorders. Nat Rev Neurosci. 5, 863-573.

93. Zeller, E. A., 1963. A new approach to the analysis of the interaction of monoamine oxidase and its substrates and inhibitors. Ann.N.Y. Acad..Sci. 107, 811-820.

94. Zeller, E. A., 1979. Classification and nomenclature of monoamine oxidase and other amine oxidases. In: Singer, T.P., Korff, I., Murphy, D. (Eds.), Monoamine Oxidase, Structure, Function and Altered Functions. Academic Press, New York, pp 531-537.

95. Zheng, H., Gal, S., Weiner, L. M., Bar Am, O., Warshawsky, A., Fridkin, M., Youdim, M. B., 2005. Novel multifunctional neuro p rotective iron chelator-monoamine oxidase inhibitor drugs for neurodegenerative diseases: in vitro studies on antioxidant activity, prevention of lipid peroxide formation and monoamine oxidase inhibition. J. Neurochem. 95, 68-78.

CHAPTER 8

RESERPINE AND THE OPENING OF THE NEUROTRANSMITTER ERA IN NEUROPSYCHOPHARMACOLOGY

Silvio Garattini

INTRODUCTION

The new generations of pharmacologists and even neuropharmacologists will hardly ever come across in their training with the properties of an old drug known as reserpine, one of the alkaloids of *Rauwolfia serpentina*. The new pharmacology texts no longer even mention this drug that was instrumental in the generation of new knowledge about the chemical mediators of the brain that gave rise to the field of psychopharmacology. Reserpine has also served as a useful tool for detecting the potential antidepressant activity of other substances. This mini-review is not meant to be exhaustive but highlights some of those early investigations with reserpine that still have significant impact on the history of the development of psychotropic drugs.

GENERAL INFORMATION ON RESERPINE

The history of the medicinal uses of the Rauwolfia serpentina root dates back to the 16th century when it was known as a remedy for insomnia and hypochondria (Curzon, 1990). In 1949 Vakil (Vakil, 1949) described the therapeutic effect of Rauwolfia serpentine in hypertensive patients and in 1952 Müller et al. (1952) isolated reserpine from the root of the plant. After Dorfman et al. (1954) established the chemical structure of reserpine (Figure 1), Woodward (1958) synthesised the substance.

From the first pharmacological studies reserpine's pleiotropic effect was apparent. Bein (1953) described a reduction of blood pressure accompanied by bradycardia, respiratory inhibition, stimulation of peristalsis, miosis and relaxation of the nictitating membrane in cats. Characteristic features of reserpine's action in rats include initial hyperthermia (Garattini and Jori, 1967) followed by a marked drop of body temperature (Usinger, 1962). In addition, reserpine has sedative and tranquillizing effects that differ from that of know hypnotics because reserpinized animals when slightly stimulated are able to react normally for a short time (Bein, 1953).

All the effects of reserpine were initially considered to be of mixed central and peripheral origin. The central effect was interpreted as a reduction of sympathetic tone and was considered to be the main action of the drug because reserpine does not inhibit the peripheral effects of catecholamines and has no ganglion-blocking activity (Bein, 1955). The predominance of the vagal system, as shown by bradycardia and miosis, was regarded not as a direct action of reserpine, but as a result of the reduction of sympathetic tone (Bein, 1957).

Figure 1. Chemical structure of reserpine and some of its derivatives.

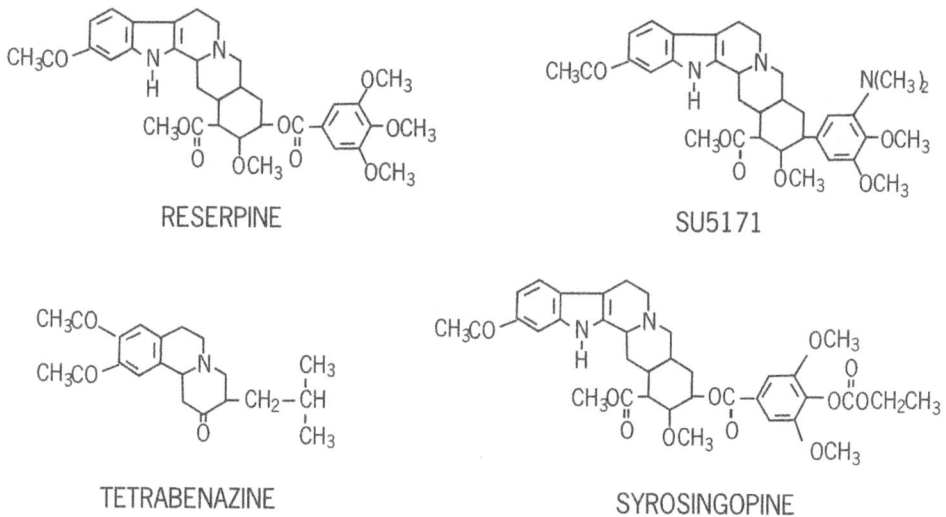

RESERPINE

SU5171

TETRABENAZINE

SYROSINGOPINE

Reserpine was initially used in man to lower blood pressure although the hypotensive effect of the drug is relatively small and too limited to treat patients with high blood pressure. Other drawbacks are sedation and a shallow dose-response curve (Green, 1962). It was the sedating effect of the drug that prompted psychiatrists to use reserpine in mentally ill patients. The results were considered revolutionary because they indicated a possibility of treating neuropsychiatric disorders pharmacologically and opened the way to the uce of other drugs such as chlorpromazine and haloperidol in these disorders (Schlittler and Plummer, 196$).

As frequently happens with a new drug, clinical conditions beported to be sensitive to reserpine blossomed, including acute and chronic psychoses, anxiety, psychomotor hyperactivity, and compulsive aggressive behavior. However, as early as in 1957 Benedetti (1957) focused attention on the limitations of reserpine therapy, and Shepherd (1957), summarizing the findings in clinical trials with reserpine, pointed out: (i) the unpredictability of individual responses and of the toxic and side effects;

(ii) the usefulness in hospital for facilitating the ward–management of excited chronic psychotic patients (Merry, 1956; Penman and Dredge, 1956; Sabshin and Ramot, 1956); (iii) that while a small proportion of chronic schizophrenic patients improve, the drug is of little value in the treatment of major depressive illnesses and senile conditions; (iv) that even among the less incapacitated inpatients and psychiatric outpatients, controlled clinical trials do not show any specific benefit (Feldberg et al., 1956; Ferguson 1956; Folkson and May, 1955).

These limitations and the toxic effects, including severe, even suicidal depression and sex hormone changes, led to the withdrawal of reserpine from the market. Yet reserpine was the cornerstone for the development of clinical psychopharmacology.

RESERPINE AND MONOAMINES

The presence of an indole in the chemical structure of reserpine, the observation that parenterally administered serotonin causes certain effects similar to those of reserpine (Shore and Brodie, 1957), the findings that in the dog reserpine increases urinary excretion of 5-hydroxyindoleacetic acid the major metabolite of serotonin (Shore et al., 1955) and in the rabbit intestine it lowers serotonin concentrations (Pletscher et al., 1955), and the availability of a sensitive and specific assay of serotonin (Bowman et al., 1955; Bogdanski et al., 1956) were probably some of the reasons that led Brodie and his associates to investigate reserpine's action on brain serotonin. Their research led to the fundamental discovery that reserpine caused marked, long-lasting depletion of brain serotonin in rabbits (Brodie et al., 1955). The decrease was evident 15 minutes after an intravenous injection of reserpine already at the dose of 0.5 mg/kg. The effect lasted about four days, then brain serotonin gradually recovered, reaching normal values after about seven days (Shore and Brodie, 1957; Shore et al., 1957a).

Simultaneously with the contributions of Brodie and his associates (Brodie et al., 1955; Shore et al., 1957a) Carlsson's group observed a depletion of catecholamines in the adrenals and heart of the rabbit within 16 hours after the injection of reserpine (Bertler et al., 1956; Carlsson and Hillarp, 1956), and Vogt (Holzbauer and Vogt, 1956) reported a decrease of noradrenaline in the hypothalamus of the cat. Reserpine also depletes brain stores of dopamine (Bertler, 1961). All these findings set the stage for a large number of studies to establish the mechanisms involved in the interaction between reserpine and monoamines, and served as a stimulus for other studies to characterize monoamines as neurotransmitters in the brain.

The almost overlapping depletion of brain serotonin, dopamine and noradrenaline in terms of time-course and dose response pattern points to a similar action of reserpine on these amines. In fact, reserpine's primary effect is the depletion of brain stores of monoamines (t1/2 in brain 7 minutes) (Costa et al., 1966) which are localized in presynaptic granules (Shore et al., 1957b). Reserpine causes the release of monoamines, rapidly metabolized by monoamine oxidase, by impairing Mg++-adenosine triphosphate-dependent monoamine uptake (Carlsson et al., 1963; Stitzel, 1977) by the membrane of storage particles (Carlsson, 1965). This block of monoamine uptake is initially competitive but later on becomes irreversible, requiring for its removal the formation of new particles that are transferred by the Golgi apparatus to the terminal varicosities of the axons (Dahlstrom, 1965; Dahlstrom and Haggendal, 1966). Since monoamines are stored in granules in association with adenine nucleotides (Hagen, 1959; Schumann, 1960) it has been suggested that reserpine acts on this intragranular complex (Bein, 1957; Green, 1962). Reserpine is different from imipramine in that it has no effect on monoamine uptake by the presynaptic membrane (Carlsson, 1966).

KINETICS OF RESERPINE

The finding that reserpine's action on brain monoamines persists after the drug has disappeared from the brain (Brodie et al., 1956) led to the suggestion that reserpine is a "hit-and-run" drug (Shore, 1966). A meaningful discussion of this suggestion calls for some pharmacokinetic information on reserpine. Reserpine is completely metabolized in most animal species. Its main metabolites are methyl-reserpate, and trimethoxybenzoic acid. Other metabolites of reserpine include reserpic acid, syringomethyl-reserpate, syringic acid and carbon dioxide (Plummer et al., 1957; Stitzel, 1977). These metabolites have not been shown to share the biological activities of reserpine. In view of the low doses of reserpine used and the rapid metabolism of the substance, highly specific and sensitive methods, such as tritium-labelled (Manara and Garattini, 1967a) or carbon-^{14} C_{14} labelled reserpine (Sheppard et al., 1955) were needed to measure brain reserpine concentrations. In 1957 Plummer et al. demonstrated that nanograms of reserpine persisted in the brain after injection of H^3 but not of C^{14}- reserpine at pharmacological doses (Plummer et al., 1957). In view of its lipid-solubility reserpine rapidly penetrates the cells and remains there for the duration of the depletion of brain monoamines (Manara et al., 1972; Manara and Garattini 1967a). These findings invalidate the "hit and run" theory of Shore et al. (1957a). The significance of the findings that low levels of reserpine persist in the cells for a long time became of interest when it was demonstrated that tetrabenazine, a short-acting reserpine analogue could protect against the brain noradrenaline depletion and the pharmacological effects of the substance (Quinn et al., 1959) if given before reserpine administration (Carlsson and Lindquist, 1966). It was also shown that tetrabenazine displaced the low brain concentrations of H^3 reserpine (Alpers and Shore, 1969; Manara and Garattini, 1967b; Wagner and Stitzel, 1972). Since tetrabenazine given after reserpine administration was not able to remove the persistent concentration of brain reserpine it was presumed that reserpine bound irreversibly to subcellular structures. Indeed it was established that 12 hours after a dose of reserpine most of the H^3-reserpine was in the brain microsomal fraction containing the granules (Manara et al., 1972; Wagner and Stitzel, 1972). It was also established that prior treatment with tetrabenazine reduced the amount of reserpine in the granules (Wagner and Stitzel, 1972). The nanogram reserpine levels in the brain granular fraction is with all probability explained by i r reversible binding since it is only partially removed by peanut oil or other solvents in which reserpine is highly soluble (Manara et al., 1974). Reserpine binding to granules is considered to be covalent because the drug cannot be removed even by p rolonged dialysis (Giachetti et al., 1974).

By using mass fragmentography it was recently validated that H^3-reserpine in the brain is not due to a redistribution of tritium (Pantarotto et al., 1976, 1977). Reserpine's persistent binding to granules containing monoamines was confirmed in experiments in which the brain serotonin and catecholamine terminals were removed respectively by lesion of the nucleus raphé dorsalis and medianus, and the administration of 6-hydroxydopamine. In both cases the levels of H^3-reserpine in some brain areas decreased after a few hours but not after 15 minutes (Mennini et al., 1977, 1980).

SEROTONIN OR NORADRENALINE?

After the early finding which indicated that reserpine reduced the stores of serotonin, noradrenaline and dopamine, different views were expressed about the role of serotonin and catecholamines in reserpine's multifaceted pharmacological actions. Bein (1957) suggested that decreased sympathetic tone led to vagal prevalence centrally and on the periphery. However, Carlsson et al. (1957) showed that by giving reserpine 16 hours before splanchnic nerve stimulation, the pressor effect of the stimulation was abolished, indicating that the depletion of noradrenaline at the end organs was responsible for the lack of functional effects. Thus, those amines that act through catecholamine release, e.g., tyramine, ephedrine and amphetamine, lose their activity while amines acting directly on catecholamine receptors maintain their effects, or their effects may even become stronger (Green, 1962).

According to Shore and Brodie (1957), because of the impairment of serotonin storage, the continuously synthesized serotonin could flow until the storage sites regain their capacity to take it up. It is this flow of "highly active" free serotonin that stimulates subcortical centers, and increases central parasympathetic activity (Brodie and Shore, 1957; Shore et al., 1957a) resulting in sedation.

It is probable that the complex activity of reserpine and especially the antipsychotic activity of the substance does not depend on a single monoamine, but is explained by the depletion of all three, serotonin, dopamine and noradrenaline. In fact most antipsychotic agents act by inhibiting more than one monoamine receptor. Already during the development of chlorpromazine, one of the early antipsychotic agents, it had been shown that it was active on dopamine and serotonin receptors (Anden et al., 1970). The so-called second-generation antipsychotics have the same action as the first generation antipsychotics, but with greater selectivity to given receptors.

RESERPINE ANALOGUES

Following the enthusiasm aroused by the initial multiple therapeutic applications of reserpine, several analogues and derivatives of the substance were synthesized and pharmacologically tested in an effort to obtain better drugs. It is beyond the scope of this review to describe the relationships between chemical structure and pharmacological effects. However, it is of interest to recall that only those derivatives of reserpine that showed pharmacological activity (hypotension and sedation) which were effective in reducing serotonin and presumably catecholamine levels (Shore and Brodie, 1957). For instance, rescinnamine and deserpidine shared the effect of reserpine, whereas methylreserpate, reserpic acid and isoreserpine did not (Shore and Brodie, 1957).

Tetrabenazine attracted some interest because it reached the market. It is a benzoquinoline derivative with shorter action than reserpine. It was characterized mostly as an antipsychotic (Pletscher, 1957). Yet, tetrabenazine had a short life on the market because, similar to reserpine it induced a depressive state together with extrapyramidal symptoms.

Substances with a small change in the trimethoxybenzoic acid moiety of reserpine usually maintain reserpine-like pharmacological activity, although this activity tends to be weaker than that of the parent substance (Karim et al., 1960). One of these derivatives, syrosingopine (see figure 1) aroused interest because of its selectivity in inducing hypotension (Bartels, 1959) more than sedation. Similarly, another derivative, SU5171 (see figure 1) was considered to be interesting because of its relative selectivity for the central nervous system compared to its hypotensive action. Interestingly, SU5171 was more potent than syrosingopine in depleting brain serotonin (Garattini et al., 1959). Syrosingopine entered clinical investigations and appeared to be better tolerated than reserpine (Bartels, 1959).

RESERPINE IN DEPRESSION STUDIES

Reserpine has played a major role in clarifying the mechanism of action of new antidepressants: both monoamine oxidase inhibitors (MAOIs) and imipramine-like drugs, also known as tricyclic antidepressants (TCAs).

The story of antidepressants starts with the observation that the antitubercular drugs isoniazid and iproniazid, improved the mood more than the infection in some tubercular patients. This observation led to investigations that showed that iproniazide inhibited the monoamine oxidase enzymes important for terminating the activity of monoamines, and subsequently to the introduction of iproniazid in the treatment of depression. It is now well known that MAOIs increase serotonin, dopamine and noradrenaline levels in several tissues including the brain.

Several years after their introduction MAOIs were withdrawn from the market because of the advent of new drugs and because of serious side effects when they interacted with food constituents, e.g., tyramine, and other drugs. However, MAOIs have been useful for understanding the mechanism of action of reserpine. When animals pre-treated with a MAOI are given reserpine there is a delay in the depletion of noradrenaline (Pletscher, 1956; Shore et al., 1957b) and reserpine instead of having a sedative has a stimulating action (Brodie et al., 1956; Chessin et al., 1957). This reversal of the effect of reserpine has been interpreted as proof for the reserpine-induced release of monoamines which in normal animals are metabolised by monoamine oxidase (MAO) and show no action, but in animals in which their breakdown is inhibited induce a variety of effects (Brodie et al., 1959; Spector et al., 1960). For instance in the MAO-inhibited animal, intravenous reserpine has a marked pressor effect in cats (Chessin et al., 1957), dogs (Eltherington and Horita, 1960), and rats (Garattini et al., 1960). This pressor effect is related to noradrenaline because it is inhibited by the administration of catecholamine antagonists.

The antidepressant agent imipramine was discovered during clinical investigations (Kuhn, 1957). Laboratory work had predicted that the drug should have a mild sedative effect (Domenjoz and Theobald, 1959). It was therefore necessary to study the mode of action of imipramine and to devise experimental methods to detect inipramine-like antidepressant activity. In this effort, reserpine was again of great help. Since reserpine was reported to induce a depressive syndrome in some patients and a peculiar sedation in animals, it was tested whether imipramine would reveal its pharmacological properties in "depressed" animals. Experimental observations showed that depending on the experimental conditions imipramine was able to prevent either partially or completely some of the symptoms induced by high doses of reserpine (Costa et al., 1960; Domenjoz and Theobald, 1959; Garattini, 1959; Sulser et al., 1960). In a short time several papers were published (Garattini and Jori, 1967) which showed that imipramine was effective in antagonizing the effects not only of reserpine, but also of its short-acting derivatives such as tetrabenazine (Garattini et al., 1962), Ro 4-1284 (Sulser et al., 1964) and P-2565 (Watts et al., 1964). In addition, all TCAs showed some kind of antagonism toward reserpine not only in the rat but also in mice (Askew, 1963), rabbits (Maxwell and Palmer, 1961) and man (Dick and Shepherd, 1965; Pöldinger 1963). Unlike MAOIs, TCAs did not change the depletion of serotonin and noradrenaline in the brain (Garattini et al., 1962; Pletscher and Gey, 1962; Sulser et al., 1962) and unlike tetrabenazine, imipramine did not change the "persistent" low concentrations of reserpine in the brain (Manara and Garattini, 1967b).

A simple parameter to measure the effect of an intravenous dose of reserpine is the biphasic change of body temperature: early hyperthermia (Jori et al., 1967) followed after a few hours by lasting hypothermia (Garattini and Jori, 1967). TCAs are effective in raising body temperature in reserpinized but not in normal rats. This action is relatively specific because TCAs have no effect on the hypothermia induced by chlorpromazine, serotonin, and α-methyldopa, or on the hyperthermia induced by injection of yeast (Jori and Garattini, 1965). TCAs increase the hyperthermia induced by dopa (3,4 –dihydroxyphenylalnine) or infusion of catecholamines. The increase of body temperature after the administration of a TCA in reserpinized animals is antagonized by adrenolytics or by α-methyl-p-tyrosine, which blocks catecholamine synthesis. All these findings are consistent with the idea that TCAs restore somehow the reserpine-induced relative deficiency of monoamines. Indeed as shown by Axelrod's group, TCAs block at the presynaptic sites the uptake of monoamines released by reserpine, and thereby render more monoamines available for the postsynaptic receptors (Glowinsky and Axelrod, 1964). The main chemical mediator is noradrenaline, because desipramine, a metabolite of imipramine and a selective noradrenaline uptake blocker with no activity on serotonin uptake, is a strong reserpine antagonist (Garattini and Jori, 1967).

CONCLUSIONS

This review aimed at showing how a drug like reserpine has revolutionized our approach to the therapy of mental illness. With the introduction of reserpine it was felt for the first time that mental illness was amenable to treatment, like any other disease, because we had an idea of possible targets for the treatment. The discovery that reserpine's effects on brain noradrenaline, dopamine and serotonin, are reflected in pharmacological effects, led to the identification of new neurochemical mediators, and ushered in an era when monoamines were to be characterized first by their specific localization in brain neurons, their synthesis, storage, release, and uptake, and later, by their receptors. For many years reserpine has served as a tool for testing new antidepressants and differentiating between various classes of drugs. Reversal of its pharmacological effects was one of the basic tests for the primary screening of new chemicals.

Reserpine failed as a drug in the treatment of schizophrenia, and as it frequently happens in science its importance for the progress of knowledge could not be forecasted when first introduced. Reserpine gave impetus to psychopharmacology and opened the gate to the introduction of modern psychotropic drugs. We now know that things are much more complex than it was thought at the time when reserpine was introduced. We are entering an era of molecular medicine based on genomic and proteomic approaches. Reserpine is no longer of interest. Most of the reserpine-era researchers are no longer active. But it is hoped that the enthusiasm of those years will be transmitted to the new generation of psychopharmacologists.

REFERENCES

1. Alpers, H.S., Shore, P.A., 1969. Specific binding of reserpine. Association with norepinephrine depletion. Biochem. Pharmacol. 18, 1363-1372.
2. Anden, N.E., Butcher, S.G., Corrodi, H., Fuxe, K., Ungerstedt, U., 1970. Receptor activity and turnover of dopamine and noradrenaline after neuroleptics. Eur. J. Pharmacol. 11, 303-314.
3. Askew, B.M., 1963. A simple screening procedure for imipramine-like antidepressant agents. Life Sci. 10, 725-730.
4. Bartels, C.C., 1959. Syrosingopine: a new Rauwolfia preparation. N. Engl. J. Med. 261, 785-788.
5. Bein, H.J., 1953. Pharmacology of reserpin, a new alkaloid from Rauwolfia serpentina Benth. Experientia 9, 107-110.
6. Bein, H.J., 1955. Significance of selected central mechanisms for the analysis of the action of reserpine. Ann. N. Y. Acad. Sci. 61, 4-16.
7. Bein, H.J., 1957. Effect of reserpine on the functional strata of the nervous system. In: Garattini, S., Ghetti, V. (Eds.), Psychotropic Drugs. Elsevier, Amsterdam, pp. 325-331.
8. Benedetti, G., 1957. Possibilita' e limiti della terapia reserpinica. In: Garattini, S., Ghetti, V. (Eds.), Psychotropic Drugs. Elsevier, Amsterdam, pp. 527-533.
9. Bertler, A., 1961. Effect of reserpine on the storage of catecholamines in brain and other tissues. Acta Physiol Scand. 51, 75-83.
10. Bertler, A., Carlsson, A., Rosengren, E., 1956. Release by reserpine of catecholamines from rabbit's hearts. Naturwissenschaften 43, 521.
11. Bogdanski, D.F., Pletscher, A., Brodie, B.B., Udenfriend, S., 1956. Identification and assay of serotonin in brain. J. Pharmacol. Exp. Ther. 117, 82-88.
12. Bowman, R.L., Caulfield, P.A., Udenfriend, S., 1955. Spectrophotofluorometric assay in the visible and ultraviolet. Science 122, 32-33.
13. Brodie, B.B., Shore, P.A., 1957. A concept for a role of serotonin and norepinephrine as chemical mediators in the brain. Ann. N. Y. Acad. Sci. 66, 631-642.
14. Brodie, B.B., Pletscher, A., Shore, P.A., 1955. Evidence that serotonin has a role in brain function. Science 122, 968-969.
15. Brodie, B.B., Hess, S.M., Shore, P.A., 1956. Persistence of reserpine action after the disappearance of drug from brain: effect on serotonin. J. Pharmacol. Exp. Ther, 118, 84-89.
16. Brodie, B.B., Spector, S., Shore, P.A., 1959. Interaction of monoamine oxidase inhibitors with physiological and biochemical mechanisms in brain. Ann. N. Y. Acad. Sci. 80, 609-616.
17. Carlsson, A., 1965. Drugs which block the storage of 5-hydroxytryptamine and related amines. In: Erspamer, V. (Ed.), Handbook of Experimental Pharmacology, vol. 19. Springer Verlag, Berlin, pp. 529-592.
18. Carlsson, A., 1966. Modification of sympathetic function. Pharmacol. Rev. 18, 541-549.
19. Carlsson, A., Hillarp, N.A., 1956. Release of adrenaline from the adrenal medulla of rabbits produced by reserpine. Kgl. Fysiograf. Sallskap. Lund. Forh. 26, 8-9.
20. Carlsson, A., Lindqvist, M., 1966. The interference of tetrabenazine, benzquinamide and prenylamine with the action of reserpine. Acta Pharmacol. Toxicol. (Copenh.) 24, 112-120.
21. Carlsson, A., Rosengren, E., Bertler, A., Nilsson, J., 1957. Effect of reserpine on the metabolism of catecholamines. In: Garattini, S., Ghetti, V. (Eds.), Psychotropic Drugs. Elsevier, Amsterdam, pp. 363-372.
22. Carlsson, A., Hillarp, N.A., Waldeck, B., 1963. Analysis of the Mg++-ATPdependent storage mechanism in the amine granules of the adrenal medulla. Acta Physiol. Scand. 59 (Suppl. 215), 1-38.
23. Chessin, M., Kramer, E.R., Scott, C.C., 1957. Modifications of the pharmacology of reserpine and serotonin by iproniazid. J. Pharmacol. Exp. Ther. 119, 453-460.
24. Costa, E., Garattini, S., Valzelli, L., 1960. Interactions between reserpine, chlorpromazine, and imipramine. Experientia 16, 461-463.
25. Costa, E., Boullin, D.J., Hammer, W., Vogel, W., Brodie, B.B. 1966. Interactions of drugs with adrenergic neurons. Pharmacol. Rev. 18, 577-597.
26. Curzon, G., 1990. How reserpine and chlorpromazine act: the impact of key discoveries on the history of psychopharmacology. Trends Pharmacol. Sci. 11, 61-63.

27. Dahlstrom, A., 1965. Observations on the accumulation of noradrenaline in the proximal and distal parts of peripheral adrenergic nerves after compression. J. Anat. 99, 677-689.
28. Dahlstrom, A., Haggendal, J., 1966. Studies on the transport and life-span of amine storage granules in a peripheral adrenergic neuron system. Acta Physiol. Scand. 67, 278-288.
29. Dick, P., Shepherd, M., 1965. A study of the interaction between desmethylimipramine and tetrabenazine in normal man. Psychopharmacologia 8, 32-40.
30. Domenjoz, R., Theobald, W., 1959. On the pharmacology of Tofranil N-(3-dimethylamino-propyl)-iminodibenzyl hydrochloride. Arch. Int. Pharmacodyn. Ther. 120, 450-489.
31. Dorfman, L., Furlenmeier, A., Huebner, C.F., Lucas, R., Macphillamy, H.B., Mueller, J.M., Schlittler, E., Schwyzer, R., St. André, A.F., 1954. Die konstitution des reserpins. 8. Mitteilung über Rauwolfia-alkaloide. Helv. Chim. Acta 37, 59-75.
32. Eltherington, L.G. , Horita, A., 1960. Some pharmacological actions of ß-phenylisopropyl-hydrazine (PIH). J. Pharmacol. Exp. Ther., 128, 7-14.
33. Feldberg, T.M., Frank, J.D., Meath, J.A., Rosenthal, D., 1956. Comparison of reserpine and placebo in treatment of psychiatric outpatients. AMA Arch. Neurol. Psychiatry 76, 207-214.
34. Ferguson, R.S., 1956. A clinical trial of reserpine in the treatment of anxiety. J. Mental Sci. 102, 30-42.
35. Folkson, A., May, A.R., 1955. Use of reserpine and Rauwolfia in psychoneuroses. Br. Med. J. 5, 1121-1122.
36. Garattini, S., 1959. Farmaci psicotropi che agiscono attraverso supposti mediatori centrali. Schweiz. Arch. Neurol. Neurochir. Psychiat. 84, 269-291.
37. Garattini, S., Jori, A., 1967. Interactions between imipramine-like drugs and reserpine on body temperature. In: Garattini, S., Dukes, M.N.G. (Eds.), Antidepressant drugs. Excerpta Medica, Amsterdam, pp. 179-193.
38. Garattini, S., Mortari, A., Valsecchi, A., Valzelli, L., 1959. Reserpine derivatives with specific hypotensive or sedative activity. Nature 183, 1273-1274.
39. Garattini, S., Fresia, P., Mortari, A., Palma, V., 1960. The pressor effect of reserpine after monoamine-oxidase inhibitors. Med. Exp. Int. J. Exp. Med. 2, 252-259.
40. Garattini, S., Giachetti, A., Jori, A., Pieri, L., Valzelli, L., 1962. Effect of imipramine, amitriptyline and their monomethyl derivatives on reserpine activity. J. Pharm. Pharmacol. 14, 509-514.
41. Giachetti, A., Hollenbeck, R.A., Shore, P.A., 1974. Localization and binding of reserpine in the membrane of adrenomedullary amine storage granules. Naunyn Schmiedebergs Arch. Pharmacol. 283, 263-275.
42. Glowinski, J., Axelrod, J., 1964. Inhibition of uptake of tritiated-noradrenaline in the intact rat brain by imipramine and structurally related compounds. Nature 204, 1318-1319.
43. Green, A.F., 1962. Antihypertensive drugs. Adv. Pharmacol. 1, 161-225.
44. Hagen, P., 1959. The storage and release of catecholamines. Pharmacol. Rev. 11, 361-373.
45. Holzbauer, M., Vogt, M., 1956. Depression by reserpine of the noradrenaline concentration in the hypothalamus of the cat. J Neurochem, 1, 8-11.
46. Jori, A., Garattini, S., 1965. Interaction between imipramine-like agents and catecholamine-induced hyperthemia. J. Pharm. Pharmacol. 17, 480-488.
47. Jori, A., Paglialunga, S., Garattini, S., 1967. Effect of antidepressant and adrenergic blocking drugs on hyperthermia induced by reserpine. Arch. Int. Pharmacodyn. 165, 384-393.
48. Karim, M.A., Linnel, W.H., Sharp, L.K., 1960. Potential reserpine analogues. Part II. 3,4,5-Trimethoxybenzoic acid derivatives. J. Pharm. Pharmacol. 12, 82-86.
49. Kuhn, R., 1957. Treatment of depressive states with an iminodibenzyl derivative (G 22355). Schweiz. Med. Wochenschr. 87, 1135-1140.
50. Manara, L., Garattini, S., 1967a. Failure of desipramine-pretreatment to modify the initial concentration of reserpine in rat tissues. Eur. J. Pharmacol. 2, 142-143.
51. Manara, L., Garattini, S., 1967b. Time course of ^{3}H-reserpine levels in brains of normal and tetrabenazine-pretreated rats. Eur. J. Pharmacol. 2, 139-141.
52. Manara, L., Carminati, P., Mennini, T., 1972. In vivo persistent binding of ^{3}H-reserpine to rat brain subcellular components. Eur. J. Pharmacol. 20, 109-113.
53. Manara, L., Mennini, T., Cerletti, C., 1974. ^{3}H-reserpine persistently bound "in vivo" to rat brain subcellular components: limited removal by peanut oil extraction. Life Sci. 14, 2267-2276.

54. Maxwell, D.R., Palmer, H.T., 1961. Demonstration of anti-depressant or stimulant properties of imipramine in experimental animals. Nature, 191, 84-85.

55. Mennini, T., Bernasconi, S., Manara, L., Samanin, R., Serra, G., 1977. The effect of intracerebral 6-hydroxydopamine on 3H-reserpine binding to diffe rent brain regions of the rat. Pharmacol. Res. Commun. 9, 857-862.

56. Mennini, T., Pataccini, R., Crunelli, V., Caccia, S., Ballabio, M., Samanin, R., Garattini, S., 1980. Localization of fenfluramine and reserpine in brain regions of rats with extensive degeneration of 5-hydroxytryptaminergic neurons. J. Pharm. Pharmacol. 32, 505-507.

57. Merry, J., 1956. An experiment in a chronic psychotic ward. Br. J. Med. Psychol. 29, 287-293.

58. Müller, J.M., Schlittler, E., Bein, H.J., 1952. Reserpine, the sedative principle from Rauwolfia serpentina B. Experientia 8, 338.

59. Pantarotto, C., Belvedere, G., Frigerio, A., Manara, L., Mennini, T., 1977. Gas chromatographic-mass fragmentographic identification and quantitative determination of reserpine in rat brain. In: Frigerio, A. (Ed.), Advances in Mass Spectrometry in Biochemistry and Medicine, Vol. 2. Spectrum Publ., New York, pp. 351-364.

60. Pantarotto, C., Belvedere, G., Frigerio, A., Mennini, T., Manara, L., 1976. Persistence of reserpine in rat brain: Gas chromatographic-mass fragmentographic identification and quantitative determination. Eur. J. Drug Metab. Pharmacokinet. 1, 25-34.

61. Penman, A.S., Dredge, T.E., 1956. Effect of reserpine and open-ward privileges on chronic schizophrenics. AMA Arch. Neurol. Psychiatry 76, 42-79.

62. Pletscher, A., 1956. Effects of isonicotinic acid hydrazide on 5-hydroxytryptamine metabolism in brain. Experientia 12, 479-480.

63. Pletscher, A., 1957. Release of 5-hydroxytryptamine by benzoquinolizine derivatives with sedative action. Science 126, 507.

64. Pletscher, A., Gey, K.F., 1962. Action of imipramine and amitriptyline on cerebral monoamines as compared with chlorpromazine. Med. Exp. Int. J. Exp. Med. 6, 165-168.

65. Pletscher, A., Shore, P.A., Brodie, B.B., 1955. Serotonin release as a possible mechanism of reserpine action. Science 122, 374-375.

66. Plummer, A.J., Sheppard, H., Schulert, A.R., 1957. The metabolism of reserpine. In: Garattini, S., Ghetti, V. (Eds.), Psychotropic Drugs. Elsevier, Amsterdam, pp. 350-362.

67. Pöldinger, W., 1963. Combined administration of desipramine and reserpine or tetrabenazine in depressive patients. Psychopharmacologia (Berl) 4, 308- 310.

68. Purves, D., Augustine, G.J., Fitzpatrick, D., Katz, L.C., Lamantia, A.S., McNamara, J.O., Williams, S.M., 2001. Box C. Biogenic amine neurotransmitters and psychiatric disorders. In: Neuroscience, 2nd edition. Sinauer Associates, Sunderland (MA).

69. Quinn, G.P., Shore, P.A., Brodie, B.B., 1959. Biochemical and pharmacological studies of Ro 1-9569 (tetrabenazine), a nonindole tranquilizing agent with reserpine-like effects. J. Pharmacol. Exp. Ther. 127, 103-109.

70. Sabshin, M., Ramot, J., 1956. Pharmacotherapeutic evaluation and the psychiatric setting. AMA Arch. Neurol. Psychiatry 75, 362-370.

71. Schlittler E., Plummer A.J., 1964. Tranquilizing drugs from Rauwolfia. XI. Clinical uses. In: Gordon, M. (Ed.), Psychopharmacological Agents. Academic Press, New York, pp. 9-34.

72. Schumann, H.J., 1960. Formation of adrenergic transmitters. In: Vane, J.R., Wolstenholme, G.E.W., O'Connor, M.. (Eds), Adrenergic Mechanisms. Churchill, London, pp. 6-16.

73. Shepherd, M., 1957. Reserpine and clinical trials. In: Garattini, S. , Ghetti, V. (Eds), Psychotropic Drugs. Elsevier, Amsterdam, pp. 565-568.

74. Sheppard, H., Lucas, R.C., Tsien, W.H., 1955. The metabolism of reserpine-C[14]. Arch. Int. Pharmacodyn. Ther. 103, 256-269.

75. Shore, P.A., 1966. The mechanism of norepinephrine depletion by reserpine, metaraminol and related agents. The role of monoamine oxidase. Pharmacol. Rev. 18, 561-568.

76. Shore, P.A., Brodie, B.B., 1957. Influence of various drugs on serotonin and norepinephrine in the brain. In: Garattini, S., Ghetti, B.(Eds.), Psychotropic Drugs. Elsevier, Amsterdam, pp. 423-427.

77. Shore, P.A., Silver, S.L., Brodie, B.B., 1955. Interaction of reserpine, serotonin, and lysergic acid diethylamide in brain. Science 122, 284-285.

78. Shore, P.A., Pletscher, A., Tomich, E.G., Carlsson, A., Kuntzman, R. , Brodie, B.B., 1957a. Role of brain serotonin in reserpine action. Ann. N. Y. Acad. Sci. 66, 609-615.
79. Shore, P.A., Mead, J.A., Kuntzman, R.G., Spector, S., Brodie, B.B., 1957b. On the physiologic significance of monoamine oxidase in brain. Science 126, 1063-1064.
80. Spector, S., Shore, P.A., Brodie, B.B., 1960. Biochemical and pharmacological effects of the monoamine oxidase inhibitors, iproniazid, 1-phenyl-2-hydrazinopropane (JB 516) and 1-phenyl-3-hydrazinobutane (JB 835). J. Pharmacol. Exp. Ther. 128, 15-21.
81. Stitzel, R.E., 1977. The biological fate of reserpine. Pharmacol. Rev. 28, 179-208.
82. Sulser, F., Watts, J. , Brodie, B.B., 1960. Antagonistic action of imipramine (Tofranil) and reserpine on central nervous system. Fed. Proc. 19, 268.
83. Sulser, F., Watts, J. , Brodie, B.B., 1962. On the mechanism of antidepressant action of imipramine like drugs. Ann. N. Y. Acad. Sci. 96, 279-288.
84. Sulser, F., Bickel, M., Brodie, B.B., 1964. The action of desmethylimipramine in counteracting sedation and cholinergic effects of reserpine-like drugs. J. Pharmacol. Exp. Ther. 144, 321- 330.
85. Usinger, W., 1962. The effect of reserpine on temperature regulation. Arzneimittelforschung 12, 435-438.
86. Vakil, R.J., 1949. Clinical trial of Rauwolfia serpentina in essential hypertension. Br. Heart J. 11, 350-355.
87. Wagner, L.A., Stitzel, R.E., 1972. The relation between the subcellular distribution of [^{3}H]reserpine and its proposed site of action. J. Pharm. Pharmacol. 24, 396-402.
88. Watts, J.S., D'Aguanno, W., Reilly, J., 1964. Comparative action of benzquinamide and P-2565 on the desmethylimipramine reversal and bradycardia. Fed. Proc. 23, 457.
89. Woodward, R.B., 1958. The total synthesis of reserpine. Tetrahedron 2, 1-57.

PART FOUR

EFFECT OF DRUGS ON NEUROTRANSMITTERS

CHAPTER 9

TRICYCLIC ANTIDEPRESSANTS, NEUROTRANSMITTERS AND NEUROPSYCHOPHARMACOLOGY

John M. Davis

INTRODUCTION

Fifty years ago, psychiatry underwent a marked paradigm shift. This was as dramatic a change as has been seen in any field of medicine, e.g., the change in surgery that came as the result of general anesthesia and sterile technique, in medicine of immunization, and in public health of water purification. Prior to this change, psychiatry was restricted to descriptive and psychoanalytic paradigms. The only effective treatment for depression was electroconvulsive therapy (ECT) for severe cases used generally as a last resort in the private practice of psychiatry and in academic medical centers. There was virtually no effort to prevent recurrences of depression and the lifetime death rate from depression was 15%.

THE BEGINNINGS

The major elements of change occurred as a consequence of the clinical discovery of three classes of drugs: antipsychotics, antidepressants, and lithium. My focus will be on the interplay between clinical research with tricyclic antidepressants (TCAs) and the practice of psychiatry.

Two of the major breakthroughs (the breakthrough with antipsychotics and the breakthrough with antidepressants) started in the pharmaceutical industry with the development of new drugs. Had the pharmaceutical industry not developed these drugs there would be no chance of finding important new indications for them.

MAJOR BREAKTHROUGHS

I think it is of fundamental importance to discover new indications for drugs. Chlorpromazine started with the search for a better adjunct to anesthesia, and it was tried in a number of different diseases just to observe what it would do. Its antipsychotic properties were discovered by chance while using the drug developed for one purpose for a new indication to see what it would do. The first TCA imipramine was developed in the effort to find and develop a chlorpromazine-like drug. Kuhn (1958) serendipitously observed that the drug has antidepressant effect in schizophrenic patients with depressive symptoms. The discovery of monoamine oxidase inhibitors (MAOIs) by George Crane (Crane, 1957), and Nathan Kline (Kline, 1958), followed observations that iproniazid had euphoric or antidepressant effect when it was used as an antituberculosis drug. The discovery of lithium by Cade (1949) in Australia was entirely serendipitous. I feel these discoveries were in a certain sense just as fundamental as many discoveries in the basic sciences. They altered the intellectual landscape of basic science, of psychiatric theory, and of clinical practice.

The term "translational research" implies that science advances by discoveries in the basic sciences, and suggests that some effort should be made for the translation of these basic science discoveries for clinicians. I believe that there are important clinical discoveries as well and the reverse, i.e., the translation of clinical discoveries to basic scientists should also be the case. The clinical discoveries in psychiatry, and the basic and clinical discoveries that occurred consequently resulted in many new fields of research. Basic science would suffer without these clinical insights. By assuming that the norepinephrine (NE) and serotonin (5-HT) theory of depression, that was based on clinical research findings, was true, basic scientists developed new drugs and made many fundamental discoveries about neurotransmitters. It would be important to find out whether psychiatric diseases are caused by abnormalities of neurotransmitters and whether the therapeutic effect of drugs in these disorders is the result of their effect on neurotransmitters. It is possible that the mechanism involved in the mode of action of a drug that was initially thought to produce the beneficial effect may actually be incorrect. There may be other mechanisms involved as well in the mode of action the drug.

It is important to understand the underlying mechanism of side effects for developing drugs without side effects. A related question is how to avoid side effects including those resulting from drug-drug interactions to be able to use drugs safely in man.

THE METHODOLOGY OF CLINICAL RESEARCH

Prior to chlorpromazine, imipramine, and lithium, there was little controlled research in psychiatry. The need for well-controlled studies to prove efficacy necessitated the development of rating scales, and the adoption of random assignment and double blind methodology in psychiatry. This led to the development of controlled research in the different areas of psychiatry: nosology, genetics, natural course of disease, and epidemiology. It also led to studies in cognitive functions, basic emotions, etc. The clinical investigators in the Early Clinical Drug Evaluation Units in the USA (Cole, Crane, Lehmann, Ban, Simpson, Sugerman, Overall, Hollister, Klerman, Rickels, Feighner, Beasley) and their equivalents in other countries (Montgomery, Asberg,

Hamilton, Coppen, Shaw, Baastroup, Schou and many others) facilitated the birth of modern quantitative psychiatry. Controlled research did not take away anything from psychology/psychoanalysis but added to it.

THE ANTIDEPRESSANTS

After the discovery of the antidepressant effect of TCAs and MAOIs, the pharmaceutical industry developed drugs that act through mechanisms which are similar to the mode of action of these drugs and several .of new TCAs and MAOIs were found to be efficacious in depression. The potentiation of the effects of NE and 5-HT by blocking their metabolism or reuptake were assumed to be involved in the mode of action of these drugs. The TCAs became the dominant mode of treatment in biological depression because they were safer and easier to use than the MAOIs.

Before the introduction of antidepressants, severe depressive episodes lasted several years with marked suffering of patients, family, and many other people. Drug treatment results in recovery in most but not in all patients in three weeks or so. In the early years of pharmacotherapy with antidepressants one-third of the patients improved with placebo, two-third with antidepressants, and switching from one to another antidepressant helped about 50% of the non-responsive patients. This is a profound difference compared to two years of near unbearable suffering.

CLINICAL RESEARCH ON TRICYCLIC ANTIDEPRESSANTS: IMPLICATIONS FOR THE PSYCHIATRIC CONCEPT OF DEPRESSION

The effectiveness of imipramine in depression and the failure of the drug to help some depressed patients led to new knowledge about depression. It provided clues for the identification of subtypes of depression with leads to their cause, treatments and natural course. The precipitation of bipolar episodes by TCAs helped to delineate the difference between bipolar and unipolar depression subtypes and led to the concept of bipolar II disease.

While studying clinical responses in patients in his research on plasma levels of antidepressants Glassman (Glassman et al., 1977) discovered that psychotically depressed patients very frequently have a poor response to TCAs (Glassman et al., 1975). Prior to this, psychotic depression was thought of just as a severe depression. This led to the discovery that combined administration of an antidepressant with an antipsychotic is needed in psychotic depression (Spiker et al., 1985) because antidepressants help to control only depressive symptoms in depression. The separation of psychotic from other depression (Chan et al., 1987) led to the demonstration that cortisol dysregulation is particularly severe in psychotic depression (Nelson and Davis, 1997).

PROPHYLACTIC RESEARCH ON DEPRESSION. THE PREVENTION OF RE-OCCURRENCE

One of the most significant advances in modern clinical psychopharmacology has been the prophylactic use of drugs to prevent relapse (Davis, 1976). This occurred roughly the same time with antipsychotics, antidepressants, and lithium. When a patient had a good response to a drug in the early years, the drug was discontinued and many clinicians observed that patients relapsed, generally not immediately but after a period of some months. I collected this information from clinicians and analyzed it statistically using a method that was to be called meta-analysis. The term "meta-analysis" had not been coined at the time. I did the first meta-analysis in psychiatry using the same methodology as is now used by the Cochrane group and in most meta-analysis in general medicine. I showed that the rate of relapse of depressed patients whose tricyclic antidepressant was discontinued was approximately 10% per month. I found the same relapse rate with the discontinuation of neuroleptics in schizophrenia, and of lithium, in mania. These findings indicated a need for prophylactic treatment in depression, schizophrenia and mania presumably for lifetime. Kupfer et al. (1992) found that in patients treated with TCA's without relapse for five years the substitution of the TCA with placebo resulted in relapse. Before the discovery of TCAs, neuroleptics and lithium there was no real preventative psychiatry. Now the recurrence of episodes can be prevented.

SIDE EFFECTS

After the introduction of TCAs it was soon apparent that they produced anticholinergic side effects such as dry mouth. When high doses are used these anticholinergic effects can produce "atropine psychosis" with loss of immediate memory, florid hallucinations and disorientation. Such psychosis is most commonly encountered in patients receiving several different pharmacological agents with atropine-like properties (El-Yousef et al., 1972). We proved that these are "atropine psychoses" by reversing the syndrome with the administration of physostigmine, a substance that increases acetylcholine and therefore overcomes the atropine blockade (El-Yousef et al., 1972).

TCAs also produce postural hypotension and cardiac toxicity. While reviewing findings with TCAs in his plasma level studies Glassman (Glassman and Roose, 1987) noted that there was substantial morbidity and mortality from postural hypotension in his sample. In several hundred patients there would be several deaths or disability from broken hips. Patients would fall because of postural hypotension, hit their heads and then die later of subdural hematoma. Regarding cardiac toxicity Glassman and his collaborators established that it was due to the quinidine like properties of TCAs (Giardina et al., 1979, 1982, 1985; Roose et al., 1986, 1987).

There are also drug-drug interactions that are mediated by NE uptake inhibition. By inhibiting the NE uptake pump that pumps guanethidine inside the neuron to be able to exert its blood pressure lowering effect, TCAs interfere with the therapeutic effect of the drug (Fann et al., 1971, 1972). In hypertensive patients successfully treated with guanethidine the addition of a TCA renders guanethidine ineffective. Guanethidine no longer works because it no longer reaches the necessary concentration at its site of action. Research in drug-drug interaction is based on findings in drug metabolism carried out by basic scientists, but it is clinical research that translates the findings of basic research for clinical practice (Glassman et al., 1983).

TOXIC OVERDOSE

Overdose toxicity of TCA's either in a suicide attempt or sometimes by a child taking his parents medication is important because even a small number of tablets could cause a fatal overdose (Davis et al., 1968). It was overdose toxicity that led to the research of the Glassman group which established the quinidine like effect of TCA's in order to be able to treat the patients in the emergency room to prevent death (Preskorn and Irwin, 1982).

BIOGENIC AMINE THEORY OF DEPRESSION

When I started my career in psychiatry, the field was heavily psychoanalytic. Psychiatric residents received virtually no training in clinical psychopharmacology, or basic science for that matter. Residents used drugs sub-rosa and rarely mentioned them in case conference. If mentioned, the faculty criticized the resident's counter-transference and questioned the ability of the resident as a therapist for having to resort to a subhuman treatment. Even today, some psychoanalysts, psychotherapists, behavior therapists, and even administrators at the National Institute of Mental Health (NIMH), doubt the importance of biological treatment in psychiatry.

When I went to the NIMH to do my military service and was assigned to a clinical research ward run by William (Biff) Bunney. I was asked to help in developing a biological theory of depression based on what was known about the biology of treatment of depression, i.e., about the effect of TCAs, MAOI's and ECT on monoamine neurotransmitters, such as NE and 5-HT. My task was to look for a common denominator in the action of treatments that help depression. We knew that Joseph Schildkraut, a brilliant young psychiatrist, who had just finished his training and was a clinical associate at NIMH in another ward, was working on the same problem He had done previous work in this area of research, establishing his priority but even so, we wanted to get our review paper out in a timely fashion. We quickly submitted our paper to Science, but it was rejected, and Schildkraut published his review (Schildkraut, 1965) about a month before our article appeared (Bunney and Davis, 1965). Since the common feature of effective treatments of d e p ression was an increase of NE and/or 5-HT, we both suggested that low levels or function of NE and/or 5-HT is the biological basis of depression. ECT increased the synthesis of both of these amines. TCA's potentiated these amines by blocking their re-uptake, and MAOIs inhibitors increased their levels by blocking their destruction. Conversely, reserpine depleted the brain from these monoamines in a dose related manner and caused depression particularly in patients who had a history of depression when treated with reserpine for hypertension (Ayd, 1958). α-Methyldopa, a false transmitter also lowered brain NE and caused depression. This theory was a radical shift in thinking about psychiatry. It suggested that mental disease could have a biological cause and a strategy of interference with the biological disturbance that is the cause of the disease. The theory does not contradict the role of psychological factors in depression because psychological events could precipitate or aggravate a biochemical disturbance. At the time we never doubted that NE was the culprit of depression, but we did note that almost all the evidence implicated 5-HT as well. The only evidence in favor of NE was that the NE effects occurred at a dose more close to the pharmacological dose. In re t rospect had we not overvalued our basic idea and focused on both momoamines we would have written a better paper. In talking about the norepinephrne-serotonin theory of depre s-sion I often hasten to add that even if drugs may act through a certain mechanism that does not mean that diseases are caused by the opposite of what the drugs do. For example, pneumococcal pneumonia is not caused by penicillin deficiency.

MECHANISM OF TRICYCLIC ANTIDEPRESSANT ACTION

Drugs have different pharmacological effects at diff e rent doses. Evidence that a drug produces a particular action at the dose desired in treatment is an indication that that particular action may be a good candidate for the study of the mode of action of the drug. Higher doses may produce effects that are not relevant to the mode of action of the drug.

Early on basic scientists showed that the 5-HT uptake pump exists also in platelets (Murphy et al., 1970). The effects of TCA's on NE uptake can also be inferred from studies of the peripheral autonomic nervous system by measuring the effects of direct noradrenergic agonists such as NE infusion or indirect agonists such as tyramine infusion which acts by releasing NE in patients on TCAs (Fann et al., 1972).

THE SEROTONIN HYPOTHESIS

Coppen (Coppen et al., 1992) and van Praag (1981) in Europe proposed a 5-HT hypothesis of depression. While it is difficult to make inferences about NE in brain, cere b rospinal fluid (CSF) 5-hydroxyindoleacetic acid (5-HIAA) concentrations reflect brain 5-HT synthesis. The observation that 5-HIAA was decreased in the CSF in depre s-sion was a critical link from animal pharmacology to human disease, and a major advance. Marie Asberg (Asberg et al., 1987) showed that 5-HIAA was decreased in depressed patients and particularly in suicidal depressed patients. She suggested that the subgroup with low (depressed) CSF-5-HIAA was a distinct entity and that 5-HIAA was bi-modally distributed in depressed patients with a peak corresponding to the suicidal depressed sub-entity. Gibbons and I (Gibbons and Davis, 1986) examined the distribution of 5-HIAA in normal subjects and depressed patients. We found that it was no mally distributed in healthy controls, whereas in depressed patients there was a mixture of two distinct normal distributions: One of the distributions was the same as in normal controls and the other was the same as in the suicidal depressed subgroup.

It is also known that homovanillic acid (HVA) concentration in the CSF reflects brain dopamine concentration. We found that CSF-HVA was normally distributed in healthy controls but that there was a subgroup of depressed patients who had low CSF-HVA. We extended the mixture distribution analysis in two dimensions and found that the same depressed patients who had low levels of 5-HIAA had also low levels of HVA. Postmortem studies in the brains of depressed patients who killed themselves also showed low 5HIAA concentrations (Bourne et al., 1968).

In favor also of the 5-HT hypothesis of depression are findings that drugs with an effect on 5-HT like lithium (Heninger et al., 1983) and pindolol (Blier and Bergeron, 1998) can either speed the action of antidepressants or augment their efficacy (Nelson and Mazure 1986). Also in favor are that percursor loading with tryptophan helps depression, tryptophane depletion can cause depression (Delgado et al., 1990), and the administration of parachlorophenylalanine (PCPA), a drug that blocks the synthesis of 5-HT can induce depression (Shopsin et al., 1976).

SELECTIVE SEROTONIN UPTAKE INHIBITORS

Eli Lilly, a pharmaceutical company, developed selective serotonin uptake inhibitors (SSRIs). This was a major breakthrough in safety (Stark et al., 1985) because TCA's caused death by overdose, plus many other side effects. The SSRI's have relatively few side effects The withdrawal syndrome that may occur with SSRI's with a short half life can be treated with SSRI's which have a longer half life (Giakas and Davis, 1997 a, b). Introduction of SSRIs facilitated the exploration of therapeutic indications for antidepressants because their use involved less risk. With the use of SSRI's many diseases were delineated in which 5-HT may play a role.

DUAL ACTION ANTIDEPRESSANTS

The Danish University Antidepressant Group (1986, 1990) noted that clomipramine (CMI) a substance with dual action, i.e., NE and 5-HT uptake inhibition, was more effective than selective uptake inhibitors. If both 5-HT and NE uptake inhibition is important in the treatment of depression or in a subtype of depression, than antidepressants with a dual action would be more effective than single transmitter inhibitors. There is evidence that combining selective NE and 5-HT uptake inhibitors is beneficial in the treatment of depression (Nelson et al., 2004). Ten years ago when venlafaxine, a drug that has dual action, was developed, I did a meta-analysis and found that venlafaxine offered advantages to selective monoamine oxidase inhibitors (Davis, 1995). New controlled trials verified my findings.

THE BIOLOGY OF SUICIDE

The correlation between low 5-HT levels and suicide stimulated interest in the biology of suicide. It was found that low CSF-5HIAA concentrations are more related to impulsivity than to depression. Linnolla et al. (1983) found that impulsive murderers and fire-setters have low 5-HIAA concentrations in their CSF. This led to investigations about the role of 5-HT in alcoholism.

There is excellent evidence from many controlled trials that lithium reduces suicide. The issue is more complicated with antidepressants. The incidence of suicide is about the same in double-blind controlled trials of antidepressants versus placebo. Possible antidepressants prevent some suicides but also some antidepressants may increase suicide. Healy (2003) suggests that SSRIs might activate the energy that may fuel a suicide, or produce akathisia. It is possible that these effects cancel out their beneficial effect. This is a difficult problem to solve. In any case, suicide occurs in a wide variety of psychiatric conditions (Weissman et al., 1989).

TRICYCLIC ANTIDEPRESSANTS IN THE DISCOVERY OF OTHER PSYCHIATRIC DISEASES

TCA's led to the discovery of several new diseases: panic disorder, social phobia, body dysmorphic disease etc. as well as provided clues to the cause and treatments of others. In the early 1960s in a clinical study imipramine, chlorpromazine or placebo was administered to hospitalized patients unresponsive to psychotherapy and it was found that some of the patients improved dramatically on imipramine. Examination of the symptoms that improved resulted in the discovery of panic disorder by Klein (Klein, 1964; Klein and Davis, 1969; Klein and Fink, 1962). This opened a completely new field in psychiatry. Antidepressants led to the discovery of social phobia. Antidepressants are helpful also in posttraumatic stress disorder (Davidson et al., 1990).

One of the most important clinical discoveries involving TCAs was their effectiveness in obsessive-compulsive disorder (OCD). The dramatic improvement with clomipramine (CMI) in patients with OCD was discovered in Spain (Lopez-Ibor 1969).

Since CMI inhibits the reuptake of both NE and 5-HT, the link between CMI and OCD was provided by the finding that the therapeutic effects of the drug were related to the plasma levels of unchanged CMI that is a more potent 5-HT uptake inhibitor than NE uptake inhibitor (Thoren et al., 1980). The effectiveness of CMI in OCD was verified in clinical investigations beyond reasonable doubt (Ananth et al., 1981; Insel et al., 1983; Karabanow 1977; Mavissakalian and Michelson, 1983; Montgomery, 1980; Pigott et al., 1990; Volavka et al., 1985; Zohar et al., 1987). CMI reduced obsessive-compulsive symptoms quite substantially in 50% of the patients, whereas placebo reduced the symptoms only by 5% in studies used in the registration of CMI in the USA. The findings that SSRI's are effective in OCD, whereas the prevailingly NE uptake inhibitor antidepressants are ineffective are supportive of the link between 5-HT and OCD (Pato et al., 1990). Responsiveness to SSRI's in OCD led to research which resulted the elucidation of body dysmorphic disease (Phillips et al., 1990) and the recognition of the link between trichotillomania and 5-HT (Swedo et al., 1989). There is also a link between 5HT and Tourette's disease (Pauls and Leckmann, 1986).

SUMMARY

I believe that the discovery of the effects of drugs developed by the pharmaceutical industry involves an interplay of basic and clinical science. Clinical research provides the necessary information on how to use a drug and in whom to use it. Clinical research has also a major role in finding the therapeutic dose and detecting side effects.

There is some evidence in favor of the norepinephrine-serotonin hypothesis of depression. It is fair to say that it has remained a viable hypothesis.

The availability of brain imaging techniques to measure in human the receptor occupancy of drugs when given in therapeutic doses makes it possible to correlate the therapeutic effect of drugs with their basic pharmacology more precisely than it was possible before. Employment of the new technology helps to establish causal connections between the pharmacological properties of a drug and its therapeutic effects.

Basic scientists made fundamental discoveries regarding the mode of action of drugs developed by the pharmaceutical industry but many of the paradigm breaking research came from clinicians all over the world, illustrating a common humanity of trying to help patients with the same disease in Australia, France, Switzerland, Spain, Belgium, Holland, USA, Sweden, Denmark, Germany, UK and so forth.

REFERENCES
1. Ananth, J., Pecknold, J.C., Van Den Steen, N., Engelsman, F., 1981. Double-blind comparative study of clomipramine and amitriptyline in obsessive neurosis. Prog. Neuropsychopharmacol. Biol. Psychiatry 5, 257–262.

2. Asberg, M., Schalling, D., Traskman-Bendy, L., Wagner A., 1987. A psychobiology of sui-
    cide, impulsivity and related phenomena. In: Meltzer, H.Y. (Ed.), Psychopharmacology:
    The Third Generation of Progress. Raven Press, New York, pp. 655-668.
3. Ayd, F.J. Jr., 1958. Drug-induced depression - fact or fallacy. N. Y. Med. J. 58, 354–356.
4. Blier, P., Bergeron, R., 1998. The use of pindolol to potentiate antidepressant medication.
    J. Clin. Psychiatry 59, 16–23, 24–25.
5. Bourne, H.R., Bunney, W.E., Jr., Colburn, R.W., Davis, J.M., Davis, J.N., Shaw, D.M.,
    Coppen, A.J., 1968. Noradrenaline, 5-hydroxytryptamine, and 5-hydroxyindolacetic acid in
    hindbrains of suicidal patients. Lancet 2 (572), 805-808.
6. Bunney, W. E., Jr., Davis, J.M., 1965. Norepinephrine in depressive reactions. Archives of
    General Psychiatry 13, 483-494.
7. Cade, J.F.J., 1949. Lithium salts in the treatment of psychotic excitement. Medical Journal
    of Australia 36, 349-352.
8. Chan, C.H, Janicak, P.G., Davis, J.M., Altman, E., Andriukaitis, S., Hedeker, D.,1987.
    Response of psychotic and non-psychotic depressed patients to tricyclic antidepressants.
    J. Clin. Psychiatry 48, 197–200.
9. Coppen, A., Prange, A.J., Hill, C., Whybrow, P.C., 1992. Abnormalities of indolamines in
    affective disorders. Arch. Gen. Psychiatry 26, 474–478.
10. Crane, G.E., 1957. Iproniazid (Marsilid) phosphate, a therapeutic agent for mental disor-
    ders and debilitating disease. Psychiatry Res. Rep. 8, 142-152.
11. Danish University Antidepressant Group, 1990. Paroxetine: a selective serotonin reuptake
    inhibitor showing better tolerance, but weaker antidepressant effect than clomipramine in
    a controlled multicenter study. J. Affect. Disord. 18, 289–299.
12. Danish University Antidepressant Group, 1986. Citalopram: clinical effect profile in com-
    parison with clomipramine: a controlled multicenter study. Psychopharmacology 90,
    131–138.
13. Davidson, J.R.T, 1997 Biological therapies for posttraumatic stress disorder: an overview.
    J. Clin. Psychiatry 58 (Suppl. 9), 29-32.
14. Davis, J.M., 1976. Overview: Maintenance therapy in psychiatry. II. Affective disorders.
    American Journal of Psychiatry 133, 1-13.
15. Davis, J.M., 1995. A comparative evaluation of the SSRIs, venlafaxine and nefazodone.
    Directions in Psychiatry 15(14) July 5, 1995.
16. Davis, J.M., Bartlett, E., Termini, B.A., 1968. Overdosage of psychotropic drugs: a review.
    II: Antidepressants and other psychotropic agents. Dis. Nerv. Syst. 29, 246-256.
17. Delgado, P.L., Goodman, W.K., Price, L.H., Heninger, G.R., Charney, D.S., 1990.
    Fluvoxamine/pimozide treatment of concurrent Tourette's and obsessive-compulsive dis-
    order. Br. J. Psychiatry 157, 762–765.
18. El-Yousef, M.K., Janowsky, D.S., Davis, J.M., Sekerke, H.J., 1972. Reversal of benzotropine
    mesylate toxicity by physostigmine. JAMA 220, 125.
19. Fann, W.E., Janowsky, D.S., Davis, J.M., Oates, J.A., 1971. Chlorpromazine reversal of the
    antihypertensive action of guanethidine. Lancet 2(721), 436-437.
20. Fann, W.E., Davis, J.M., Janowsky, D.S., Cavanaugh, J.H., Kaufmann, J.S., Griffith, J.D.,
    Oates, J.A., 1972. Effects of lithium on adrenergic function in man. Clin. Pharm. and
    Therap. 13, 71-77.
21. Giakas, W.J., Davis, J.M., 1997a. Intractable withdrawal from venlafaxine treated with flu-
    oxetine. Psychiatric Annals 27, 85- 85.
22. Giakas, W.J., Davis, J.M., 1997b. SSRI withdrawal symptoms. Psychiatric Annal 27, 335-
    335.
23. Giardina, E.G.V., Bigger, J.T. Jr., Glassman, A.H., Perel, J.M., Kantor, S.J., 1979. The elec-
    trocardiographic and antiarrhythmic effects of imipramine hydrochloride at therapeutic
    plasma concentrations. Circulation 60, 1045– 1052.
24. Giardina, E.G.V., Johnson, L.L., Vita, J., Bigger, J.T. Jr., Brem, R.F., 1985. Effect of
    imipramine and nortriptyline on left ventricular function and blood pressure in patients
    treated for arrhythmias. Am. Heart J. 109, 992–998.
25. Gibbons, R.D., Davis, J.M., 1986. Consistent evidence for a biological sub-type of depres-
    sion characterized by low CSF monoamine levels. Acta Psychiatr. Scand. 74, 8-12.

26. Glassman, A.H., Roose, S.P., 1987. Cardiovascular effects of tricyclic antidepressants. Psychiatric Annals 17, 340-347.

27. Glassman, A.H., Kantor, S.H., Shostak, M., 1975. Depression, delusions, and drug response. American Journal of Psychiary 132, 716-719.

28. Glassman, A.H., Perel, J.M., Shostak, M., Kantor, S.J., Fleiss, J.L., 1977. Clinical implications of imipramine plasma levels for depressive illness. Archives of General Psychiatry 34, 197-204.

29. Glassman, A.H., Johnson, L.L., Giardina, E.G.V.,Walsh, B.T., Roose, S.P., Cooper, T.B., 1983. The use of imipramine in depressed patients with congestive heart failure. JAMA 250, 1997–2001.

30. Healy, D., 2003. Let Them Eat Prozac. James Lorimer & Company, Toronto, 1-462.

31. Heninger, G.R, Charney, D.S,, Sternberg, D.E., 1983. Lithium carbonate augmentation of antidepressant treatment. Arch. Gen. Psychiatry 40, 1335–1342.

32. Insel, T.R., Murphy, D.L., Cohen, R.M., Alterman, I., Kilts, C., Linnolla, M., 1983. Obsessive-compulsive disorder: a double-blind trial of clomipramine and clorgyline. Arch. Gen. Psychiatry 40, 605–612.

33. Janowsky, D.S., el-Yousef, M.K., Davis, J.M., Sekerke, H.J., 1972. A cholinergic-adrenergic hypothesis of mania and depression. Lancet 2 (7778), 632-635.

34. Karabanow, O., 1977. Double-blind controlled study in phobias and obsessions. J. Int. Med. Res. 5 (Suppl. 5), 42–48.

35. Klein, D.F., 1964. Delineation of two drug-responsive anxiety syndromes. Psychopharmacologia 5, 397–408.

36. Klein, D.F., Davis, J.M., 1969. Diagnosis and Drug Treatment of Psychiatric Disorders. Williams and Wilkins, Baltimore, pp. 1-480.

37. Klein, D.F., Fink, M., (1962) Psychiaric reaction patterns to imipramine. American Journal of Psychiatry 119, 432-438.

38. Kline, N.S., 1958. Clinical experience with iproniazid (Marsilid). J. Clin. Exp. Psychopath. 19 (Suppl. 1), 72-78.

39. Kuhn, R., 1958. The treatment of depressive states with G-22355 (imipramine hydrochloride). American Journal of Psychiatry 115, 459-464.

40. Kupfer, D.J., Frank, E., Perel, J.M., Cornes, C., Mallinger, A.G., Thase, M.E., McEachran, A.B., Grochocinski, V.J., 1992. Five year outcome for maintenance therapies in recurrent depression. Arch. Gen. Psychiatry 49, 769–773.

41. Linnolla, M.V., Virkkunen, M., Scheinin, M., Nuutula, A., Rimon, R., Goodwin, F.K., 1983. Low cerebrospinal fluid 5-hydroxyindoleacetic acid concentration differentiates impulsive from nonimpulsive violent behavior. Life Sci. 33, 2609-2614.

42. Lopez-Ibor, J.J. 1969: Intravenous Infusions of Monochlorimipramine. In: Proceedings of the 6th International Congress of the CINP, Taragona, April 2668. Excepta Medica Foundation Inc. Congress Series No. 180. Amsterdam 1969 529-521.

43. Mavissakalian, M., Michelson, L., 1983. Tricyclic antidepressants in obsessive-compulsive disorder. Anti-obsessional or anti-depressant agents. J. Nerv. Ment. Dis. 171, 301–306.

44. Montgomery, S.A., 1980. Clomipramine in obsessional neurosis: a placebo controlled trial. Pharm. Med. 1, 189–192.

45. Murphy, D., Colburn R., Davis, J.M., Bunney, W., 1970. Imipramine and lithium effects on biogenic amine transport in depressed and manic depressed patients. American Journal of Psychiatry 127, 339-345.

46. Nelson, J.C., Davis, J.M., 1997. DST studies in psychotic depression: a meta-analysis. Am. J. Psychiatry 154, 1497-1503.

47. Nelson, J.C., Mazure, C.M., 1986. Lithium augmentation in psychotic depression refractory to combined drug treatment. Am. J. Psychiatry 143, 363–366.

48. Nelson, J.C., Mazure, C.M., Jatlow, P.I., Bowers, M.B., Jr., Price, L.H.,. 2004. Combining norepinephrine and serotonin re-uptake inhibition mechanisms for treatment of depression: a double-blind, randomized study. Biol. Psychiatry 55, 296–300.

49. Pauls, D.L., Leckman, J.F., 1986. The inheritance of Gilles de la Tourette's syndrome and associated behaviors: evidence for autosomal dominant transmission. N. Engl. J. Med. 315, 993–997.

50. Pato, M.T., Pigott, T.A., Hill, J.L., Grover, G.N., Bernstein, S., Murphy, D.L., 1991. Controlled comparison of buspirone and clomipramine in obsessive-compulsive disorder. Am. J. Psychiatry 148, 127–129.

51. Phillips, K.A., McElroy, S.L.,Keck, P.E., Jr., Pope, H., 1993. Body dysmorphic disorder: 30 cases of imagined ugliness. Am. J. Psychiatry 150, 302-308.
52. Pigott, T.A., Pato, M.T., Bernstein, S.E., Grover, G.N., Hill, J.L., Tolliver, T.J., Murphy, D.L., 1990. Controlled comparisons of clomipramine and fluoxetine in the treatment of obsessive-compulsive disorder. Arch. Gen. Psychiatry 47, 926–932.
53. Preskorn, S.H., Irwin, H., 1982. Toxicity of tricyclic antidepressants: kinetics, mechanisms, intervention: a review. Clinical Psychiatry 143, 151-156.
54. Roose, S.P., Glassman, A.H., Giardina, E.G.V, Johnson, L.L., Walsh, B.T., Woodring, S., Bigger, J.T., Jr., 1986. Nortriptyline in depressed patients with left ventricular impairment. JAMA 256, 3253–3257.
55. Roose, S.P., Glassman, A.H., 1989. Cardiovascular effects of TCAs in depressed patients with and without heart disease. J. Clin. Psychiatry Monogr. Ser. 7, 1–18.
56. Roose, S.P., Glassman, A.H., Giardina, E.G., Walsh, B.T., Woodring, S., Bigger, J.T., 1987. Tricyclic antidepressants in depressed patients with cardiac conduction disease. Archives of General Psychiatry 44, 273-275.
57. Shopsin, B., Freedman, E., Gershon, S., 1976. PCPA reversal of tranylcypromine effects in depressed patients. Arch. Gen. Psychiatry 33, 811–819.
58. Schildkraut, J.J., 1965. The catecholamine hypothesis of affective disorders: a review of supporting evidence. American Journal of Psychiatry 122, 509-522.
59. Spiker, D.G., Weiss, J.C., Dealy, R.S. Griffin, S.J., Hanin, I., Neil, J.F., Perel, J.M. Rossi, A.J., Soloff, P.H., 1985. The pharmacological treatment of delusional depression. American Journal of Psychiatry 142, 430-436.
60. Stark, P., Fuller, R., Wong, D., 1985. The pharmacologic profile of fluoxetine. J. Clin. Psychiatry 46, 7–13.
61. Swedo, S.E., Leonard, H.L., Rapoport, J.L., Lenane, M.C., Goldberger, E.L., Cheslow, D.L., 1989. A double-blind comparison of clomipramine and desipramine in the treatment of trichotillomania (hair pulling). N. Engl. J. Med. 321, 497–501.
62. Thoren, P., Asberg, M., Cronholm, B., Jornestedt, L., Traskman, L., 1980. Clomipramine treatment of obsessive-compulsive disorder. A controlled clinical trial. Arch. Gen. Psychiatry 37, 1281–1285.
63. Van Praag, H.M., 1981. Management of depression with serotonin precursors. Biological Psychiatry 16, 291-310.
64. Volavka, J., Neziroglu, F., Yaryura-Tobias, J.A., 1985. Clomipramine and imipramine in obsessive-compulsive disorder. Psychiatry Res. 14, 83–91.
65. Weissman, M.M., Klerman, G.L., Markowitz, J.S.V. 1989. Suicidal ideation and suicide attempts in panic disorder and attacks. N. Engl. J. Med. 321:1209-1214.
66. Zohar, J., Mueller, E.A., Insel, T., Zohar-Kadouch, R.C., Murphy, D.L., 1987. Serotonergic responsivity in obsessive-compulsive disorder. Comparison of patients and healthy controls. Arch. Gen. Psychiatry 44, 946-951.

CHAPTER 10

NEUROLEPTICS, NEUROTRANSMITTERS AND NEUROPSYCHOPHARMACOLOGY

Elliott Richelson

In his Nobel Prize review paper (Carlsson, 2001), Arvid Carlsson, called it "A paradigm shift in brain research." He was referring back to the time in the late 1950s, when researchers started thinking about chemical messengers - neurotransmitters - as being the key elements in the communication between neurons in the brain, rather than electricity *per se*.

However, it was Carlsson who caused a paradigm shift in our thinking about the pharmacology of neuroleptics. This came from the paper by Carlsson and Lindqvist in 1963 (Carlsson and Lindqvist, 1963) in which it was proposed on the basis of experimental data with mice that drugs like chlorpromazine and haloperidol worked by blocking monoaminergic receptors. They treated animals with low doses of these antipsychotic drugs, measured brain levels of dopamine, norepinephrine, and their respective metabolites (3-methoxytyramine and normetanephrine), and found increases in the metabolites, with minimal or no effect on the parent compounds. They hypothesized as the most likely explanation that these chemically distinct neuroleptic drugs increased the release of dopamine and norepinephrine as a compensatory mechanism due to monoaminergic receptor blockade in brain. It took another decade before other researchers using in vitro radioligand binding techniques largely confirmed and extended these results.

In vitro radioligand binding studies themselves caused a paradigm shift in the way researchers gathered pharmacological data on neuroleptics, as well as other classes of psychiatric drugs. Many of the advances in our understanding of the pharmacological effects of psychotherapeutic drugs have resulted from the application of this important technological advance. A more recent extension of this technology has been the use of radioactively labeled psychotropic drugs to identify receptors and transporters for neurotransmitters and drugs in living human brain by positron emission tomography or PET scanning. One of the first of these studies looked at dopamine receptors in brains of schizophrenic patients (Wong et al., 1986). Furthermore, this technology has helped to find new psychiatric drugs, which are being sought by high-throughput screening assays utilizing radioligand binding. Finally, the molecular cloning of neurotransmitter receptors and transporters has been facilitated by the use of radioligand binding methods.

Although researchers had conceived the notion that a radioactively labeled drug could be used to identify the receptor to which it bound at an earlier date (Paton and Rang, 1965), it was not until the 1970s that radioligand binding technology really took off and changed our understanding of the pharmacology of antipsychotic and other psychiatric drugs.

Back in the mid-1960s Paton and Rang (1965) were among the first to perform in vitro radioligand binding studies, which presaged the work done in the following decade by such laboratories as those of Solomon Snyder at The Johns Hopkins University School of Medicine (Creese et al., 1976; Snyder et al., 1974) and of Philip Seeman at the University of Toronto (Seeman et al., 1976). Paton and Rang (1965) made use of relatively intact tissue - the smooth muscle of guinea pig small intestine. The radioligand was tritiated atropine that was shown to bind with all the specificity expected of this muscarinic receptor antagonist.

With the advent of the batch technique of rapid filtration under vacuum to separate bound from free radioligand in binding assays (Cuatrecasas, 1971a, b), as well as the availability of highly specific compounds of high specific activity, it has become possible for researchers to obtain rapidly a wealth of data on the receptor binding properties of neuroleptics.

What were the exciting findings that were learned? Among the earliest of the exciting findings were the results from studies on the antimuscarinic properties of neuroleptics and how these properties relate to their propensity to cause extrapyramidal side e ffects (Miller and Hiley, 1974; Snyder et al., 1974). There was a lot that was intere s ting about this research, aside from the fact that two laboratories (Miller and Hiley, 1974; Snyder et al., 1974) separated by the Atlantic Ocean published similar results and d rew similar conclusions almost simultaneously. Like Paton and Rang (1965) nearly one decade earlier, both groups (Miller and Hiley, 1974; Snyder et al., 1974) focused on the muscarinic receptor. However, in these more recent studies, the muscarinic receptors were in brain homogenates and the radioligands were highly potent and highly specific antimuscarinics that came from chemical warf a re research.

In case of the work from Snyder's laboratory, the radioligand was 3-quinuclidinyl benzilate (QNB). QNB came from the chemical warfare division of the United States military following World War II. QNB, which has been called a "superhallucinogen," may still be stockpiled somewhere around the world by various governments and regimes. (For some interesting reading on QNB, it is suggested that the reader view the following websites: http://en.wikipedia.org/wiki/3-quinuclidinyl_benzilate, and http:// www. levity. com/ aciddreams/samples/bz.html). Henry ("Hank") Yamamura, when he was in the military worked at Edgewood Arsenal in Maryland, the headquarters of the US Army Chemical Corps. Afterwards he was a special research fellow with Solomon Snyder at Johns Hopkins in Baltimore, Maryland. Snyder knew about the work of Paton and Rang (1965) and thought that a higher affinity cholinergic antagonist would result in greater specific binding. He remembered that one of his Yale colleagues, who had previously been in the military at Edgewood Arsenal, had done some experiments with a very potent anticholinergic agent. Yamamura asked his former boss at Edgewood Arsenal, John O'Leary, who suggested the use of QNB, that Yamamura obtained and had radiolabeled by a commercial firm. Thus, [³H]QNB was used to identify muscarinic receptors in homogenates of rat brain tissue (Yamamura and Snyder, 1974 a, b). Furthermore, with this methodology Snyder and colleagues were able to determine the affinities of a series of neuroleptics for muscarinic acetylcholine receptors (Snyder et al., 1974). They concluded that they could predict the likelihood that a neuroleptic would cause extrapyramidal side effects from its affinity at these receptors. Thus, the higher the affinity of a neuroleptic for muscarinic receptors, the less likely it will cause these side effects.

Similar results and conclusions were reported by Miller and Hiley (1974) that same year. However, for a radioligand these researchers did not use QNB, but a related compound called propylbenzilylcholine mustard (PrBCM). Unlike QNB, PrBCM binds irreversibly to muscarinic receptors. Miller and Hiley (1974) predicted this result in the conclusion of their paper: "Combination of the method used here with an in vitro measure of dopamine receptor blockade, such as the dopamine-sensitive adenyl cyclase, should ensure improved and rapid selection of potentially useful neuroleptic agents."

With respect to dopamine-sensitive adenyl cyclase, Miller and Hiley were referring to a discovery made a few years earlier (Kebabian and Greengard, 1971) in the laboratory of a person that shared the Nobel Prize with Carlsson, namely Paul Greengard, then of the Department of Pharmacology, Yale University School of Medicine, New Haven, Connecticut. (This Nobel Prize in Physiology or Medicine was awarded in 2000 to Arvid Carlsson, Paul Greengard, and Eric R. Kandel "for their discoveries concerning signal transduction in the nervous system").

Back in the 1970s there were skeptics of radioligand binding as a way to identify receptors. The concerns were related to the fact that what was being detected was only a binding site for a drug, with no guarantee that it was in fact the pharmacologic receptor for that drug. This skepticism prevailed, even though researchers were careful in their selection of radioligand and careful in demonstrating that the binding of the radioligand had the expected pharmacologic specificity and tissue specificity. Pharmacological specificity was determined from deriving binding data for a series of drugs that, from independent experiments, were known to interact with the receptor of interest. Drugs not known to interact were also tested and were expected not to affect binding of the radioligand. For tissue specificity, for example, a radioligand identifying muscarinic receptors would be expected to bind to brain tissue, but not to liver tissue.

Nonetheless, in all receptor-binding studies it is essential to demonstrate that binding data reflect a drug-receptor interaction in a pharmacological sense (Hollenberg and Cuatrecasas, 1975). Ideally, such correlations should be determined using the same tissue for binding and for biological studies as was done for certain polypeptide hormone receptors (Hollenberg and Cuatrecasas, 1975) and for the ∃-adrenergic receptor (Mukherjee et al., 1976). A direct correlation of binding data with pharmacological data had not been shown for the muscarinic acetylcholine receptor of nervous tissue (Miller and Hiley, 1974; Snyder et al., 1974). Therefore, because there was a question whether competition by psychotropic drugs of a radioactively labeled muscarinic receptor antagonist from brain homogenates reflected blockade by these drugs of this receptor, we set out to show this by another approach.

Our approach was to measure a second messenger response mediated by the muscarinic receptor. We would use a specific agonist of the muscarinic receptor (carbachol) in dose-response studies done in the absence and in the presence of a fixed dosage of the antagonist. This, after all, was the classical approach to defining receptors put forth by Schild (1957). Thus, we made use of a cellular clone of murine neuroblastoma, namely N1E-115 (Amano et al., 1972), which we had derived from work in the laboratory of Marshall Nirenberg, at National Institutes of Health (NIH), Bethesda, Maryland in the early 1970s, soon after he had shared the Nobel Prize for his work on the genetic code. (The Nobel Prize in Physiology or Medicine in 1968 was shared by Marshall Nirenberg from the NIH, Gobind Khorana from the University of Wisconsin, Madison, Wisconsin, and Robert W. Holley, from Cornell University, Ithaca, New York. It was "for their interpretation of the genetic code and its function in protein synthesis").

We discovered that N1E-115 cells, which became the most widely studied murine neuroblastoma cell line, had muscarinic receptors that mediated the formation of the second messenger cyclic GMP (cGMP) (Richelson and Divinetz-Romero, 1977). These cells also possess many other receptors that can be studied by agonist-mediated second messenger synthesis (Pfenning and Richelson, 1990). In our studies (Richelson and Divinetz-Romero, 1977) we showed that neuroleptics, and other drugs, blocked the cGMP response mediated by carbachol. From dose-ratio analyses (Schild, 1957), we were able to obtain equilibrium dissociation constants that correlated well with previously published data derived from radioligand binding techniques. We were becoming less skeptical of this newer technology (radioligand binding).

Earlier in the 1970s, the first dopamine receptor (D_1) was identified from studies that measured the second messenger cyclic AMP (cAMP) in response to low doses of dopamine (Clement-Cormier et al., 1974; Kebabian and Greengard, 1971). Thus, dopamine activated the enzyme adenyl cyclase to form cAMP. This work was very important and exciting, but somewhat disappointing.

Initially discovered in bovine superior cervical ganglia (Kebabian and Greengard, 1971), dopamine-sensitive adenyl cyclase was quickly found to be present in brain of several different species of animal (Clement-Cormier et al., 1974). Specifically, dopamine stimulated cAMP formation in superior cervical ganglia (Kebabian and Greengard, 1971) and in brain regions rich in dopamine nerve endings, such as the caudate nucleus, olfactory tubercle, and nucleus accumbens (Clement-Cormier et al., 1974). Thus, these researchers discovered the first dopamine receptor (D_1).

These researchers also showed that this effect of dopamine was competitively antagonized by low concentrations of antipsychotic drugs (Clement-Cormier et al., 1974). Several psychotropic drugs without antipsychotic efficacy were ineffective at antagonizing the effects of dopamine. In addition, there was a reasonable correlation between the potency of a neuroleptic as an inhibitor of dopamine-sensitive adenyl cyclase and its potency as an antipsychotic drug in patients.

However, the disappointment came with the one major discrepancy: the potency of haloperidol in this system. This drug is clinically many times more potent than is chlorpromazine at treating schizophrenia on a mg/kg basis, but it was much less potent than chlorpromazine in this in vitro system. Specifically, the Ki (inhibitor constant) for haloperidol was 0.22 ΦM, while it was over 3 times lower for chlorpromazine (Clement-Cormier et al., 1974). Thus, this dopamine receptor did not predict clinical potency of all neuroleptics.

Researchers, therefore, began the search for the second dopamine receptor (D_2) that would correlate more strongly with the known clinical potencies of neuroleptic drugs. Since haloperidol was relatively weak at the D_1 receptor compared to its clinical potency, researchers decided to use radiolabeled haloperidol as the radioligand to identify a binding site for which haloperidol had high affinity. With this approach two different laboratories once again independently and simultaneously found the D_2 receptor (Creese et al., 1976; Seeman et al., 1976). Competition binding studies with [³H]haloperidol or [³H]dopamine and a series of antipsychotic drugs showed an incredibly strong correlation of the affinity of these drugs for [³H]haloperidol binding sites and the daily dosage for treating schizophrenia. As in the studies of the D_1 receptor (Clement-Cormier et al., 1974), there was not a good correlation for the affinity of these drugs for [³H]dopamine binding sites and the daily dosage for treating schizophrenia.

Thus, with a test tube assay, researchers had identified the site of therapeutic action of antipsychotic drugs. The strong correlation between the *in vitro* affinity for [³H]haloperidol binding sites in (non-human) brain and the *in vivo* daily dosage for treating schizophrenia was truly remarkable, because the correlation was so strong in the absence of any consideration of the pharmacokinetics of the neuroleptic drugs. There is wide variation in oral bioavailability, rate of penetrance into brain, and elimination half-lives of antipsychotic drugs. These differences do not seem to matter with respect to this assay that predicts clinical effects of these drugs. It also predicts the likelihood that these compounds will cause extrapyramidal and certain endocrinologic side-effects, unless the compound possesses some other mitigating property (e.g., antimuscarinic property).

Now, the pharmaceutical industry had a tool to obtain new neuroleptic drugs by screening their huge libraries of compounds for "hits" at [³H]haloperidol binding. Assuming that a "hit" would be absorbed in the gut and penetrate into brain, one could immediately establish the daily dosage to treat schizophrenia in a clinical trial by interpolating the graph of affinity versus dosage (Richelson and Nelson, 1984b; Seeman et al., 1976). This was a truly remarkable result, predicted by Carlsson and Lindqvist over one decade earlier (Carlsson and Lindqvist, 1963).

As a curious aside in the history of neuropsychopharmacology, we should not have been surprised that neuroleptics block dopamine receptors. Phenothiazines, the class of compounds from which the prototypical neuroleptic chlorpromazine was derived, were used as anthelminthics, antihistaminics, and antiemetics, long before they were used to treat psychosis in the 1950s. Because of the effectiveness of chlorpromazine in treating psychosis and because of its antiemetic property, pharmaceutical companies routinely screened for antiemetic agents in the hopes of finding new neuroleptics. One of these screening tests used the dopamine agonist apomorphine to elicit emesis in dogs. Thus, neuroleptics were selected because of their ability to block this emesis and hence block dopamine receptors.

There was a lot more to learn about the pharmacology of neuroleptics beyond their ability to block dopamine or muscarinic receptors. With the availability of many more specific radioligands of high specific activity we, and also others, thought it might be useful to learn more about the receptor pharmacology of these compounds, particularly as it relates to their adverse effects. When Snyder et al. (1974) and Miller and Hiley (1974) first reported on the muscarinic receptor binding properties of neuroleptics, their emphasis was on the therapeutic benefits (fewer extrapyramidal side effects) of having this property in a drug that blocked dopamine receptors. Similarly for the D_2 receptor binding data, the emphasis was on the therapeutic aspects of this binding (Creese et al., 1976; Seeman et al., 1976).

We had a different emphasis that related the receptor binding properties to adverse effects of these compounds in patients. This emphasis was influenced by the fact that I was treating a large number of patients with these drugs and I wanted to understand the mechanisms of their side effects. This would allow me to minimize or avoid certain side effects in my patients.

Since there was always the potential for species differences in the way drugs bind to receptors and since we were interested in the clinical application of our data, we decided to study the binding of neuroleptics to human receptors. Since this work (Lin et al., 1986; Richelson and Nelson, 1984a; Wander et al., 1987) preceded the molecular cloning of human receptors, we decided to use human brain tissue as the source of receptors. At that time (early to mid-1980s) few researchers around the world were able to get normal human brain tissue at autopsy as readily as we could at Mayo Clinic in Rochester, Minnesota, through the good graces of our neuropathologist, Haruo Okazaki. With these data early on, we introduced practicing clinicians to clinical utility of receptor binding data for neuroleptics, as well as other psychotherapeutic drugs (Richelson, 1980, 1983).

A recurring quest with respect to neuroleptics, neurotransmitters, and neuropsychopharmacology over the past several decades has been the search for the mechanism by which a neuroleptic is atypical. The prototypical atypical neuroleptic clozapine, which was first used clinically in the mid-1970s, has yet to be improved upon with respect to its therapeutic actions, although newer compounds are clearly devoid of its serious side effect of agranulocytosis. The original definition of an atypical neuroleptic was an antipsychotic drug that caused few or none of the extrapyramidal side-effects that are common to neuroleptics (e.g., dystonia, parkinsonism, akathisia, and tardive dyskinesia). The definition has been modified over the years to include especially good efficacy in treatment-resistant patients, as well as in the treatment of the so-called negative signs and symptoms of schizophrenia (e.g., apathy, anhedonia, and cognitive blunting).

The early work on muscarinic receptor antagonism by neuroleptics (Miller and Hiley, 1974; Snyder et al., 1974) suggested that this property conferred atypicality on neuroleptics. However, with some newer-generation drugs that lacked this property (e.g., sertindole), it was clear that no single factor could explain atypicality for all neuroleptics and, so, other mechanisms were involved. In the late 1980s, from the laboratory of Herbert Meltzer, came the notion that a more potent blockade of 5-HT$_{2A}$ receptors than of D$_2$ receptors conferred atypicality on antipsychotic drugs (Meltzer et al., 1989). Although in recent years there has been a debate in the literature about this hypothesis (Kapur and Meltzer, 2001), it should be no surprise that most, if not all, of the newer generation atypical antipsychotics are very potent antagonists of 5-HT$_{2A}$ receptors (Richelson and Souder, 2000).

Where do we go from here? In the future researchers will again be writing historical pieces about neuroleptics, neurotransmitters, and neuropsychophamacology. However, rather than the emphasis being on the classical neurotransmitters, there will be a shift in emphasis toward the newer generation neurotransmitters and neuromodulators, namely, the neuropeptides. One peptide in particular, neurotensin, which was hypothesized many years ago to be the endogenous neuroleptic (Nemeroff, 1980), may be the target of future atypical neuroleptic drugs (Boules et al., 2005).

REFERENCES
1. Amano, T., Richelson, E., Nirenberg, M., 1972. Neurotransmitter synthesis by neuroblastoma clones. Proc. Natl. Acad. Sci. USA 69, 258-263.
2. Boules, M., Fredrickson, P., Richelson, E., 2005. Neurotensin agonists as an alternative to antipsychotics. Expert Opin. Investig. Drugs 14, 359-369.
3. Carlsson, A., 2001. A paradigm shift in brain research. Science 294, 1021-1024.
4. Carlsson, A., Lindqvist, M., 1963. Effect of chlorpromazine or haloperidol on formation of 3-methoxytyramine and normetanephrine in mouse brain. Acta Pharmacol.Toxicol. (Copenh.) 20, 140-144.
5. Clement-Cormier, Y.C., Kebabian, J.W., Petzold, G.L., Greengard, P., 1974. Dopamine-sensitive adenylate cyclase in mammalian brain: a possible site of action of antipsychotic drugs. Proc.Natl. Acad. Sci. USA 71, 1113-1117.
6. Creese, A., Burt, D.R., Snyder, S.H., 1976. Dopamine receptor binding predicts clinical and pharmacological potencies of antischizophrenic drugs. Science 192, 481-483.
7. Cuatrecasas, P., 1971a. Insulin—receptor interactions in adipose tissue cells: direct measurement and properties. Proc. Natl. Acad. Sci. USA 68, 1264-1268.
8. Cuatrecasas, P., 1971b. Properties of the insulin receptor of isolated fat cell membranes. J. Biol. Chem. 246, 7265-7274.
9. Hollenberg, M.D., Cuatrecasas, P., 1975. Biochemical identification of membrane receptors: principles and techniques. In: Iversen, L.L., Iversen, S.D., Snyder, S.H. (Eds.), Handbook of Psychopharmacology. Plenum Press, New York, pp. 129-177.
10. Kapur, S., Meltzer, H., 2001. Serotonin and atypicality. Journal of Psychotic Disorders: Reviews & Commentaries V, 3, 12-15.
11. Kebabian, J.W., Greengard, P., 1971. Dopamine-sensitive adenyl cyclase: possible role in synaptic transmission. Science 174, 1346-1349.
12. Lin, S.C., Olson, K.C., Okazaki, H., Richelson, E., 1986. Studies on muscarinic binding sites in human brain identified with [^{3}H]pirenzepine. J. Neurochem. 46, 274-279.

13. Meltzer, H.Y., Matsubara, S., Lee, J.C., 1989. Classification of typical and atypical antipsychotic drugs on the basis of dopamine D_1, D_2 and serotonin$_2$ pKi values. J. Pharmacol. Exp. Ther. 251, 238-246.

14. Miller, R.J., Hiley, C.R., 1974. Anti-muscarinic properties of neuroleptics and drug-induced parkinsonism. Nature 248, 596-597.

15. Mukherjee, C., Caron, M.G., Mullikin, D., Lefkowitz, R.J., 1976. Structure-activity relationships of adenylate cyclase-coupled ß-adrenergic receptors: determination by direct binding studies. Mol. Pharmacol. 12, 16-31.

16. Nemeroff, C.B., 1980. Neurotensin: perchance an endogenous neuroleptic? Biological Psychiatry 15, 283-302.

17. Paton, W.D., Rang, H.P., 1965. The uptake of atropine and related drugs by intestinal smooth muscle of the guinea-pig in relation to acetylcholine receptors. Proc. R. Soc. Lond. B. Biol. Sci. 163, 1-44.

18. Pfenning, M.A., Richelson, E., 1990. Methods for studying receptors with cultured cells of nervous tissue origin. In: Enna, S.J., Kuhar, M.J. (Eds.), Methods in Neurotransmitter Receptor Analysis. Raven Press, New York, pp. 147-175.

19. Richelson, E., 1980. Neuroleptics and neurotransmitter receptors. Psychiatric Annals 10, 21-40.

20. Richelson, E., 1983. Are receptor studies useful for clinical practice? J Clin Psychiatry 44, 4-9.

21. Richelson, E., Divinetz-Romero, S., 1977. Blockade by psychotropic drugs of the muscarinic acetylcholine receptor in cultured nerve cells. Biol. Psychiatry 12, 771-785.

22. Richelson, E., Nelson, A., 1984a. Antagonism by neuroleptics of neurotransmitter receptors of normal human brain in vitro. Eur. J. Pharmacol. 103, 197-204.

23. Richelson, E., Nelson, A., 1984b. Antagonism by neuroleptics of neurotransmitter receptors of normal human brain in vitro. Eur. J. Pharmacol. 103, 197-204.

24. Richelson, E., Souder, T., 2000. Binding of antipsychotic drugs to human brain receptors focus on newer generation compounds. Life Sci. 68, 29-39.

25. Schild, H.O., 1957. Drug antagonism of pAx. Pharmacol. Rev. 9, 242-246.

26. Seeman, P., Lee, T., Chau-Wong, M., Wong, K., 1976. Antipsychotic drug doses and neuroleptic/dopamine receptors. Nature 261, 717-719.

27. Snyder, S., Greenberg, D., Yamamura, H.I., 1974a. Antischizophrenic drugs and brain cholinergic receptor-affinity for muscarinic sites predicts extrapyramidal effects. Arch. Gen. Psychiatry 31, 58-61.

28. Snyder, S., Greenberg, D., Yamamura, H.I., 1974b. Antischizophrenic drugs and brain cholinergic receptor-affinity for muscarinic sites predicts extrapyramidal effects. Arch. Gen. Psychiatry 31, 58-61.

29. Wander, T.J., Nelson, A., Okazaki, H., Richelson, E., 1987. Antagonism by neuroleptics of serotonin 5-HT$_{1A}$ and 5-HT$_2$ receptors of normal human brain in vitro. Eur. J. Pharmacol. 143, 279-282.

30. Wong, D.F., Wagner, H.N., Jr., Tune, L.E., Dannals, R.F., Pearlson, G.D., Links, J.M., Tamminga, C.A., Broussolle, E.P., Ravert, H.T., Wilson, A.A., Toung, J.K., Malat, J., Williams, J.A., O'Tuama, L.A., Snyder, S.H., Kuhar, M.J., Gjedde, A., 1986. Positron emission tomography reveals elevated D_2 dopamine receptors in drug-naive schizophrenics. Science 234, 1558-1563.

31. Yamamura, H.I., Snyder, S.H., 1974. Muscarinic cholinergic binding in rat brain. Proc. Natl. Acad. Sci. USA 71, 1725-1729.

CHAPTER 11

LITHIUM AND THE EARLY
NEUROTRANSMITTER ERA

Gordon F. Johnson

Lithium is the lightest metal known. It was discovered in 1818. Its name is derived from the Greek word for stone. It belongs to the alkali metal group that includes sodium and potassium. It occurs widely in nature and is found in trace amounts in plants, animals and man. It has been shown to produce a wide variety of biological effects. However, lithium is not known to possess any physiological function in man (Schou, 1957).

The discovery of the anti-manic effects of lithium by John Cade preceded the neurotransmitter era in psychiatry (Cade, 1949). In telling his story, Cade (1970) commented that lithium's effect is so specific, that it inevitably leads to speculation as to the possible aetiological significance of lithium deficiency. At that time, the dominant theories of how the brain worked were electrophysiological. As lithium is a monovalent cation chemically related to sodium and potassium, both of which are known to play a critical role in neuronal excitability, initial studies in its mechanism of action focussed on its effects on the metabolism and function of these ions. Trautner et al. (1955) studied the effects of lithium on the ionic balance in patients with mania compared to healthy controls. They found transient early increases in the excretion of sodium and potassium following lithium ingestion, and were the first to report a different pattern of retention and excretion of the lithium ion in mania and normal subjects. While normal subjects retained lithium, reaching equilibrium between intake and output during the first five to six days, manic patients continued to retain a large proportion of lithium until the manic symptoms disappeared whereupon lithium excretion then exceeded intake until equilibrium between intake and output was reestablished. These findings supported the initial suggestion of the therapeutic specificity of lithium in mania.

In the following decade, further research work was reported on water and electrolyte balance and the effect of lithium in manic-depressive patients, but the findings did not provide information about changes in electrolyte metabolism in the central nervous system that might underlie the drug's therapeutic effects (Coppen and Shaw, 1967). Research has continued however on the effect of the substance on ions critical to neuronal excitability, such as sodium, potassium and calcium, but their importance for lithium's therapeutic effect remains an open question.

Following the discovery of neurotransmitters in brain and the technology to measure them, exploring the effects of psychotropic drugs on neurotransmitters assumed centre stage in the hypotheses explaining their mechanism of action (Healy, 2002). It was at this time that clinical and research interest in lithium accelerated.

Initial research on lithium focussed on presynaptic effects such as synthesis, release and reuptake of monoamine neurotransmitters. Evidence from studies in animals and man on the effects of reserpine and two classes of antidepressant drugs; the monoamine oxidase inhibitors and tricyclic antidepressants on monoamine neurotransmitters suggested that the amount, distribution or metabolism of norepinephrine might be altered in patients with depression (Bunney and Davis, 1965). Schildkraut (1965) proposed a catecholamine hypothesis of affective disorders that stated that some, if not all depression was associated with an absolute or relative decrease in catecholamines, particularly norepinephrine available at central adrenergic receptor sites. Elation conversely may be associated with excess of such amines. To assess the effects of lithium on norepinephrine metabolism Schildkraut et al. (1966) injected H^3-norepinephrine intracisternally into rats before acute lithium administration. They reported that lithium produced a shift in intra-neuronal inactivation of norepinephrine, decreasing the norepinephrine available to adrenergic receptors. Colburn et al. (1967) showed that synaptosomes from the brain of rats pre-treated with lithium, within the time frame of five to seven days, at plasma levels of 1 to 2 mEq/L, similar to plasma levels in the treatment of mania, took up norepinephrine to a significantly greater extent than controls. Corrodi et al. (1967) reported an increase in noradrenaline neurone activity after intraperitoneal administration of lithium in rats. In their experiment, lithium alone did not alter noradrenergic content of the brain but when lithium was combined with an inhibitor of tyrosine hydroxylase it produced a fall in brain noradrenaline, which was significantly more rapid than that produced by the inhibitor alone. These findings supported the assumption for a role of norepinephrine in mania and in the mechanism of action of lithium. The specific mechanisms by which lithium exerted its action had been unclear. It may alter the membrane directly, interact with an enzyme and/or transport mechanisms, affect adrenergic binding sites or interact with cations as they affect amine uptake. Schou (1968) in his review of lithium commented that the evidence for the role of norepinephrine in the mode of action of lithium is derived from drugs that affect the mood in one direction only. Lithium prevents both manic and depressive relapses and therefore may suggest that it counteracts manic-depressive disorder at a different level.

While interest in the USA centred on catecholamines, in Europe an hypothesis implicating the neurotransmitter serotonin (5-HT) in mood was proposed, based on observations that conventional antidepressants, both tricyclics and monoamine oxidase inhibitors (MAOIs) increase the availability of 5-HT in the brain and that substances that reduce 5-HT availability, such as reserpine may produce depressive episodes in some individuals. The earliest formulation of the indoleamine hypothesis of depression postulated that a deficiency of central 5-HT could lead to the emergence of depression. (Coppen et al., 1965). This was extended to a "permissive" hypothesis that stated that an essential deficit of 5-HT coupled with increased noradrenergic transmission would lead to mania (Prange et al., 1974). Findings in clinical studies were supportive of this hypothesis. Tryptophan was reported to have antidepressant activity when given in combination with antidepressants and to enhance the efficacy of antidepressants. The drug parachlorophenylalanine, which decreases 5-HT synthesis, was shown to induce a recurrence of depressive symptoms in recovered patients receiving antidepressant treatment (Shopsin et al., 1976). Consistent with these findings was the demonstration that lithium treatment in animals led to an increased rate of uptake of L-tryptophan into synaptosomal preparations and an increased rate of synthesis of 5-HT (Knapp and Mandell, 1973). Lithium was also shown to increase 5-HT release in the hippocampus. The finding that lithium increases 5-HT release in the hippocampus provided the rationale for the use of lithium to augment antidepressant drugs in treatment refractory depression (Blier and de Montigny, 1985). This is one of the few successful clinical strategies based on preclinical pharmacological evidence.

Acetylcholine was the first central nervous system neurotransmitter discovered but it was not until 1972 that a link between a disturbance in cholinergic function and affective disorder was proposed with mania characterised by a predominance of brain noradrenergic activity relative to cholinergic activity and depression by the converse (Janowsky et al., 1972). Some of the most striking evidence suggesting a role of central cholinergic influences in the regulation of mood comes from observations on the acetylcholine enhancing effect of choline esterase inhibitors. In the 1950s and the 1960s, several groups of investigators studied healthy volunteers, depressed patients, manic patients as well as normal subjects accidentally exposed to insecticide poisonings and observed that choline esterase inhibitors induced depressive symptoms (Gershon and Shaw, 1961). The choline esterase inhibitor physostigmine was claimed to cause a dramatic but brief reduction in hypomanic and manic symptoms in bipolar patients. It was also reported to produce depression in the majority of a group of euthymic bipolar patients maintained on lithium (Janowsky et al., 1972). Choline is the precursor of acetylcholine. Its availability and uptake into the neurone are important determinants of acetylcholine synthesis and cholinergic function. An increase in choline concentration and acetylcholine was shown in rat synaptosomal preparations following 10 days treatment with lithium (Jope, 1979). Studies in man using the red blood cell as a model of neuronal membrane transport mechanism showed that lithium produced a tenfold increase in intracellular choline concentrations. (Johnson et al., 1980). Other psychotropic drugs have no effect on red blood cell choline content or transport. In addition, choline transport in red blood cells appears to be irreversible. A prospective study of red blood cell choline levels using nuclear magnetic resonance spectroscopy over 11 months in manic-depressive patients on lithium maintenance reported that significant changes in mood were not accompanied by changes in red blood cell choline levels. In addition, red blood cell choline levels did not differ between normal volunteers and newly admitted lithium free patients with either mania or depression (Kuchel et al., 1984). While lithium produced a specific accumulation of choline the increased levels appeared to be unrelated to clinical changes and did not distinguish between lithium responders and non-responders. However, there a re diff erences in the type and functional significance of choline transport systems between the neurone and the red blood cell. Only cholinergic neurones possess a high affinity choline transport system coupled to acetylcholine synthesis. Other cells in the body as well as neurones possess a low affinity system linked to phosphatidylcholine synthesis. The effect of lithium on the choline membrane transport system is unclear.

These early studies of lithium's action on monoamine neurotransmitters identified a number of effects that may contribute to lithium's mechanism of action. But the findings were inconclusive in explaining the specific effects of lithium in mood disorders.

The expectations generated by the initial research of lithium's action on neurotransmitters was not fulfilled and an exhaustive review of the biochemical and neuropharmacological effects of lithium came to the conclusion "that the pharmacological actions central to the therapeutic effect of lithium have not yet been established despite almost 40 years of clinical use and scientific investigation" (Wood and Goodwin, 1987).

In the 1970s a shift in research focus from presynaptic to postsynaptic events that paralleled the advances in neurochemistry led to identification of postsynaptic receptors and their coupling to second messenger systems, such as cyclic adenosine monophosphate (cAMP) and phosphoinositide. The early monoamine hypotheses of too much or too little gave way to more complex models of drug action. Lithium's effects on adenyl cyclase activity and cAMP mediated action at a number of tissue sites, including kidney and thyroid led to a focus on signal transduction systems as a model for lithium action. The discovery that lithium is a potent inhibitor of inositol monophosphatase, the enzyme that converts inositol monophosphate to free inositol led to an inositol "depletion hypothesis" of lithium action (Sherman et al., 1986). The following downstream effects on intracellular signalling identified effects on "third messengers" - protein kinases and their role in complex processes involving membrane phosphoproteins effecting long-term neuronal activity and plasticity.

It is currently thought that the effect of lithium on the spectrum of neurotransmitter systems may be mediated through its actions at intracellular sites, with the net effect of long-term lithium attributed to its ability to alter the balance among neurotransmitter/neuropeptide signalling pathways (Lenox and Frazer, 2002).

In summarising the extensive and sometimes conflicting research on the effects of lithium on signal transduction systems Jope (1999) concluded that lithium has a bimodal mechanism of action achieving a balance between negative and positive modulating effects. This explanatory bipolar model would come closer to what Schou (1957) had speculated many years previously.

REFERENCES
1. Blier, P., de Montigny, C., 1985. Short-term lithium administration enhances serotonergic neurotransmission: Electrophysiological evidence in rat. CNS Eur. J. Pharmacol. 113, 69-77.
2. Bunney, W., Davis, J., 1965. Norepinephrine in depressive reactions. A review. Arch. Gen. Psychiat. 13, 483-494.
3. Cade, J.F.J., 1949. Lithium salts in the treatment of psychotic excitement. Med. J. Austr. 36, 349-352.
4. Cade, J.F.J., 1970. The story of lithium. In: Ayd, F.J., Blackwell, B. (Eds.), Discoveries in Biological Psychiatry. Lippincott, Philadelphia/Toronto, pp. 219-229.
5. Colburn, R., Goodwin, F., Bunney, W., Davis, J., 1967. Effect of lithium on the uptake of noradrenaline by synaptosomes. Nature 215, 1395-1397.
6. Coppen, A., Shaw, P., 1967. The distribution of electrolytes and water in patients after taking lithium carbonate. Lancet 11, 805-806.
7. Coppen, A., Shaw, D., Malleson, A., Egglestone E., 1965. Tryptamine metabolism in depression. Brit. J. Psychiat. 111, 993-998.
8. Corrodi, H., Fuxe, K., Hökfelt, T., Schou, M., 1967. The effect of lithium on cerebral monoamine neurons. Psychopharmacologia 11, 345-353.
9. Gershon, S., Shaw, F., 1961. Psychiatric sequelae of chronic exposure to organophosphorus insecticides. Lancet 1, 1371-1374.
10. Healy D., 2002. The Creation of Psychopharmacology. Harvard University Press, Cambridge (Massachusetts)/ London (England), pp. 1-469.
11. Janowsky, D., El-Yousef, M., Davis, J., Sererke, H., 1972. A cholinergic-adrenergic hypothesis of mania and depression. Lancet 2, 6732-6735.
12. Johnson, G., Kuchel, P., Singh, B., Hunt G,. Begg W., Jones A., 1980. Red cell choline in manic-depressive patients taking lithium. New Eng. J. Med. 303, 705
13. Jope, R., 1979. Effects of lithium treatment in vitro and in vivo on acetylcholine metabolism in rat brain. J. of Neurochem. 33, 487-495.
14. Jope R., 1999. Antibipolar therapy: Mechanism of action of lithium. Mol. Psychiatry 4, 117-128.
15. Knapp, S., Mandell, A., 1973. Short and long-term lithium administration effects on the brain serotonergic biosynthetic systems. Science 180, 645-647.
16. Kuchel, P., Hunt, G., Johnson, G., Beilharz G. Chapman B. Jones A. Singh B., 1984. Lithium, red blood cell choline and clinical state A prospective study in manic depressive patients J. Aff. Dis. 6, 83-94.
17. Lennox, R., Frazer, A., 2002. Mechanism of action of antidepressants and mood stabilisers in neurophychopharmacology. In: Davis, K., Charney, J., Coyle, J, Nemeroff, C. (Eds.), The Fifth Generation of Progress. Lipincott Williams & Wilkins, Baltimore, pp 1139-1165.
18. Prange, A.J., Wilson, I.C., Lynn, C.W., Alltop, L.B., Stikelather, R.A., 1974. L-tryptophan in mania, contribution to a permissive hypothesis of affective disorders. Arch. Gen. Psychiat. 30. 56-62.
19. Schildkraut, J., 1965. The catecholamine hypothesis of affective disorders: A review of supporting evidence. Amer. J. Psychiat. 122, 509-522.
20. Schildkraut, J., Schanberg, S., Kopin, I., 1966. The effects of lithium ion on H^3 – norepinephrine metabolism in brain. Life Sciences 5, 1479-1483.
21. Schou, M., 1957. Biology and pharmacology of the lithium ion. Pharmacol. Rev. 9, 17-58.
22. Schou, M., 1968. Lithium in Psychiatry. In: Efron, D., Cole, J., Levine, J., Wittenborn, R. (Eds.), Psychopharmacology A Review of Progress 1957-1967. U.S. Publ. Hlth. Serv. Publ., Washington DC., pp.701-718.
23. Sherman, W., Gish, B., Honchar, M., Munsell, L., 1986. Effects of lithium on phosphoinositide metabolism in vivo. Fed. Proc. 45, 2639-2646.
24. Shopsin, B., Friedman, E., Gershon, S., 1976. Paracholorophenylalanine reversal of tranylcypromine effect in depressed patients Arch. Gen. Psychiat, 33, 811-822.
25. Trautner, E., Gershon, S., Morris, R., Noack, C., 1955. The excretion and retention of ingested lithium and its effect on the ionic balance of man. Med. J. Aust. 2, 280-291.
26. Wood, A., Goodwin, G., 1987 A review of the biochemical and neuropharmacological actions of lithium. Psychol. Med. 17, 579-600.

CHAPTER 12

THE NEUROTRANSMITTER ERA IN PSYCHIATRY

MONOAMINES AND DEPRESSION - A RETROSPECTIVE

Herman M. Van Praag

ANTIDEPRESSANTS: A THERAPEUTIC REVOLUTION

1958 was a revolutionary year in modern psychopharmacology, as 1952 had been. In 1952 chlorpromazine (Largactil), the first antipsychotic, was introduced, representing a completely novel class of therapeutics. 1958 was the year that the antidepressants appeared on the scene, not one, but two compounds, structurally completely different, both discovered by pure chance and originating from different research domains. One was iproniazid (Marsilid), the first monoamine oxidase inhibitor (MAOI). It was derived from research into tuberculostatic drugs. It turned out to have mood-elevating properties that went beyond its ability to ameliorate tubercular lesions. The other was imipramine (Tofranil), the first tricyclic antidepressant (TCA). Structurally it is closely related to chlorpromazine. Initially it was therefore offered to clinicians as a potential antipsychotic.

Antidepressants were a completely novel therapeutic option. The only biological treatment modality available at the time for (certain types of) depression was electroconvulsive treatment (ECT). Since the 1930s we had at our disposal amphetamine derivatives and some of them were used in depression. They exerted psychomotor stimulant effects but had no lasting effects on mood. Hence, they did not deserve the qualification antidepressant. The appearance of drugs that truly deserved that name was revolutionary. Much of the psychiatric community, however, failed to appreciate that, particularly in Europe. Antidepressants were for quite some time considered to be pure symptom-suppressors, sops, distracting attention from the true causes of depression, thought to be purely psychological, thus depriving patients from the only effective treatment: psychotherapy (on analytic lines). Since they were thought to obscure the real origins of depression, antidepressants were considered in essence anti-therapeutic. It was only in the 1970s and 1980s that psychiatrists learned to appreciate the therapeutic significance of antidepressants.

ANTIDEPRESSANTS: A SCIENTIFIC REVOLUTION

At the time of its introduction it was known that iproniazid was an inhibitor of the enzyme monoamine oxidase (MAO), involved in the degradation of certain amines localized in the brain. It was the first of the modern psychotropic drugs that came along with some information about its action mechanism in the brain. This was of fundamental importance. The body/soul problem so far had been a purely philosophical problem. Now the notion loomed up that an empirical component could be added. Psychotropic drugs exercise influence on abnormal behaviour and they do impact on certain neuronal systems in the brain. This dual action prompted three interrelated questions:

1. Is there a relation between their biological and behavioural effects?
2. Are the brain systems influenced by a psychotropic drug disturbed in those psychiatric disorders responding favourably to the drug?
3. If so, are these brain dysfunctions corrected by the drug in question?

In other words, it seemed likely that psychotropic drugs could become points of crystallization for hypotheses on relationships between (abnormal) brain functions and (abnormal) behaviour.

Shortly before the introduction of the antidepressants a hypothesis of this nature had been introduced. It related to lysergic acid diethylamide (LSD), not a therapeutic agent, in fact a compound producing psychotic symptoms in clear consciousness. Psychotic symptoms without clouding of consciousness were considered typical for schizophrenia. LSD was shown to influence serotonergic (5-HTergic) transmission, at least peripherally. Woolley and Shaw (1954) hypothesized that serotonin (5-hyroxytryptamine, 5-HT) was involved in LSD psychoses and, by inference, in schizophrenia.

As said, in 1958 iproniazid was the only psychotropic drug of which some actions on the brain were known. It inhibits MAO leading to increased extra-cellular concentration of catecholamines (CA) and 5-HT. This prompted the question whether increased monoamine (MA) concentration and antidepressant action were related and whether disturbances in MAergic systems were demonstrable in depression responsive to the drug. These were the questions I studied from the introduction of iproniazid in 1958 on, together with the biochemist Bart Leijnse. This research resulted four years later my thesis (Van Praag, 1962). One of my conclusions was, that there were reasons to assume a relationship between MAO inhibition and antidepressant actions and between 5-HTergic dysfunctions and the occurrence of certain types of vital depression. The term vital depression stands for the syndrome described at the time under the heading of endogenous depression and presently under that of major depression, melancholic type.

THE WAYS CENTRAL MONOAMINES WERE STUDIED

Initially central MAs could be studied only post-mortem and via peripheral indices, such as urinary excretion of MA metabolites, and activity of enzymes involved in MA metabolism in plasma or blood cells. 5-HT was studied in blood platelets, considered to be models of 5-HTergic nerve endings.

In the 1960-s and 1970s methods were developed to study MA metabolites in cerebrospinal fluid (CSF). CSF concentrations of MA metabolites were considered to be (crude) indicators of MA metabolism in the central nervous system (CNS).

From the 1970s on the challenge test won favour. Particular MA receptors were stimulated with an agonist (or antagonist) of one of the MAs. A function regulated by that receptor system was measured, e.g., the release of a pituitary hormone, or body temperature. An excessive response signifies increased receptor responsivity, a subnormal response down-regulation of that system. First indirect agonists were used such as the CA precursor L-dopa and the 5-HT precursor L-tryptophan, activating that particular receptor system in its entirety. Later agonists more or less selective for a particular receptor sub-population became available, providing more specific information about a particular receptor type.

Finally from the 1980s on, brain imaging techniques were introduced in biological depression research, making it feasible to study blood flow, glucose metabolism, density of certain MA receptors and metabolic rate of certain MAs in the living brain.

The database thus established is impressive. In the following I will present a summary, focusing on the question to what extent the available data suggest a role of central MAs in the pathophysiology of depression.

SEROTONIN AND DEPRESSION

The 5-HT hypothesis of depression, formulated in the 1960s, hypothesized a causal connection between disturbances in central 5-HTergic systems and depression (Coppen, 1967; Van Praag, 1962). Studies of peripheral 5-HT related variables, however, did not produce sufficiently supportive evidence. It is true, some disturbances were found, for instance in platelet 5-HT and in the activity of some enzymes involved in 5-HT metabolism, but it remained uncertain whether these abnormalities could be extrapolated to the state of the 5-HT system in the CNS.

Not until techniques were developed to measure 5-HT metabolites in CSF and to measure the density of 5-HT receptors in the CNS, was evidence generated supporting the 5-HT hypothesis.

5-HT METABOLISM

The major degradation product of 5-HT, 5-hydroxyindoleacetic acid (5-HIAA), is found in the CSF as well as in the brain itself. 5-HIAA in lumbar CSF originates partly in the brain, partly in the spinal cord. However, both animal studies (Mignot et al., 1985) and human (post- mortem) studies (Stanley et al., 1985), have revealed a close correlation between brain and CSF 5-HIAA. Furthermore the 5-HIAA concentration in the brain is to a large extent a function of 5-HT metabolism. Therefore CSF 5-HIAA can be considered as an indicator, albeit it is a crude indicator, of 5-HT metabolism in (certain parts of) the brain.

Several studies reported that in (a subgroup of) depression the CSF concentration of 5-HIAA is lower than in a non-depressed control group. This applied both to baseline, and to post-probenecid concentrations (Asberg et al., 1976; Van Praag and Korf, 1971a; Van Praag et al., 1970). Probenecid is a blocker of 5-HIAA transport from the CSF to the blood stream. The rise of 5-HIAA concentration in CSF after probenecid is (again, a crude) indicator of the production rate of 5-HT in the brain (Korf and Van Praag, 1971).

Low baseline and post-probenecid CSF 5-HIAA suggest a diminution of 5-HT metabolism in the CNS. Several lines of evidence were supportive of this tentative conclusion.

First, there is abundant data that the various classes of antidepressants as well as electroconvulsive treatment (ECT) improve the efficiency of 5-HTergic transmission particularly of 5-HT$_{1A}$ receptor-mediated transmission. This happens either by sensitisation of postsynaptic receptors or by desensitisation of presynaptic receptors that normally reduce the release of 5-HT in the synaptic cleft or inhibit the firing rate of the 5-HT nerve cell (Blier and de Montigny, 1994).

A second group of data is derived from the so-called tryptophan-depletion strategy (Young et al., 1985). Tryptophan is an essential amino acid and the precursor of 5-HT. A shortage of tryptophan will lead to a deficiency of 5-HT. Such a shortage can be generated by ingesting a mixture of amino acids competing with tryptophan for the same transport mechanism from the blood stream into the CNS. This leads to rapid decrease of tryptophan in the blood stream (Delgado et al., 1990), lowering of 5-HIAA in the CSF (Williams et al., 1999) and, in animals, to substantial lowering of brain 5-HT (Moja et al., 1989). Applied to normal volunteers this procedure leads to the occurrence of mood lowering (Young et al., 1985), in particular in those individuals with a family history of depression (but without having gone through depressive episodes themselves) (Benkelfat et al., 1994; Klaasen et al., 1999). Patients in remission from an episode of major depression, who responded to tryptophan depletion with mood lowering, showed an increased relapse risk in the next 12 months (Moreno et al., 2000). Depletion of 5-HT but not of noradrenaline (NA) induces a relapse in depressed patients in remission after treatment with 5-HT specific antidepressants (Delgado and Moreno, 2000). Conversely, treatment with the 5-HT precursor 5-hydroxytryptophan (5-HTP), in combination with a peripheral decarboxylase inhibitor, led to amelioration of depression, particularly in patients with low CSF 5-HIAA (Van Praag and de Haan, 1980a, b). Furthermore (some) depressed patients exhibit reduced tryptophan availability in plasma (Maes et al., 1990), reduced increase in plasma 5-HTP after an oral load with L-tryptophan (Deakin et al., 1990) and decreased uptake of 5-HTP across the blood-brain barrier (Agren et al., 1991). These data, too, suggest a defect in the synthesis of 5-HT.

Direct measurement of 5-HT synthetic capacity is presently possible by positron emission tomography (PET), measuring the trapping of the tracer α-[11C]methyl-L-tryptophan (α-MTrp) into the synthesis of 5-HT. α-MTrp is a synthetic analog of L-tryptophan. Its methyl group prevents incorporation of the tracer in protein metabolism, but does not interfere with its incorporation in the synthesis of 5-HT. The rate of trapping of α-MTrp is considered to be an index of 5-HT synthetic capacity (Chugani and Muzig, 2000). Low 5-HT synthesis capacity has been found in impulsive subjects with borderline personality disorder (Leyton et al., 2001) a disorder often complicated by depressive symptoms, as well as in depression in particular in those patients with high impulsivity (Benkelfat et al., 2002).

A polymorphism of the gene expressing tryptophane hydroxylase 2 (TPH2) is deficient in converting tryptophane to 5-hydroxy-tryptophane. This polymorphism is more frequent in depressed patients and their relatives than in controls. It is also p redictive of low CSF 5-HTAA. This suggests a shortage of 5-HT in the CNS (Zhou et al., 2005).

These data combined, point to a central 5-HT deficit in (certain types of) depression. Interestingly, lowering of CSF 5-HIAA in a subgroup of depression, appears to be a trait-related phenomenon: it does not disappear after remission of the depression (Träskman-Bendz et al., 1984; Van Praag, 1977, 1992). Marginal 5-HT production possibly represents a vulnerability factor, increasing the risk of depression in times of mounting stress (Van Praag, 1988). This hypothesis is supported by the finding that treatment with L-5-HTP, has not only therapeutic but likewise prophylactic efficacy in depression, in particular in those with signs of deficient 5-HT metabolism (Van Praag and De Haan, 1980 a, b).

5-HT RECEPTORS AND DEPRESSION

The 5-HT system operates via a great number, at least 15, probably function-specific receptors. They are subdivided in 7 subtypes, named 5-HT₁, 5-HT₂, 5-HT₃ ,5-HT₄ 5-HT₅ 5-HT₆, and 5-HT₇ receptors. The 5-HT₁ receptor family is subdivided into 4 subgroups 5-HT₁A up to 5-HT₁D, the 5-HT₂ family counts 3 subtypes: 5-HT₂A up to 5-HT₂C receptors.

5-HT₁A receptors are located both pre- and postsynaptically. The presynaptic 5-HT₁A receptor is located on the cell bodies and involved in negative feedback regulation of the 5-HT neuron. Its activation leads to reduction of its firing rate. Stimulation of a 5-HTergic nerve cell leads to release of 5-HT not only in the synaptic cleft but also in the region of the cell body. The 5-HT₁D receptor (analogous with the 5-HT₁B receptor in rodents) is also found pre- and postsynaptically. The presynaptic receptor is located on the presynaptic membrane and functions likewise as a "5-HT brake": its activation leads to diminution of 5-HT release.

For years challenge tests were the only way to study 5-HT receptors *in vivo*. In most 5-HT receptor studies indirect 5-HT agonists have been used such as the 5-HT precursors tryptophan and 5-HTP, fenfluramine, a 5-HT releaser and inhibitor of its reuptake (Newman et al., 1998), and selective serotonin re-uptake inhibitors (SSRI's). The secretion of prolactin and adrenocorticotrope hormone (ACTH) by the pituitary gland and of cortisol by the adrenal cortex have been mostly used as serotonergically mediated variables.

Most of those studies reported blunting of the hormonal responses to indirect 5-HT agonists in a subgroup of depression (Ansseau, 1997), indicating down-regulation of 5-HT receptors. The prolactin responses to fenfluramine and to the SSRI's citalopram and clomipramine remain blunted in recovered patients (Bhagwagar et al., 2002; Golden et al., 2002). The cortisol response to citalopram on the other hand does normalize. These findings suggest, that some aspects of impaired 5-HTergic transmission are trait-markers, just as low CSF 5-HIAA is.

Indirect 5-HT agonists act presynaptically and hence increase 5-HT availability throughout the entire 5-HT system. They do not provide information on which of the some 15 different subtypes of 5-HT receptors are actually down regulated. To this end one needs selective and direct agonists (or antagonists) of each of the receptor subtypes. Those are not available for use in humans.

The best studied of the 5-HT receptors is the 5-HT$_{1A}$ receptor, to which I will restrict myself. Challenge tests have been carried out with some azapirone derivatives, i.e., ipsaperone, giperone and buspirone. Those compounds are partial agonists of the 5-HT$_{1A}$ receptor and not very selective ones: their main metabolite 1–phenyl-piperazine, for instance, is also an α_2-adrenergic antagonist (De Vrij, 1995). Blocking of this presynaptically located adrenergic receptor, present on both 5-HTergic and NAergic neurons, could lead to increased 5-HT and NA release and thus contribute to hormonal effects. In addition these drugs activate the dopamine$_2$ (D$_2$) receptor, particularly buspirone.

Several studies reported blunted hormonal responses after an ipsaperone challenge in (a subgroup of) depression as well as attenuation of buspirone-induced hypothermia, suggesting abnormal functioning of the 5-HT$_{1A}$ receptor (Lesch et al., 1990). Blunted hormonal responses to ipsaperone could mean: hyporesponsivity of the postsynaptic 5-HT$_{1A}$ receptor or hyperresponsivity of its presynaptic equivalent. Since, normally, after administration of ipsaperone, the release of hormones like prolactin and cortisol increases, activation of the postsynaptic receptor evidently supersedes that of the presynaptic receptor and hence blunting of the ipsaperone response can be regarded as an indication of down-regulation of the postsynaptic 5-HT$_{1A}$ receptor.

Studies with positron emission tomography (PET) provided direct evidence for 5-HT$_{1A}$ receptor pathology in depression. A widespread reduction in 5-HT$_{1A}$ receptor binding was reported in patients with major depression, both presynaptically in the raphé nuclei – and postsynaptically, i.e., in several cortical regions (Drevets et al., 1999; Sargent et al, 2000). After remission an increase failed to occur. Apparently 5-HT$_{1A}$ receptor disturbances in depression carry trait-character, possibly representing risk factors for depression.

5-HT₁ₐ RECEPTORS AND ANTIDEPRESSANT RESPONSE

If 5-HT$_{1A}$ receptor pathology were to be involved in the pathophysiology of depression, one would expect selective, full, postsynaptic 5-HT$_{1A}$ agonists and presynaptic 5-HT$_{1A}$ antagonists with the same qualifications, to exert antidepressant effects, at least in patients with signs of 5-HT$_{1A}$ receptor pathology (Van Praag, 1996). A (small) number of studies do report antidepressant activity of the azapirone type of partial 5-HT$_{1A}$ agonists (Pecknold, 1994). The same type of drugs exert anxiolytic effects. This dual efficacy is explained by their partial agonistic properties (Olivier et al., 1999). In anxiety states, presumed to be associated with over-stimulation of 5-HT receptors, the azapirones displace 5-HT from the postsynaptic 5-HT$_{1A}$ receptor and thus act as antagonists. In depression, supposedly associated with 5-HT deficiency, the azapirones do not have to compete with 5-HT and act as agonists. The azapirones, however, are not very selective drugs. Highly selective, postsynaptic 5-HT$_{1A}$ agonists have not yet been studied in humans.

The non-selective presynaptic 5-HT$_{1A}$ receptor antagonist pindolol (being also a β-adrenergic blocker) has been shown by some (Blier and Bergeron, 1998), but not all (Berman et al., 1997) authors to speed up and augment the therapeutic effect of SSRI's and some other antidepressants. The variable results are possibly caused by sub-optimal dosages. There is no indication of its therapeutic activity given as monotherapy.

In animal models of depression (particularly the forced swimming test and the learned helplessness test), highly selective 5-HT$_{1A}$ receptor agonists possess antidepressant properties (Mayorga et al., 2001). In addition they exert anti-aggressive and anxiolytic effects (Borsini et al., 1999). Mice lacking the 5-HT$_{1A}$ receptor show increased anxiety (Parks et al., 1998). Several lines of evidence indicate that these are postsynaptic effects. This was most elegantly demonstrated by Gross et al. (2002). They developed a method to knock out and restore the 5-HT$_{1A}$ receptor and demonstrated that anxiety-like behaviour was only produced if 5-HT$_{1A}$ receptors in the forebrain were deleted, but not if their presynaptic counterpart in the raphé nuclei were knocked out.

SSRI's increase neurogenesis in the dentate gyrus and this effect is hypothesized to be associated with their antidepressant potential (Jacobs et al., 2000). In the adult brain neurogenesis continues in two regions: subventricular zone and dentate gyrus (Taupin and Gage, 2002). 5-HT, in addition to some trophic factors, do increase this neurogenesis and for this action the 5-HT$_{1A}$ receptor is required (Banasr et al., 2004; Santarelli et al., 2003).

Thus, various observations point to the 5-HT$_{1A}$ receptor system as a key factor in the therapeutic action of antidepressant drugs.

GENETIC STUDIES

Genetic studies, investigating possible associations between polymorphisms of 5-HT related genes and (components of) the depressive syndrome, have been disappointingly contradictory.

The most promising genetic data pertaining to depression so far concern the gene expressing the 5-HT transporter protein (5-HTT) (Caspi et al., 2003). This gene shows a functional polymorphism in the promoter region; that is, it exists with a long (l) and short (s) allele in the promoter region. Individuals may carry two copies of the l-allele, two of the s-allele or one copy of each. They can be, in other words, homozygous or heterozygous for this length variation. The s-promoter is less active than the l-promoter, resulting in lower levels of 5-HT uptake.

Mice with one or two copies of the s-allele show more intense fearful reactions to stressors than their counterparts with the l-allele(s) (Murphy et al., 2001). Monkeys with the s-allele show decreased levels of CSF 5-HIAA, but only if they were reared in stressful conditions. This phenomenon was absent in normally raised monkeys (Bennett et al., 2002). Humans with one or two copies of the s-allele show, if stressed, more intense activation of the amygdala than individuals with two l-alleles (Hariri et al., 2002).

The tentative conclusion drawn from these data, that polymorphisms of the 5-HTT gene determine in some manner the strength of the stress response was notably strengthened by the data of Caspi et al. (2003). In a prospective study, they showed that individuals with one or two copies of the short allele exhibited more depressive symptoms, more 'case-depression', and more suicidality than individuals homozygous for the l-allele. Moreover they found that abuse as a child predicted depression after the age of 18 only in those individuals with at least one s-allele.

Supporting the conclusions of Caspi et al. (2003) is the observation that the ss and sl alleles are over-represented in individuals who had committed (violent) suicide attempts. The highest rates were found in those who also had a history of major depression (Courtet et al., 2001).

The study of Caspi et al. (2003) is important for two reasons. It provides additional evidence for the involvement of the 5-HT system in the pathophysiology of depression. Secondly, it demonstrates most elegantly, that the impact of environmental stimuli, i.e., adversity, is modulated by genetic factors, i.e. polymorphisms of the 5-HTT gene.

CONCLUSIONS

Several lines of evidence suggest the occurrence of disturbances in 5-HT metabolism in (certain types of) depression. Reducing 5-HT metabolism elicits depressive symptoms, in particular in individuals with a family history of depression, while increasing 5-HT availability exerts antidepressant effects. Hence, disturbances in 5-HT metabolism have probably pathogenic significance rather than being consequences of the depression.

These metabolic disturbances have trait character and are possibly risk factors for depression increasing the risk of depression in times of mounting stress.

Furthermore, disturbances in 5-HT receptors function have been established most notably in the 5-HT$_{1A}$ receptor system. It seems to be down regulated; like the diminution of 5-HT metabolism, in a trait-related manner. Tentative evidence suggests that most antidepressants increase the efficiency of 5-HT$_{1A}$ receptors and that more or less selective 5-HT$_{1A}$ receptor agonists possess antidepressant properties. Dysfunction of the 5-HTT gene, finally, is associated with increased stressor sensitivity and depression vulnerability.

All in all, these data strongly suggest that reduced 5-HT metabolism and 5-HT$_{1A}$ receptor down regulation play a causative role in the occurrence of certain types of depression.

NORADRENALINE

In 1965 Schildkraut suggested a causal relationship between a central NA deficit and depression (Schildkraut, 1965). The so-called NA hypothesis of depression set in motion an avalanche of studies into the functioning of the NA system in depression.

NA METABOLISM

Initially studies of the NA hypothesis have focussed on urinary secretion of NA metabolites. Those studies seemed relevant because vanillylmandelic acid (VMA) was shown to be the major metabolite of NA peripherally while 3-methoxy-4-hydroxyphenylglycol (MHPG) is its major metabolite in the CNS. Renal MHPG thus would reflect to a large degree NA metabolism in the CNS.

These excretion studies have not been very revealing. In unipolar depression urinary MHPG concentration varies over a wide range of values. In bipolar I depressed patients urinary MHPG was found to be reduced, compared with unipolar and bipolar II patients. The low MHPG patients may respond better to antidepressants than patients with high urinary MHPG excretion (Schildkraut, 1965). These findings, however, have not been uniformly confirmed (Janicak et al., 1986). The supposition that urinary MHPG reliably reflects central NA metabolism, moreover, was challenged by Blomberg et al. (1980) who calculated that actually no more than 20% of urinary MHPG is derived from the CNS.

CSF MHPG studies have likewise produced equivocal results. Not surprisingly, because MHPG in lumbar CSF stems mainly from the spinal cord, and only to a minor degree from the brain.

In fact, subsequent studies showed that most data point to an *increase* of CA metabolism in depression, rather than to a decrease, at least in the periphery (Table 1).

Table 1. Data indicative of disturbed NAergic functioning in (a subgroup) of depression

Data indicative of NAergic hypofunctioning	Data indicative of NAergic hyperfunctioning
↓ Urinary MHPG in some patients	↑ Plasma concentration of NA and adrenalin
CA depletion may cause depressive symptoms	↑ Urinary excretion of NA and NA metabolites
CA depletion may cause recurrence in remitted depressed patients	↑ CSF NA concentration around the clock
↓ Arterio-venous NA gradient	
↓ Responsivity of the ß-adrenergic receptor	

The sympatho-adrenal system - comprising the adrenal medulla and the sympathetic nervous system – often shows signs of hyperactivity, such as increased plasma concentration of adrenalin and NA, increased urinary excretion of NA, MHPG and other NA metabolites and around the clock increases in NA concentration in CSF (Potter et al., 1993; Wong et al., 2000).

Sympatho-adrenal activation is an integral component of Cannon's (1929) "fight and flight reaction" and the "general adaptation syndrome" described by Selye (1936). It occurs in many conditions threatening homeostasis; physical (intensive motor activity; illness, such as a myocardial infarction) or mental (stress) in nature. In case of depression it is an important but unresolved question whether this activation relates to depression as such or rather to the emotional turmoil the depression leads to or that preceded the depression (Van Praag et al., 2004).

The approaches mentioned so far have thus produced little evidence that NA metabolism is indeed reduced in depression. A recent study by Lambert et al. (2000) threw new light on this issue. They determined the arterio-venous NA gradient between the vena jugularis interna and the arteria brachialis in depressed patients. They found this gradient to be decreased in depression. This is a strong indication that central NA t u mover may be decreased in depression. This observation awaits confirmation.

CA depletion studies also provide some evidence for reduced CA availability as a pathogenic factor in depression. Neither in normals without a history of major depression nor in depressives did CA depletion cause any (increase in) depressive symptoms (Miller et al., 1996a). Euthymic, medication–free subjects, with a history of major depression, however, did show depressive symptoms after administration of α-methyl-para-tyrosine (α-MPT), an inhibitor of tyrosine hydroxylase, the enzyme that katalyzes the first step in CA syntesis (Berman et al., 1999). Furthermore, CA depletion studies provided evidence for the involvement of CA in the action mechanism of antidepressants. α-MPT administered to depressed patients in remission, caused recurrences in those treated with and improved on NA reuptake inhibitors. This was not the case in those who had responded to SSRI's (Miller et al., 1996b).

NORADRENALINE RECEPTOR STUDIES

NA receptors are subdivided into 3 groups, i.e., α_1, α_2 and β-adrenergic receptors. The α_1 and α_2 groups are subdivided into 4 subtypes, named α_{1A} up to α_{1D} receptors, and α_{2A} up to α_{2D} receptors. The group of β-adrenergic receptors is subdivided into 3 subgroups, i.e. $ß_1$ – $ß_3$ adrenergic receptors.

As far as the adrenergic receptor system is concerned the α_2 and the β-adrenergic receptors have been the main focus of research in depression. α_2-Adrenergic receptors are located both pre- and postsynaptically. The presynaptic receptor mediates a negative feedback system: when stimulated NA release is diminished. The β-receptor is predominantly localized on postsynaptic sites.

The growth hormone response to clonidine has been used to study the functionality of the α_2 receptor. Clonidine is a α_2-receptor agonist, which in the higher dose range predominantly activates the postsynaptic α_2-receptor. Blunting of the growth hormone response, therefore, is understood to be a sign of down-regulation of the α_2-receptor system. This phenomenon was found to occur in depression (Matussek, 1988) and seemed to be trait-related (Siever et al., 1992), i.e., not to disappear after lifting of the depression. However, it has been demonstrated that the growth hormone response is diminished after various MA agonists, such as apomorphine, a dopamine (DA) agonist; amphetamine, a DA and NA agonist, and m-chlorophenylpiperazine (MCPP), a 5-HT agonist (Asnis et al., 1992; Schatzberg and Schildkraut, 1995). Blunting of the growth hormone response, thus, seems to point to a defect in the growth hormone production or release rather than to a specific NA receptor defect.

In low doses clonidine is thought to stimulate predominantly the presynaptic α_2-adrenergic receptor, leading to reduction of NA release. In normal conditions low doses clonidine lower plasma MHPG levels; in depression the decrease is greater than normal. This phenomenon has been interpreted as an indication of hypersensitivity of the presynaptic α_2 receptor. Such condition would lead to a decreased efficiency of NAergic transmission. It has however not been consistently confirmed (Anand and Charney, 1997).

Direct measurement of the α_2 receptor on blood platelets or post mortem in the brain, also produced contradictory results.

The status of the β-adrenergic receptor system in the brain of depressed patients is equally uncertain. Most antidepressants, chronically administered, produce a down-regulation of ß-receptors (Hosada and Duman, 1993). ECT has the same effect. Some selective SSRIs, however, defy this rule (Palvimaki et al., 1994). The inference based on these observations, that in depression the β-adrenergic receptor system might be upregulated, has not been substantiated. The relevant data are controversial. Post-mortem studies of suicide victims yielded contradictory results (Crow et al., 1984; Mann et al., 1986) and the same is true for measuring β receptors in blood platelets and lymphocytes (Healy et al., 1985).

The cortisol response to the NA reuptake inhibitor desipramine is, at least in part, mediated via β-adrenergic receptors. This response has been found blunted in depression (Asnis et al., 1986), a sign of diminished responsivity of the β-receptor. The nocturnal increase in melatonin secretion – considered to be a β-receptor mediated effect because it is blocked by β-blockers – is likewise blunted (Frazer et al., 1986). It cannot be excluded, however, that β-receptor down-regulation is a phenomenon secondary to stress-induced increase of plasma NA.

Down-regulation of the β-receptor system in depression is hard to reconcile with the findings that most antidepressants down-regulate the β-receptor system, assuming that this effect forms part of their mechanism of action.

Be this as it may, different strategies resulted in different conclusions regarding the state of the β-adrenergic receptor system in depression.

CONCLUSIONS

It is clear that NA metabolism may be disturbed in depression. Most data, however, point to an *increase*, conceivably stress-induced; a *decrease* in NA metabolism has not been convincingly demonstrated, though subgroup-specificity hidden by calculating overall measures for major depression (a utterly heterogeneous construct,) remains a distinct possibility. The study by Lambert et al. (2000), reporting reduced arteriovenous NA gradient in depressed individuals, is a notable exception, in that it does suggest reduced NA utilisation in the CNS of depressed individuals.

If a NAergic deficit would indeed play a role in the pathogenesis of depression, one would expect antidepressants to facilitate NAergic transmission. It is, however, by no means clear that this happens. NA reuptake inhibition by TCA's and inhibition of NA degradation through MAOI's indeed lead to a rapid increase of NA availability in NAergic synapses. This, however, cannot be a crucial mechanism because therapeutic effects of antidepressants do not generally occur before two to four weeks of treatment. The effect of most antidepressants and of ECT on adrenergic receptors is one of down-regulation. This holds both for β-receptors and for α_2-receptors. This suggests reduction, rather than an increase in efficiency of NAergic transmission. Receptor down-regulation may be an adaptation to increased NA availability, rather than a primary component of the action mechanism of antidepressants. CA depletion studies, on the other hand, do provide evidence that CA do indeed play a role in the therapeutic activity of antidepressants, at least in those with specific actions on the NAergic system.

The conclusion cannot be other than that the role of NA in the pathogenesis of depression is not yet clear.

DOPAMINE AND DEPRESSION

Dopamine (DA) for many years has been a stepchild of biological depression research. On the one hand this is understandable. TCA's have no or only modest influence on the DA system and, before the introduction of SSRI's, TCA's occupied almost monopoly position in pharmacological depression treatment. Because of side effects MAOI were only used sporadically.

On the other hand the neglect of DA was puzzling. Motor retardation and anhedonia may be prominent symptoms in depression and it became known not long after introduction of the TCA's that dopaminergic (DAergic) neurons are involved in the regulation of motoricity and of reward/motivational systems. This time lag has not yet been completely recovered.

DOPAMINE METABOLISM

In humans homovanillic acid (HVA) is the main degradation product of DA. Most HVA in lumbar CSF originates from the nigrostriatal DA pathways and to a much lesser extent from the mesocorticolimbic DA system and the spinal cord. The explanation is, that the caudate nucleus is a large, DA-rich structure located close to the ventricles.

Several investigators found CSF HVA concentration to be lowered in a subgroup of depressed patient. This appeared to be so for both baseline values and for postprobenecid concentrations (Van Praag and Korf, 1971a; Van Praag et al., 1973; Willner, 1983). In mania levels of CSF HVA were found to be increased (Willner, 1995). The same is true for delusional melancholic depression (Gjerris et al., 1987). Tremblay et al. (2002) found the rewarding effects of dextroamphetamine to be increased in depressive patients, relative to controls. They hypothesized the enhanced response to reflect decreased DAergic output resulting in secondary up-regulation of DA receptors.

DA RECEPTOR STUDIES

DA receptors are divided into two groups: the DA_1 (D1) and DA_2 (D2) receptors. The D1 group is subdivided in two subgroups: the D_1 and D_5 receptors; the D2 group in 3 subgroups: the D_2, D_3 and D_4 receptors. D_3 and D_5 receptors are richly represented in the limbic domain; the D_4 receptor is concentrated in the frontal cortex, midbrain and amygdala. Agonists are available for the D1 and the D2 group, not for each receptor subtype separately. This holds for animal work. For human studies selective D1 and D2 agonists are not yet available.

The D1 and D2 receptors were reported to exert opposite effects on reward systems (Self et al., 1996). In animals, D1 receptor agonists attenuate, D2 receptor agonists augment reward seeking behaviour. Disturbances in reward experiences (translated into the human situation: as anhedonia) could conceivably be related to increased D1 receptor activity or to hypoactivity of the D2 receptor system.

The results of DA receptor studies in depression have not been unequivocal. The growth hormone (GH) response to apomorphine in major depression was reported to be blunted (Ansseau et al., 1988), but these findings were contradicted by earlier reports (Meltzer et al.,1984). Since apomorphine stimulates both pre- and postsynaptic DA receptors (mostly the D_2 type), results with this test are hard to interpret. Challenge tests with other DA agonists, particularly the DA precursor L-dopa, bromocriptine and amphetamine, did not reveal diffe rences between depressed patients and control subjects (Matussek, 1988). Sulpiride a dopamine D_2 receptor antagonist, reportedly caused a significantly greater rise in plasma prolactin levels in depression as compared to controls (Verbeeck et al., 2001); possibly an indication of receptor hypersensitivity secondary to DA deficiency. In a single photon emission tomography (SPECT) study with the $D_{2/3}$ ligand ^{123}I-IBZM, Shah et al. (1997) indeed found indications of increased IBZM binding.

Spontaneous eye blinking – a phenomenon mediated by D_2 receptors – was found to be increased in depressed patients with seasonal affective disorder (Depue et al., 1990). The super-sensitivity of D_2 receptors that this phenomenon suggests, might be secondary to a central DA deficit. In accordance with these findings D 'Haenen and Bossuyt (1994) and Ebert et al. (1996), using SPECT methodology, reported a bilateral increase in D_2 receptors in the basal ganglia. In PET studies this findings could not be re p roduced (Klimek et al., 1999). Using SPECT methodology, Laasonen-Balk et al. (1999) found the density of the DA transporter in the striatum significantly higher in depressed patients than in controls. It was hypothesized that this is a primary phenomenon leading to DA deficiency. The finding that the uptake of DA precursors in the CNS is diminished in depression (Agren and Reibring, 1994)., also points to a DA shortage.

CONCLUSIONS

CSF HVA, indicator of DA metabolism in the (nigro-striatal) DA system may be reduced in depression. The evidence for that is quite firm. Receptor studies, on the other hand, are controversial and no conclusive evidence exist of disturbed DA recep-tor function in depression. One has to take into account, however, that selective agonists for the various subtypes of DA receptors are wanting and that dopamine D_1 and D_2 receptors supposedly exert opposite effects, at least in the mesolimbic and mesocortical systems. Hence one has to have the disposal of truly selective receptor agonists to sort out whether and which DA receptors might be dysfunctional in depression.

Present-days antidepressants lack pronounced effects on DAergic transmission. Hence they cannot provide evidence in favour or against involvement of the DA system in the pathophysiology of depression.

BEHAVIORAL CORRELATES OF THE MONOAMINERGIC DISTURBANCES IN DEPRESSION

Disturbances in MA metabolism and MA receptor functioning are by no means characteristic for depression as such, but only demonstrable in subgroups of depression. It became apparent that these subgroups do not coincide with any of the depressive subcategories being distinguished in the present classification of the Diagnostic and Statistical Manual of the American Psychiatric Association (1994) nor with any syndromal category presently distinguished (Van Praag et al., 1987, 1990).

Much evidence indicates that MAergic disturbances are not so much associated with syndromes or categorically defined disorders, but with disturbances in the regulation of particular psychic functions (Table 2). In other words they were shown to be *functionally specific* rather than nosologically or syndromally specific (Van Praag et al., 1987). Low CSF 5-HIAA, indicator of diminished central 5-HT metabolism, appeared to be correlated with heightened anxiety as well as with disturbed aggression regulation. The latter may become manifest in suicidal behaviour and/or in various manifestations of increased outward directed aggression such as irritability, anger outbursts, and violence against others (Linnoila et al., 1983; Van Praag et al., 1990). These relationships were not only demonstrable in depression but in other diagnostic categories as well. They seemed to occur independent of nosological diagnosis (Van Praag et al., 1987).

Table 2. Behavioral correlates of MA-ergic disturbances in depression

	(Auto) aggressivity	Anxiety	Vigilance	Apathy	Motor-retardation	Cognition disturbances
↓ 5-HT1A	X	X				X
↑ 5-HT2C		X				
↓ DA metabolism				X	X	
↓ NA metabolism				X	X	X
↑ NA metabolism		X	X			

A relation of 5-HT metabolism/suicidality was confirmed by Oquendo et al. (2003) who studied regional brain 5-HTergic function in depressed patients with a history of high-lethality suicide attempts. They found glucose uptake to be decreased in the (ventromedial) prefrontal cortex, relative to controls and low-lethality depressed suicide attempters. This effect was most pronounced after administration of fenfluramine, a compound facilitating 5-HT release and inhibiting its re-uptake.

Tryptophan depletion in normal individuals provokes aggressive impulses in those who had high aggression scores to begin with (Cleare and Bond, 1995). Tryptophan administration, on the other hand, enhances the ability to participate productively in group-related tasks, to display, in other words, affiliative behaviours (Moskowitz et al., 2001).

The blunting of the prolactin response to d-fenfluramine in depression is significantly correlated with the level of state anxiety, not with the severity of the depression (O'Keane and Dinan, 1991). A significant correlation has also been established between blunting of the prolactin response to fenfluramine and suicidal behaviour (Corrêa et al., 2000). In depressed patients a positive correlation has been found between cortex 5-HT$_2$ receptor binding potential (a variable proportional to receptor density and affinity) and dysfunctional attitudes (Meyer et al., 2003). Dysfunctional attitudes were defined as negatively biased views of oneself, the world, and the future.

Lowered CSF HVA, indicator of reduced DA metabolism in (at least certain parts of) the CNS, was shown to correlate with motor retardation (Van Praag and Korf, 1971a,b). Increased IBZM binding in the striatum as observed in depression was also correlated with signs of motor retardation (Shah et al., 1997). PET studies revealed a decrease of [18 F] DOPA in the caudate nucleus in retarded depression, particularly on the left side, observations likewise suggestive for a link between DA hypofunction and psychomotor retardation.

Low CSF HVA appeared not to be restricted to retarded depression but to occur also in other diagnostic categories with motor retardation, such as in Parkinson's disease and certain forms of schizophrenia (Van Praag et al., 1973; Willner, 1995). In accordance with these observations, L-dopa administered in depression exerted activating effects, particularly in low CSF HVA patients, while mood was not significantly altered (Van Praag, 1974). Antidepressants with pronounced DA potentiating effects, moreover, are most potent in retarded depression (Brown and Gerston, 1993).

A relationship between low CSF HVA and anhedonia has not been demonstrated. This is not surprising because HVA concentration in lumbar CSF is largely a reflection of DA metabolism in the nigro-striatal DA system (a predominantly motor regulating system) and not of activity in the mesolimbic and mesocortical DA system, which are considered to be involved in affective pathology.

The behavioural correlates of the NAergic disturbances are complex. Hyperactivity of this system leads first of all to arousal, increased vigilance and ultimately to anxiety. In addition cognitive changes appear. Hippocampal function is switched from a state of lowered memory formation to a state of enhanced stimulus detection and encoding when aroused with novelty or stressed with aversion (Ressler and Nemeroff, 2000). NAergic over-activity, thus, will result in excess hippocampal functioning in the stressed/aroused state, with enhanced or oversensitive memory to aversive stimuli (Mongeau et al., 1997). The NA system, moreover, facilitates the relay of adverse memories from temporary to long term storage (Van Praag et al., 2004).

NAergic hypoactivity, as seems likely to occur in some depressed patients, has been hypothesized to be linked to deficits in "emotional memory" (Van Praag et al., 1990). Perception in these patients is undisturbed but they are unable to link perceptions to the corresponding emotions. For instance, a patient goes to church, but it does not touch him anymore, while previously such visits used to evoke a sense of devotion. These hypotheses are supported by the studies of O'Carroll et al. (1999), demonstrating that, in humans, stimulation of the NAergic system results in enhancement, and blockade of this system in a reduction of recall and recognition of emotional material.

The cognitive effects of 5-HTergic stimulation are opposite to those of NAergic activation. It leads to decreased learning of aversive stimuli and an increase in tolerance toward aversive experiences (O'Carroll et al., 1999). A deficit in 5-HTergic "tone" will thus reinforce the anxiety / frustration proneness resulting from NAergic over-activity. Since the locus coeruleus (LC) (being the major locus of NAergic neurons) and raphé nuclei (the major loci of 5-HTergic neurons) are anatomically interconnected and on a functional level mutually inhibitory, activation of the LC system will induce inhibition of the raphé-system, thus further enhancing the cognitive effects of NAergic dominance.

All in all, MAergic disturbances seem to be function-specific. Since psychic dysfunctions are seldom specific for a particular syndrome or nosological entity, it is understandable that the corresponding biological variables, too, are nosologically and syndromally non-specific. By the same token it is explicable that MAergic disturbances are demonstrable only in some depressive patients, for the corresponding behavioural variables can be pronounced in one patient and subordinate in the other. In the former case, the MAergic disturbances are expected to be present, in the latter case to be absent.

CONCLUSIONS

The data collected over the past 45 years, collectively, constitute strong evidence that MAergic disturbances are involved in the pathophysiology of certain mood disorders, or, more accurately in the pathophysiology of some psychopathological features that may or may not be pronounced in depression. They correlate with psychic dysfunctions, are in other words *functionally specific*, rather than syndromally or nosologically specific.

Broadly speaking, most data pertaining to 5-HT and DA point to functional deficits, while those related to the NAergic system are mixed. Some indicate NAergic overdrive, while others are suggestive of hypoactivity of that system. As to the 5-HT system, both metabolic and receptor disturbances have been ascertained. The 5-HT$_1$ receptor system seems to be particularly involved. Since the 5-HT disturbances precede a depressive episode and pharmacological interventions geared towards amelioration of the 5-HT disturbances produce antidepressant effects, it seems likely that the 5-HT disturbances may play a role in the pathophysiology of depression. It has been hypothesized that they represent vulnerability factors that increase the risk of affective disturbances in times of mounting stress.

The disturbances in the CA systems are more likely to be state-related, but available evidence is insufficient for definitive statements. .

To disclose functional specificity of biological variables the categorical way of diagnosing, common in present-day's psychiatry, is insufficient. It should be complemented with functional analysis of the psychiatric condition. Functional analysis implies 1) dissection of the syndrome(s) in its (their) component parts, i.e., the symptoms, and 2) analysis of the psychic dysfunctions underlying the psychopathological symptoms. We have named this approach functional psychopathology (Van Praag, 1997).

The relationship between MAergic disturbances and mood disorders, of course, does not exclude causal involvement of other biological systems. The CRH/cortisol and substance P systems, for instance, are serious candidates. Both interact with MAergic systems. It is uncertain whether MA pathology drives the other systems or vice versa.

The yield of MA research in depression has been considerable. It threw light on the pathophysiology of depression and has opened ways for goal-directed search for new antidepressant agents.

SUMMARY

In biological depression research MA studies have occupied central position for more than 40 years. This paper reviews its yield over the years. It is considered to be considerable, and of great practical significance. Yet, we have to proceed, both psychopathologically - 'functionalizing' our diagnostic system - and biologically, studying non-MAergic systems in their own right and in the way they interact with MA. There remains a lot to be elucidated.

Partly derived from a chapter in: H.M. van Praag, R. de Kloet, J. van Os, Stress, the Brain and Depression. Cambridge: Cambridge University Press, 2004, and in: Historia de la Psicofarmacología, edited by F. López-Muñoz, 2006, Editorial Médica Panamericana. To be published.

REFERENCES
1. Agren, H., Reibring, L., 1994. PET studies of presynaptic monoamine metabolism in depressed patients and healthy volunteers. Pharmacopsychiat. 27, 2-6.
2. Agren, H., Reibring, L., Hartvig, P., Tedroff, J., Bjurling, P., Hornfeldt, K., et al., 1991. Low brain uptake of L [¹¹C]5-hydroxytryptophan in major depression: a positron emis-

sion tomography study on patients and healthy volunteers. Acta Psychiat. Scand. 83, 449-455.

3. American Psychiatric Association, 1994. Diagnostic and Satistical Manual of Mental Disordesr. American Psychiatric Association, Washington.

4. Anand, A., Charney, D.S., 1997. Catecholamines in depression. In: Honig, A., Van Praag, H.M. (Eds.), Depression. Neurobiological, Psychopathological and Therapeutic Advances. Chichester: John Wiley, Chichester, pp. 147-178.

5. Ansseau, M., 1997. Hormonal disturbances in depression. In: Honig, A., Van Praag, H.M. (Eds.), Depression. Neurobiological, Psychopathological and Therapeutic Advances. John Wiley, Chichester, pp. 235-250.

6. Ansseau, M., Von Frenckell, R., Cerfontaine, J.L., Papart, P., Franck, G., Timsit-Berthier, M., et al., 1988. Blunted response of growth hormone to clonidine and apomophine in endogenous depression. Brit. J. Psychiat. 153, 65-71.

7. Asberg, M., Thorén, P., Träskman, L., Bertilsson, L., Ringbergen, V., 1976. Serotonin depression – a biochemical subgroup within the affective disorders. Science 191, 478-480.

8. Asnis, G.M., Halbreich, U., Rabinovich, H, Ryan, N.D., Sacher, E.J., Nelson, B., Puig-Antich, Y., Novacenko, H., et al., 1986. The cortisol response to desipramine in endogenous depressives and normal controls: preliminary findings. Psychiat. Res. 14, 225-233.

9. Asnis, G.M., Wetzler, S., Sanderson, W.C., Kahn, R.S., Van Praag, H.M., 1992. Functional interrelationship of serotonin and norepinephrine: cortisol response to MCPP and DMI in patients with panic disorder, patients with depression and normal control subjects. Psychiat. Res. 43, 65-76.

10. Banasr, M., Hery, M., Printemps, R., Daszuta, A., 2004. Serotonin-induced increases in adult cell proliferation and neurogenensis are mediated through different and common 5-HT receptor subtypes in the dentate gyrus and the subventricular zone. Neuropsychopharmacol. 29, 450-460.

11. Benkelfat, C., Ellenbogen, M., Dean, P., Palmour, R, Young, S., 1994. Mood-lowering effect of tryptophan depletion. Enhanced susceptibility in young men at genetic risk for major affective disorders. Arch. Gen. Psychiat. 51, 687-697.

12. Benkelfat, C., Young, S.N., Leyton, M., Diksic, M., 2002. Impulsivity: serotonergic mechanisms. Int. J. Neuropsychopharm. 5 (Suppl. I), S13 –S15.

13. Bennett, A.J., Lesch, K.P., Heils, A., Long, J.C., Lorenz, J.G., Shoaf, S.E., Champoux, M., Suomi, S.Y., Linnoila, M. V., Higley, Y. D., 2002. Early experience and serotonin transporter gene variation interact to influence primate CNS function. Mol. Psychiat.7, 118-122.

14. Berman, R.M., Darnell, A.M., Miller, H.L., Anand, R.A., Charney, P.S., 1997. Effect of pindolol in hastening response to fluoxetine in the treatment of major depression: a double blind, placebo controlled trial. Am. J. Psychiat.154, 37-43.

15. Berman, R.M., Narasimhan, M., Miller, H.L., Anand, A., Cappiello, A., Oren, D.A., Heninger, R., Charney, D. S., 1999. Transient depressive relapse induced by catecholamine depletion. Arch. Gen. Psychiat. 56, 395-403.

16. Bhagwagar, Z., Whale, R., Cowen, P.J., 2002. State and trait abnormalities in serotonin function in major depression. Brit. J. Psychiat. 180, 24-28.

17. Blier, P., Bergeron, R., 1998. The use of pindolol to potentiate antidepressant medication. J. Clin. Psychiat. 59, 16-23.

18. Blier, P., de Montigny, C., 1994. Current advances and trends in the treatment of depression. Trends Pharm. Sci. 15, 220-226.

19. Blomberg, P.A., Kopin, I.J., Grodon, E.K., Markey, S.P., Ebert, M.H., 1980. Conversion of MHPG to vanillylmandelic acid. Arch. Gen. Psychiat. 37, 1095-1098.

20. Borsini, F., Brambilla, A., Grippa. N., Pitsikas, N., 1999. Behavioral effects of flibanserin (BIMT 17). Pharmacol. Biochem. Behav. 64, 137-146.

21. Brown, A.S., Gerston, S., 1993. Dopamine and depression. J. Neural. Transm. 91, 75-109.

22. Cannon, W.B., 1929. Body changes in pain, hunger, fear, and rage. Appleton, New York.

23. Caspi, A., Sugden, K., Moffitt, T., Taylor, A., Craig, I.W., Harrington, H., McClay, Y., Mill, Y., Martin, Y., Braith-Waite, A., Poulton, R., 2003. Influence of life stress on depression : moderation by a polymorphism in the 5-HTT gene. Science 301, 386-389.

24. Chugani, D.C., Muzig, O., 2000. a-[^{11}C]methyl-l-tryptophan PET maps brain serotonin synthesis and kynurenine pathway metabolism. J. Cereb. Blood Flow Metab. 20, 2-9.

25. Cleare, A.J., Bond, A.J., 1995. The effect of tryptophan depletion and enhancement on subjective and behavioural aggression in normal male subjects. Psychopharmacol. 118, 72-81.
26. Coppen, A.J., 1967. The biochemistry of affective disorders. Brit. J. Psychiat. 113, 1237-1264.
27. Corrêa, H., Duval, F., Mokrani, M.C., Bailey, P., Trémeau, F., Staner, L., 2000. Prolactin response to D-fenfluramine and suicidal behaviour in depressed patients. Psychiat. Res. 93, 189-199
28. Courtet, P., Baud, P., Abbar, M., Boulenger, J.P., Castelnau, D., Mouthon, D., Malafasse, A., Buresi, C., 2001. Association between violent suicidal behavior and the low activity allele of the serotonin transporter gene. Mol. Psychiat. 6, 338-341.
29. Crow, T.J., Cross, A.J., Cooper, S.J., Deakin, J.F., Ferrier, I.N., Johnson, J.A., et al., 1984. Neurotransmitter receptors and monoamine metabolites in the brains of patients with Alzheimer-type dementia and depression, and suicides. Neuropharmacol. 23, 1561-1569.
30. Deakin, J.F.W., Pennell, I., Upadhyaya, A.J., Lofthouse, R., 1990. A neuroendocrine study of 5-HT function in depression: evidence for biological mechanisms of endogenous and psychosocial causation. Psychopharmacol. 101, 85-92.
31. D'Haenen, H., Bossuyt, A., 1994. Dopamine D_2 receptors in the brain measured with SPECT. Biol. Psychiat. 35, 128-132.
32. Delgado, P.L., Charney, D.S., Price, L.H., Landis, H., Heninger, G.R., 1990. Neuroendocrine and behavioural effects of dietary tryptophan restriction in healthy subjects. Life Sci. 45, 2323-2332.
33. Delgado, P., Moreno, F., 2000. Role of norepinephrine in depression. J. Clin. Psychiat. 61 (Suppl), 5-12.
34. Depue, R.A., Arbisi, P., Krauss, S., Iacono, W.G., Leon, A., Muir, R., et al., 1990. Seasonal independence of low prolactin concentration and high spontaneous eye blink rates in unipolar and bipolar II seasonal affective disorder. Arch. Gen. Psychiat. 47, 356-364.
35. De Vrij, J., 1995. 5-HT$_{1A}$ agonists: recent developments and controversial issues. Psychopharmacol. 121, 1-32.
36. Drevets, W.C., Frank, E., Price, J.C., Kupfer, D.J., Holt, D., Greer, P.J., et al., 1999. PET imaging of Serotonin$_{1A}$ receptor binding in depression. Biol. Psychiat. 46, 1375-1387.
37. Ebert, D., Feistel, H., Loew, T., Pimer, A., 1996. Dopamine and depression – striatal dopamine D_2 receptor SPECT before and after antidepressant therapy. Psychopharmacol. 126: 91-94.
38. Frazer, A., Brown, R., Kocsis, J., Caroff, S., Amsterdam, J., Winokur, A., 1986. Patterns of melatonin rhythms in depression. J. Neural. Transm. 67, 215-224.
39. Gjerris, A., Werdelin, L., Rafaelson, O.J., Ailing, C., Christensen, N.J., 1987. CSF dopamine increased in depression: CSF dopamine, noradrenalin and their metabolites in depressed patients and in controls. J. Affect. Disord. 13, 279-286.
40. Golden, R.N., Durr Heine, A., Ekstrom, R.D., Bebchuk, J.M., Leatherman, M.E., Garbutt, J.C., 2002. A longitudinal study of serotonergic function in depression. Neuropsychopharmacol. 26, 653-659.
41. Gross, C., Zhuang, X., Stark, K., Ramboz, S., Oosting, R., Kirby, L. et al., 2002. Serotonin$_{1A}$ receptor acts during development to establish normal anxiety-like behavior in the adult. Nature 416, 396-400.
42. Hariri, A.R., Mattay, V.S., Tessitore, A., Kolachana, B., Fera, F., Goldman, D., et al., 2002. Serotonin transporter genetic variation and the response of the human amygdala. Science 297, 400-403.
43. Healy, D., Carney, P.A., O'Halloran, A., Leonard, B.E., 1985. Perpheral adrenoceptors and serotonin receptors in depression: changes associated with response to treatment with trazodone or amitriptyline. J. Affect. Disord. 9, 285-296.
44. Hosada, K., Duman, R.S., 1993. Regulation of β_1-adrenergic receptor mRNA and ligand binding by antidepressant treatment and norepinephrine depletion in rat frontal cortex. J. Neurochem. 60, 1335-1343.
45. Jacobs, B.L., Van Praag, H.M., Gage, F.H., 2000. Adult brain neurogenesis and psychiatry: a novel theory of depression. Mol. Psychiat. 5, 262-269.
46. Janicak, P.G., Davis, J.M., Chan, C., Altman, E., Hedeker, D., 1986. Failure of urinary MHPG levels to predict treatment response in patients with unipolar depression Am. J. Psychiat. 143, 1398-1402.

47. Klaassen, T., Riedel, W.J., Van Someren, A., Deutz, N.E.P., Honig, A., Van Praag, H.M., 1999. Mood effects of 24-hour tryptophan depletion in healthy first-degree relatives of patients with affective disorders. Biol. Psychiat. 46, 489-497.

48. Klimek, V., Rajkowska, G., Luker, B.S., Dilley, G., Meltzer, H.J., Overholser, J.C., et al., 1999. Brain noradrenergic receptors in major depression and schizophrenia. Neuropsychopharm. 21, 69-81.

49. Korf, J., Van Praag, H.M., 1971. Amine metabolism in the human brain: further evaluation of the probenecid test. Brain Res. 35, 221-230.

50. Laasonen-Balk, T., Kuikka, J., Viinamäki, H., Husso-Saastamoinen, M., Lehtonen, J., Tiihoen, J., 1999. Striatal dopamine transporter density in major depression. Psychopharmacol. 144, 282-285.

51. Lambert, G., Johansson, M., Ågren, H., Firberg, P., 2000. Reduced brain norepinephrine and dopamine release in treatment-refractory depressive illness. Arch. Gen. Psychiat. 57, 787-793.

52. Lesch, K.P., Mayer, S., Disselkamp-Tietze, J., Hoh, A., Wiesmann, M., Osterheider, M., Schulte, H. M., 1990. 5-HT$_{1A}$ receptor responsivity in unipolar depression evaluation of ipsapirone-induced ACTH and cortisol secretion in patients and controls. Biol. Psychiat. 28, 620-628.

53. Leyton, M., Okazawa, H., Diksic, M., Paris, J., Rosa, P., Mzangeza, S., Young, S. N., Blier, P., Benkelfat, C., 2001. Brain regional α-[^{11}C]methyl-l-tryptophan trapping in impulsive subjects with borderline personality disorder. Am. J. Psychiat. 158, 775-782.

54. Linnoila, M., Virkkunen, M., Scheinin, M., Nuutila, A., Rimon, R., Goodwin, F.K., 1983. Low cerebrospinal fluid 5-hydroxyindoleacetic acid concentration differentiates impulsive from nonimpulsive violent behaviour. Life Sci. 33, 2609-2619.

55. Maes, M., Jacobs, M.P., Suy, E., Minner, B., Leclercq, C., Christiaens, F., Raus, J., 1990. Suppressant effects of dexamethasone on the availability of plasma l-tryptophan and tyrosin in healthy controls and in depressed patients. Acta Psychiat. Scand. 81, 19-23.

56. Mann, J.J., Stanley, M., McBride, P.A., McEwen, B.S., 1986. Increased serotonin$_2$ and β- adrenergic receptor binding in the frontal cortex of suicide victims. Arch. Gen. Psychiat. 43, 954-959.

57. Matussek, N., 1988. Catecholamines and mood: neuroendocrine aspects. Current Topics Neuroendocrinol. 8, 145-182.

58. Mayorga, A., Dalvi, A., Page, M., Zimov-Levinson, S., Hen, R., Lucki, I., 2001. Antidepressant-like behavioural effects in 5-hydroxytryptamine$_{1A}$ and 5-hydroxytryptamine$_{1B}$ receptor mutant mice. J. Pharmacol. Exper. Ther. 298, 1101-1107.

59. Meltzer, H.Y., Kolakowska, T., Fang, V.S., Fogg, L., Robertson, A., Lewine, R., et al., 1984. Growth hormone and prolactin response to apomorphine in schizophrenia and major affective disorders: relation to duration of illness and affective symptoms. Arch. Gen. Psychiat. 41, 512-519.

60. Meyer, J.H., McMain, S., Kennedy, S.H., Korman, L., Brown, G.M., DaSilva, J.N., 2003. Dysfunctional attitudes and 5-HT$_2$ receptors during depression and self-harm. Am. J. Psychiat. 160, 90-99.

61. Mignot, E., Seffano, A., Laude, D., Elghozi, J.L., Dedek, J., Scatton, B., 1985. Measurement of 5-HIAA levels in ventricular CSF (by LCEC) and in striatum (by in vivo voltametry) during pharmacological modification of serotonin metabolism in the rat. J. Neural. Transm. 62, 117-124.

62. Miller, H.L., Delgado P.L., Salomon, R.M., Heninger, G.R., Charney, D.S., 1996a. Effects of AMPT in drug free depressed patients. Neuropsychopharmacol. 14, 151-157.

63. Miller, H.L., Delgado, P.L., Salomon, R.M., Heninger, G.R., Charney, D.S., 1996b. Clinical and biochemical effects of catecholamine depletion on antidepressant-induced remission of depression. Arch. Gen. Psychiat. 53, 117-128.

64. Moja, E., Cipolla, P., Castoldi, D., Tofanetti, O., 1989. Dose-response decrease in plasma tryptophan and in brain tryptophan and serotonin after tryptophan-free amino acid mixtures in rats. Life sci. 44, 971-976.

65. Mongeau, R., Blier, P., De Montigny, C., 1997. The serotonergic and noradrenergic systems of the hippocampus: their interactions and the effects of antidepressant treatments. Brain Res. Rev. 23, 145-195.

66. Moreno, F.A., Heninger, G.R., McGahuey, C.A., Delgado, P.L., 2000, Tryptophan depletion and risk of depression relapse: a prospective study of tryptophan depletion as a potential predictor of depressive episodes. Biol. Psychiat. 48, 327-329.

67. Moskowitz, D.S., Pinard, G., Zaroff, D.C., Annable, L., Young, S.H., 2001. The effect of tryptophan on social interaction in everyday life: a placebo controlled study. Neuropsychopharmacol. 25: 277-289.
68. Murphy, D.L., Li, Q., Engel, S., Wichems, C., Andrews, A., Lesch, K.P., et al., 2001. Genetic perspectives on the serotonin transporter. Brain Res. Bull. 56, 487-494.
69. Newman, M.E., Shapiro, B., Lerer, B., 1998. Evaluation of central serotonergic function in affective and related disorders by the fenfluramine challenge test: a critical review. Int. J. Neuropsychopharmacol.1, 49-69.
70. O'Carroll, R.E., Drysdale, E., Cahill, L., Shajahan, P., Ebmeier, K.P., 1999.. Stimulation of the noradrenergic system enhances and blockade reduces memory for emotional material in man. Psychol. Med. 29, 1083-1088.
71. O'Keane, V., Dinan, T.G., 1991. Prolactin and cortisol responses to δ-fenfluramine in major depression: evidence for diminished responsivity of central serotonergic function. Am. J. Psychiat. 148, 1009-1015.
72. Olivier, B., Soudijn, W., Van Wijngaarden, I., 1999. The 5-HT$_{1A}$ receptor and its ligands: structure and function. Progr. Drug Res. 52, 104-165.
73. Oquendo, M.A., Placidi, G.P.A., Malone, K.M., Campbell, C., Keilp, J., Brodsky, B., Kegeles, L. S., Cooper, T. B., Parsey, R. V., Van Heertum, R. L., Mann, Y. J., 2003. Positron emission tomography of regional brain metabolic responses to a serotonergic challenge and lethality of suicide attempts in major depression. Arch. Gen. Psychiat. 60, 14-22.
74. Palvimaki, E.P., Laakso, A., Kuoppamaki, M., Sylvalahti, E., Hietala, J., 1994. Up-regulation of β$_1$-adrenergic receptors in rat brain after chronic citalopram and fluoxetine treatments. Psychopharmacol. 115, 543-546.
75. Parks, C., Robinson, P., Sibille, E., Shenk, Th., Toth, M., 1998. Increased anxiety of mice lacking the serotonin$_{1A}$ receptor. Proc. Natl. Acad. Sci. USA 95, 10734-10739.
76. Pecknold, J.C., 1994. Serotonin 5-HT$_{1A}$ agonists a comparative review. CNS drugs 2, 235-251.
77. Potter, W.Z., Grossman, F., Rudorfer, M.V., 1993. Noradrenergic function in depressive disorders. In: Mann, J.J., Jupter, D.J. (Eds.), Biology of Depressive Disorders, Part A: A Systems Perspective. Plenum Press, New York, pp. 1-27.
78. Ressler, K.J., Nemeroff, Ch.B., 2000. Role of serotonergic and noradrenergic systems in the pathophysiology of depression and anxiety disorders. Depression and Anxiety 12, 2-19.
79. Santarelli, L, Saxe, M., Gross, C., Surget, A., Battaglia, F., Dulawa, S., et al., 2003. Requirement of hippocampal neurogenesis for the behavioral effects of antidepressants. Science 301, 805-809.
80. Sargent, P.A., Husted, Kjaer, K., Bench, Chr. J., Rabiner, E.A., Messa, C., Meyer, J., Gunn, Y., Grasley, P. M., Cowen, Ph. Y., 2000. Brain serotonin$_{1A}$ receptor binding measured by positron emission tomography with [^{11}C]WAY-100635. Effects of depression and antidepressant treatment. Arch. Gen. Psychiat. 57, 174-180.
81. Schatzberg, A.F., Schildkraut, J.J., 1995. Recent studies on norepinephrine systems in mood disorders. In: Bloom, F.E., Kupfer, D.J., (Eds,), Psychopharmacology: The Fourth Generation of Progress. Raven Press, New York, pp. 911-920.
82. Schildkraut, J.J., 1965. The catecholamine hypothesis of affective disorders: a review of supporting evidence. Am. J. Psychiat. 122, 509-522.
83. Self, D.W., Barnhart, W.J., Lehman, D.A., Nestler, E.J., 1996. Opposite modulation of cocaine-seeking behaviour by D$_1$- and D$_2$-like dopamine receptor agonist. Science 271, 1586-1589
84. Selye, H., 1936. Syndrome produced by nocuous agents. Nature138, 32-33.
85. Shah, P.J., Ogilvie, A.D., Goodwin, G.M., Ebmeier, K.P., 1997. Clinical and psychometric correlates of dopamine D$_2$ binding in depression. Psychol. Med. 27, 1247-1256.
86. Siever, L.J., Trestman, R.L., Coccaro, E.F., Bernstein, D., Gabriel, S.M., Owen, K., et al., 1992. The growth hormone response to clonidine in acute and remitted depressed male patients. Neuropsychopharmacol. 1992. 6, 165-177.
87. Stanley, M., Traskman, L., Dorovine, K., 1985. Correlation between animergic metabolites simultaneously obtained from human CSF and brain. Life Sci. 37, 1279-1286.
88. Taupin, P., Gage, F.H., 2002. Adult neurogenesis and neural stem cells of the central nervous system in mammals. J. Neurosci. Res. 69, 745-749.

89. Träskman-Bendz, L., Åsberg, M., Bertilsson, L., Thorén, P., 1984. CSF monoamine metabolites of depressed patients during illness and after recovery. Acta Psychiat. Scand. 69, 333-342.

90. Tremblay, L.K., Naranjo, C.A., Cardenas, L., Herrmann, N., Busto, U.E.. 2002. Probing brain reward system function in major depressive disorder. Arch. Gen. Psychiat. 59, 409-416.

91. Van Praag, H.M., 1962. A critical investigation of the significance of monoamine oxidase inhibition as a therapeutic principle in the treatment of depression (dissertation). University of Utrecht, Utrecht.

92. Van Praag, H.M.,. 1974. Towards a biochemical typology of depressions. Pharmacopsychiat. 7, 281-292.

93. Van Praag, H.M., 1977. Significance of biochemical parameters in the diagnosis, treatment and prevention of depressive disorders. Biol. Psychiat. 12, 101-131.

94. Van Praag, H.M., 1988. Serotonergic mechanisms and suicidal behavior. Psychiat. Psychobiol. 3, 335-346.

95. Van Praag, H.M., 1992. About the centrality of mood lowering in mood disorders. Eur. Neuropsychopharmacol. 2, 393-404.

96. Van Praag, H.M., 1996. Faulty cortisol/serotonin interplay, psychopathological and biological characterisation of a new hypothetical depression subtype (SeCa depression). Psychiat. Res. 65, 143-157.

97. Van Praag, H.M., 1997. Over the mainstream: diagnostic requirements for biological psychiatric research. Psychiat. Res. 72, 201-212.

98. Van Praag, H.M., De Haan, S., 1980a. Central serotonin deficiency. A factor which increases depression vulnerability? Acta Psychiat. Scand. 61, 89-95.

99. Van Praag, H.M., De Haan, S., 1980b. Depression vulnerability and 5-hydroxytryptophan prophylaxis. Psychiat. Res.3, 75-83.

100. Van Praag, H.M., Korf, J., 1971a. Endogenous depressions with and without disturbances in 5-hydroxytryptamine metabolism: a biochemical classification? Psychopharmacol. 19, 148-152.

101. Van Praag, H.M., Korf, J., 1971b. Retarded depression and dopamine metabolism. Psychopharmacol. 19, 199-203.

102. Van Praag, H.M., Korf, J., Puite, J., 1970. 5-Hydroxyindoleacetic acid levels in the cerebrospinal fluid of depressive patients treated with probenecid. Nature 225, 1259-1260.

103. Van Praag, H.M., Korf, J., Schut, T., 1973. Cerebral monoamines and depression. An investigation with the probenecid technique. Arch. Gen. Psychiat. 28, 827-831.

104. Van Praag, H.M., Kahn, R., Asnis, G.M., Wetzler, S., Brown, S., Bleich, A., Korn, M., 1987. Denosologization of biological psychiatry of the specificity of 5-HT disturbances in psychiatric disorders. J. Affect. Disord. 13, 1-8.

105. Van Praag, H.M., Asnis, G.M., Kahn, R.S., Brown, S.L., Kron, M., Harkavy, Wetzker, S., 1990. Monoamines and abnormal behavior. A multi-aminergic perspective. Brit. J. Psychiat. 157, 723-734.

106. Van Praag, H.M., De Kloet, R., Van Os, J., 2004. Stress, the Brain and Depression. Cambridge, University Press, Cambridge.

107. Verbeeck, W.J.C., Berk, M., Paiker, J., Jersky, B., 2001. The prolactin response to sulpiride in major depression: the role of the D_2 receptor in depression. Euro. Neuropyschopharmacol. 11, 215-220.

108. Williams, W.A., Shoaf, S.E., Hommer, D., Rawlings, R., Linnoila, M., 1999. Effects of acute tryptophan depletion on plasma and cerebrospinal fluid tryptophan and 5-hydroxyindoleacetic acid in normal volunteers. J. Neurochem. 72, 1641-1647.

109. Willner, P., 1983. Dopamine and depression: a review of recent evidence. Brain Res. Rev. 6, 211-246.

110. Willner, P., 1995. Dopaminergic mechanism in depression and mania. In: Bloom, F.E., Kupfer, D.J., (Eds.), Psychopharmacology - The Fourth Generation of Progress. Raven Press, New York, pp. 921-930.

111. Wong, M.H., Saam, J.R., Stappenbeck, T.S., Rexer, C.H., Gordon, J.I., 2000. Genetic mosaic analysis based on Cre recombinase and navigated laser capture microdissection. Proc. Natl. Acad. Sci. USA. 97, 12601-12606.

112. Woolley, D.W., Shaw, E., 1954. A biochemical suggestion about certain mental disorders. Proc.Nat. Acad. Sci. 40, 228-231.
113. Young, S., Smith, S., Pihl, R., Ervin, F., 1985. Tryptophan depletion causes rapid lowering of mood in normal males. Psychopharmacol. 87, 173-177.
114. Zhou, Z., Roy, A., Lipskey, R., Kuchipadi, B. S., Zhu, G., Tauleman, Y., Enoch, M. A., Virkkunen, M., Goldman, D., 2005. Haplotype-based linkage of tryptophan hydroxylase 2 to suicide attempt, major depression, and cerebrospinal fluid 5-hydroxyindoleacetic acid in 4 populations. Arch. Gen. Psychait. 62, 1109-1118.

PART FIVE

REFLECTIONS

THE NEUROTRANSMITTER ERA IN NEUROPSYCHOPHARMACOLOGY
REFLECTIONS OF A NEUROPSYCHOPHARMACOLOGIST

Norbert Matussek

In 1961 I applied for a postdoctoral research fellowship from the Public Health Service (PHS) of the United States Department of Health, Education and Welfare (US-DHEW). Prior to that I had spent four years in trying to isolate and define the structure of substance P. However, three Swiss pharmaceutical research teams were more successful than I. In my despair, I lost interest in substance P, although my process for its enrichment had already been patented by the Bayer corporation. The correct structure of substance P was not discovered until much later, in 1989.

When I received word from the U.S. that the National Institutes of Health (NIH) had accepted me as a postdoctoral research fellow, I asked Alfred Pletscher which research group he would recommend for me. He suggested that I join Bernard B. Brodie, with whom he had worked several years previously.

I eagerly set sail for the New World, leaving my wife and three children behind. On September 26, 1961 I arrived to New York and viewed the splendid skyline of Manhattan, with the impressive Statue of Liberty in the foreground. I purchased from a colleague who was returning to Germany an old Dodge for $ 25, that took me to Bethesda, the Mecca of medical research. A year later I would resell my trusty vehicle for $ 25 prior to flying home from New York.

IN B.B. BRODIE'S LABORATORY OF CHEMICAL PHARMACOLOGY AT THE NIH

Brodie received me for our first talk in his apartment, on his sickbed. He had injured his leg while vacationing in Switzerland. We discussed which field I should select for my research. I would have preferred to study antidepressants, but he already had Fridolin Sulser and Marcel Bickel in that group. I was assigned to his deputy chief, Mimo Costa. First I had to learn the spectrofluorometric determination of serotonin (5-HT). Costa was a very strict teacher, who often sharply reprimanded me when I did something wrong, or when a result was not the desired one. I was then assigned to Roger Maickel's team, which was studying the "sympathetic nervous system as a homeostatic mechanism" (Maickel et al., 1967).

Whenever I could find time between my experiments I also collaborated with

E. O. Titus. He was working with heart and brain sections in Brodie's laboratory, studying the uptake of isotopic norepinephrine (NE). His findings with Dengler had just been published in Nature (Dengler et al., 1961). About the same time Axelrod and Herrting presented similar findings in *The Journal of Pharmacology and Experimental Therapeutics* (Herrting et al., 1961). Dengler was German, Herrting Austrian, and both being postdoctoral fellows at the NIH, they knew each other well. Whether they exchanged results during this period, I cannot say. Both had left the NIH by the time I arrived. It was not until later that I got to know them personally.

I also visited the laboratory of the two Swiss fellows, Fridolin Sulser and Marcel Bickel, who were studying the action of desmethylimipramine (DMI) in counteracting the sedation of reserpine-like drugs. It was fascinating to watch as the reserpine-sedated rats, upon receiving DMI, immediately started moving again on the floor, or how these rats, when placed by Sulser and Bickel on the laboratory door, would leap down. These "suicidal rats" were often shown to guests. Learning the methodology of NE uptake and observing the research with reserpine induced sedation, were very important to my subsequent scientific career.

During my time at the NIH I found Brodie not only a scientist with a broad scope of interests but also a hospitable teacher. He frequently invited me to dinner at his house. Around 7 P.M. he would come into the laboratory and ask: "Would you like to have dinner with me tonight?" I considered this a great honor. None of my German teachers ever invited me to dinner after work. I then drove him home in my old Dodge. Mrs. Brodie had already prepared dinner. I was surprised that she called her husband Doctor and not Bernard. After dinner Brodie retired with me to his study. Mimo Costa then usually joined us. Our intense brainstorming about our experiments lasted until after midnight. I was usually allowed to go home earlier than Mimo, who also spent the night at Brodie's house more often than me.

I sometimes wondered why Brodie invited me over to dinner so often. It certainly was not because of my scientific qualifications. I was a beginner in all the areas we were working in. Did he feel sorry for my poor single existence, since my wife was not with me? What would seem to be in favor of this possibility is that, during the final three months, when my wife joined me, we hardly had an invitation to dinner from him. At any rate, to this day I am grateful to Brodie for having a decisive influence on my scientific career.

BACK AT THE MAX PLANCK INSTITUTE FOR PSYCHIATRY

After returning to Munich, I was allowed to set up a small team to carry out neuropharmacological reserach. I was glad that I did not have to continue natural products chemistry. I could finally do the research I was interested in. I believed at the time that the study of the mechanism of action of antidepressants would help me to get a better understanding of the neurobiological causes of depression. Numerous scientists considered reserpine induced sedation in the rat an animal model for depression in humans. It was based on findings that hypertensive patients often experienced a depressive syndrome when treated with reserpine.

Applying the knowledge I had gained at the NIH, I began to unravel the mysteries of the release and uptake of NE. I was helped by Eckart Rüther, a party loving but dedicated graduate student. In addition to reserpine induced sedation, similar to Pletscher and Gey (1962), we also induced sedation with the benzo(a)quinolizine, Ro 4-1284, in our studies of depression.

Our findings indicated that cocaine was similar to DMI in that it inhibited NE uptake. But unlike DMI, it also caused NE release. In view of this we hypothesized that cocaine should be a better antidepressant than the ones in clinical use. We did not test this hypothesis on depressed patients because of the risk of developing cocaine addiction. I performed only one self-experiment with cocaine in which I felt nothing probably because I took it orally. Since I used some findings from my collaboration with E.O. Titus in our German publication, I included Titus as a co-author of the paper (Matussek et al., 1964). Two years later Titus published our work in English, with Brodie and myself as co-authors (Titus et al., 1966).

5-HT AND SLEEP

I was also interested in the relationship between sleeping-waking rhythms and NE and 5-HT levels in the central nervous system (CNS). W.R. Hess, the Swiss physiologist and Nobel Laureate, had divided the central autonomous nervous system into an ergotropic and a trophotropic system (Hess, 1954). Brodie and Shore (1957) had postulated that 5-HT was the neurohormone of the trophotropic system. We decided to explore in golden hamsters the relationship between sleep and NE and 5-HT levels in the brain. We found, as we had hoped, higher 5-HT and reduced NE levels in sleep than in waking state (Matussek and Patschke, 1964). We had similar findings in the mice as in hamsters (Matussek et al, 1966a). Later on we became interested in the effect of light (continuous illumination for 30 days) and total darkness on neurohormone levels and locomotor activity in rats (Rüther et al., 1967). I presented our results at several sleep symposiums in Germany.

Angelos Halaris, who had been involved in our continuous illumination and darkness studies, had been interested in electron microscopy. He examined the pineal bodies of rats that had been subjected to continuous illumination for morphological changes in the mitochondria, and found them deformed with extreme swelling. We attributed the changes to increased 5-HT metabolism in the pineal bodies (Halaris and Matussek, 1969).

SWIMMING TEST

In addition to Rüther, I also had Manfred Ackenheil, a young graduate student on my research team. As a pharmacy student he had acquired some knowledge of biochemistry. Rüther and Ackenheil got along well. One day, when I entered the laboratory, I was horrified. Without asking me in advance they were making Sprague-Dawley rats swim in a pool of water to the point of exhaustion in order to observe their behaviour afterward under a variety of conditions. To me this was cruelty to animals. It was only later that I recognised the scientific merit of the findings that in the rat swimming stress caused sedation or catalepsy similar to that seen after the administration of reserpine or Ro 4-1284. They had also shown that the catalepsy induced by swimming stress could be counteracted by DMI and L-dopa. Administration of DL-5-hydroxytryptophan (5-HTP) had no effect on the swimming stress-induced catalepsy (Rüther et al., 1966).

Until the mid-1960s our studies had all been published in German and received little international attention. However Arvid Carlsson, who speaks German well, had noticed some of our publications. On a trip from Göteborg, Sweden, to a meeting in Italy he visited me in Munich. Of course we were familiar with the publications of his team, one of the foremost research groups in the world. During his visit Carlsson and I had an intense exchange of scientific ideas, for which I was very grateful.

We expanded our swimming stress experiments to other substances which inhibit NE uptake, such as N 7001 and N 7049, developed by the Lundbeck Corporation (Møller-Nielsen et al., 1966). I presented our results at the First International Symposium on Antidepressant Drugs, organized by Silvio Garattini, at the Mario Negri Institute in Milan, Italy. My presentation was published in English in the proceedings of the symposium (Matussek et al., 1966b).

This swimming test, also referred to as the "swimming survival test," was adopted by other group of investigators in the screening for antidepressants. Roger Porsolt, a pharmacologist working for a Parisian pharmaceutical corporation, propagated the swimming survival test to the extent that some authors have referred to it as the Porsolt test. Porsolt knew of our work and told me that the swimming survival test should be called the Ackenheil-Rüther test, since Ackenheil and Rüther were the first researchers to come up with the idea of making rats swim.

NE DEFICIT IN DEPRESSION

Based on findings in our animal experiments we were convinced that depression in humans can be attributed to a deficiency of NE, and not of 5-HT, in the CNS, as the catalepsy in the swimming test was counteracted by L-dopa and was not counteracted by 5-HTP. By mid-1965 I had submitted my manuscript of "Neurobiologie und Depression" (Neurobiology and depression) in which I described our findings relevant to NE deficiency in depression to a German medical journal, but the paper was not published until the spring of 1966 (Matussek, 1966). In the meantime, two groups in the USA had independently published similar findings indicating the important role of NE in depression (Bunney and Davis, 1965; Schildkraut, 1965). Prior to these reports, as early as in 1959, Everett and Toman, on the basis findings in studies on the reversal of reserpine induced sedation, pointed out that an imbalance in catecholamine metabolism may play a decisive role in depression (Everett and Toman, 1959).

LITHIUM AND ECT

In order to achieve a better understanding of catecholamine metabolism in the brain under various physiological and pharmacological conditions, we developed a quantitative detection method for labelled $7H^3$-NE using thin-layer chromatography with cellulose (Giese et al., 1967). Until that time our only available method for NE detremination had been the time-consuming column chromatography (Kopin et al.,1961).

Little was known at that time about the mechanism of action of lithium in the therapy of manic states and in the prophylactic treatment of depression, or about the sedative action of amphetamine in hyperactive children. In view of this we decided to study the effect of these two substances on DMI and Ro 4-1284-induced hyperactivity in the rat. We found that lithium and amphetamine both inhibited the hyperactivity induced by these substances. But we also found that lithium has no effect on the amphetamine-induced excitation. Unfortunately we were unable to relate our findings to changes in catecholamine metabolism (Matussek and Linsmayer, 1968).

Since electroconvulsive therapy (ECT) has antidepressant effects we studied the effect of chronic administration of ECT on NE metabolism in different parts of the rat brain, and on behavior after the administration of Ro 4-1284 and DMI. Although ECT inhibits the hyperactivity induced by these drugs, our analyses of NE and six of its metabolites failed to yield a clear picture that would explain this effect. I presented our findings at the 6th CINP Congress in Taragona in 1968, and published them in an expanded form one year later (Matussek and Ladisich, 1969).

L-DOPA IN DEPRESSION

Since L-dopa decrease the duration of catalepsy in the rat after reserpine administration (Carlsson et al., 1957) and in the swimming test (Rüther et al., 1966), we studied the effect of L-dopa treatment in combination with a decarboxylase-inhibitor in a three-week, placebo-controlled study in 31 patients with retarded depression (Matussek et al., 1970). About the same time Goodwin (Goodwin et al., 1970) reported on findings of a similar study in which 3 of 9 patients with retarded depression showed "clear-cut improvement". In our study there was only a slight clinical improvement with the combined tretament without a statistically significant difference between the active tretament group and the placebo group. Our expectations from L-dopa in the treatment of depression were not fulfilled. In animal pharmacological studies L-dopa was shown to increase dopamine in the brain, an effect that plays an important role in the treatment of Parkinson's disease, but without an increase in NE, that would be necessary for effective treatment in depression, if the NE-deficit hypothesis of depression is correct. There were no clearaut changes in NE metabolites in the blood, urine and cerebrospinal after the adminsitartion of L-dopa. Postmortem studies did not show changes in NE metabolites that would indicate NE deficit in depressive states. I therefore chose a different course to investigate the postulated imbalance of NE metabolism in the brain in depression.

NEUROENDOCRINE STUDIES

In 1971 I switched from the Max-Planck Institute to the Psychiatric Clinic of the University of Munich. It was the year when Hanns Hippius became the director of the clinic. His focus of interest was biological psychiatry. He asked me to set up, with his support, a department of neurochemistry at the clinic. It was unfortunately no longer possible to perform animal experiments at the clinic. From this point in time I carried out my research in depressed patients exclusively. The introduction of neuroendocrine methods in psychiatric research during the late 1960s and early 1970s opened up the possibility of using insulin and other specific drugs that affect catecholaminergic neurons as tools for exploring neuroendocrine functions. The hormones of the pituitary gland would later be called the window to the brain.

We focused our research on the growth hormone (GH) response to amphetamine first and clonidine subsequently. With both drugs we found a blunted GH-response in patients with endogenous depression in comparison to patients with non-endogenous depression and healthy control subjects. Several European and American research teams confirmed our findings. Our report became a "citation classic" in 1989 (Matussek, 1989).

Since clonidine is preferentially an α_2-adrenoreceptor agonist, we suggested that patients with endogenous depression have a sub-sensitivity of these receptors. We also suggested that the blunted GH-response to clonidine is a trait marker of endogenous depression and not a state marker of depression (Matussek, 1988).

In view of the close connections between α_2-adrenoreceptors and μ-opiate receptors we also investigated the effect of fentanyl, a rather specific μ-opiate agonist, in depressed patients and healthy controls. We found that depressed patients showed a significantly lower GH-response to fentanyl than control subjects. We also found that only in healthy subjects did fentanyl induce euphoria (Matussek and Höhe, 1989). In my opinion, current biological psychiatric research still focuses too little attention on the opiate system. This is especially difficult to understand if one considers that opiates were used effectively in the treatment of depression at least in some European countries before the introduction of the new antidepressants in the late 1950s (Weber, 1987).

REFERENCES
1. Brodie, B.B., Shore, P.A., 1957. A concept for a role of serotonin and norepinephrine as chemical mediators in the brain. Ann. N.Y. Acad. Sci. 66, 631–642.
2. Bunney, W.E., Davis, J.M., 1965. Norepinephrine in depressive reactions. Arch. Gen. Psychiatry 13, 483-494.
3. Carlsson, A., Lindqvist, M., Magnusson, T., 1957. 3,4-Dihydroxyphenylalanine and 5-hydroxytryptophan as reserpine antagonists. Nature 180, 1200.
4. Dengler, H.I., Spiegel, H.E., Titus, E.O., 1961. Effects of drugs on uptake of isotopic norepinephrine by cat tissues. Nature 191, 816-817.
5. Everett, G.M., Toman, J.E.P., 1959. Mode of action of Rauwolfia alkaloids and motor activity. In: Giese, J, Ruther, E., Matussek, N. (Eds.), Biological Psychiatry. Vol. 1. Grune & Stratton, New York/London.
6. Giese, J., Rüther, E., Matussek, N., 1967. Quantitative estimation of ^{3}H-norepinephrine and its metabolites by thin-layer chromatography. Life Science 6, 1975-1982.
7. Goodwin, F.K., Brodie, H.K.H., Murphy, D.L., Bunney, W.E., 1970. Administration of a peripheral decarboxylase inhibitor with L-DOPA to depressed patients. Lancet 1, 908-911.
8. Halaris, A., Matussek, N., 1969. Effect of continuous illumination on mitochondria of the rat pineal body. Experientia 25, 486-487.
9. Hertting, G., Axelrod, J., Whitby, G., 1961. Effect of drugs on the uptake and metabolism of ^{3}H-norepinephrine. J. Pharmacol. Exp. Therap. 134, 146-153.
10. Hess, W.R., 1954. Das Zwischenhirn. Schwabe, Basel.
11. Kopin, I.J., Axelrod, J., Gordon, E., 1961. The metabolic fate of ^{3}H –epinephrine and ^{14}C –metanephrine in the rat. J. Biol. Chem. 236, 2109–2113.
12. Maickel, R.P., Matussek, N., Stern, D.N., Brodie, B.B., 1967. The sympathetic nervous system as a homeostatic mechanism: I. Absolute need for sympathetic nervous function in body temperaturemaintenance of cold-exposed rats. J. Pharmacol. Exp. Therap. 157, 103-110.
13. Matussek, N., 1966. Neurobiologie und Depression. Medizinische Monatsschrift 3, 109-112.
14. Matussek, N., 1988. Catecholamines and mood: Neoroendocrine aspects. In: Ganten, D., Pfaff, D. (Eds.), Current Topics in Neuroendocrinology, Vol. 8, Neuroendocrinology of Mood. Springer, Heidelberg, pp. 141-182.
15. Matussek, N., 1989. α_2-Adrenoceptor subsensitivity in depression. Current Contents – Life Sciences 32, 16.
16. Matussek, N., Hoehe, M., 1989. Investigations with the specific µ-opiate receptor agonist fentanyl in depressive patients: growth hormone, prolactin, cortisol, noradrenaline and euphoric responses. Neuropsychobiology 21, 1-8.
17. Matussek, N., Ladisich, W., 1969. Chronic administration of electroconvulsive shock and norepinephrine metabolism in the rat brain. 3. Influence of acute and chronic electroshock upon drug induced behavior. Psychopharmacologia 15, 305-309.
18. Matussek, N., Linsmayer, M., 1968. The effect of lithium and amphetamine on desmethylimipramine-Ro 4-1284 induced motor hyperactivity. Life Science 7, 371-375.
19. Matussek, N., Patschke, U., 1964. Beziehungen des Schlaf- und Wachrhytmus zum Noradrenalin- und Serotoningehalt im Zentralnervensystem von Hamstern. Med. exp. 11, 81-87.
20. Matussek, N., Rüther, E., Titus, E.O., 1964. Einfluß und Wirkmechanismus adrenalinpotenzierender Pharmaka auf die Reserpin sedation. Arzneimittelforschung 14, 503-505.
21. Matussek, N., Schuster, I, Mantey, S.v., 1966a. Noradrenalin- und Serotonin-Stoffwechsel im Zentralnerwensystem in Beziehung zum Schlaf- und Wachrhytmus. Arzneimittelforschung 16, 259-261.

22. Matussek, N., Rüther, E., Ackenheil, M., Giese, J., 1966b. Amine metabolism in the CNS during exhaustion after swimming and the influence of antidepressants on this syndrome. Excerpta Medica International Congress Series 122, 70-74.

23. Matussek, N., Benkert, O., Schneider, K., Otten, H., Pohlmeier, H., 1970. L-DOPA plus decarboxalase inhibitor in depression. The Lancet 2, 660-661.

24. Møller-Nielsen, I., Nymark, M., Hougs, W., Pedersen, V., 1966. The pharmacological properties of melitracen (N 7001) and litracen (N 7049). Arzneimittelforschung 16, 135-140.

25. Pletscher, A., Gey, K.F., 1962. Action of imipramine and amitriptyline on cerebral monoamines as compared with chlorpromazine. Med. Exp. 6, 165-168.

26. Rüther, E., Ackenheil, M., Matussek, N., 1966. Beitrag zum Noradrenalin- und Serototninstoffwechsel im Rattengehirn nach Stresszuständen. Arzneimittelforschung 16, 261-263.

27. Rüther, E., Halaris, A., Matussek, N., 1967. Norepinephrine and 5-hydroxytryptamine in the CNS of rats under continuous illumination and total darkness. Med. Pharmacol. Exp. 17, 139-143.

28. Schildkraut, J.J., 1965. The cathecolamine hypothesis of affective disorders: a review for supporting evidence. Am. J. Psychiat. 122, 509-522.

29. Titus, E.O., Matussek, N., Spiegel, H.E., Brodie. B.B., 1966. The effect of desmethylimipramine on uptake of DL-norepinephrine-7-^{3}H in the heart. J. Pharmacol. Exp. Therap. 152, 469-477.

30. Weber, M.M., 1987. Die "Opiumkur" in der psychiatrie. Ein Beitrag zur Geschichte der Psychopharmakotherapie. Sudhoffs Archiv. 71, 31-61.

THE NEUROTRANSMITTER ERA IN NEUROPSYCHOPHARMACOLOGY
REFLECTIONS OF A CLINICIAN

Oldřich Vinař

One of the most prominent Czech internists, Joseph Marek declared (Discussion at the 21st Annual Psychopharmacology Meeting, Jeseník Spa, January 9-13, 1979) that psychopharmacology is the endocrinology of the brain. In my professional experience the use of endocrine preparations preceded psychotropic drugs in the treatment of psychotic patients. Hormones had played the role of neurotransmitters.

In 1952, soon after my graduation from medical school, while working in a regional mental hospital I had to treat a young girl suffering from her first episode of hebephrenia. The ususal procedure would have been a series of regressive electroconvulsive treatment (ECT). The patient was a student at an agricultural high school. When I informed her parents that she will have memory problems from the treatment, they asked me for a possible alternative therapy to ECT. Being under the influence of a paper by Sackler et al. (1952) in which they suggested that schizophrenia is a disease in which "catabolism" and "cortisol" play an important role I recived their consent to treat the girl with a combination of 100 mg. of testosterone and 3 mg. of estrogen daily for about two months. My rational for this tretament was that anabolic steroids which are cortisol-antagonists should provide for an effective tretatment. She practically recovered and gained about 17 kilograms. The successful treatment made a great impression on the staff of the hospital because hebephrenia was considered to be a relatively treatment-resistant condition. Aftrewards, I treated somewhat less successfully about 15 schizophrenic patients with steroid hormones. My belief in the importance of steroid hormones in the pathogenesis of schizophrenia was strengthened by observing a schizophrenia-like psychosis induced by treatment with adrenocorticotropine for lupus erythematosus.

When we were studying the mechanism of action of chlorpromazine we were among the first who abandoned the rational of hibernation in its mode of action (Laborit and Huguenard, 1951; Vinař, O., 1998). The antihistaminic properties of chlorpromazine (Courvoisier, 1956) are supportive of the view that Bleuler's "secondary symptoms" (Bleuler, 1930) of schizophrenia such as hallucinations, agitation and delusions which would be called "positive symptoms" today (Andreasen and Olsen, 1982) are an expression of a defense against the devastating disease process expressed in the "fundamental symtoms," i.e., autism, emotional blunting and apathy (Bleuler, 1911), which would be called "negative symptoms" today (Andreasen and

Olson, 1982). The simple idea was: if positive symptoms are a pathologic defense, they are comparable to allergy, which is a pathologically increased reaction to an antigen.. As allergy can be treated with antihistaminics, also positive symptoms respond to antihistaminic drugs (Introductory lecture by Oldřich Vinař with the title "Progress in clinical psychopahrmacology in 1960" delivered at the 3rd Annual Psychopharmcological Meeting, Jeseník Spa, January 5-7, 1961).

In my opinion histamine was the first neurotransmitter contributing to the pathogenesis of the disorder and suppressing the action of histamine by chlorpromazine could explain the therapeutic effect of the drug. Before the advent of antipsychotic drugs we treated schizophrenic patients with high doses of histamine. We encountered intensive red flushes, perspiration and somnolence with emotional changes and a mild euphoria, after histamine administration. To certain extent these "histamine shocks" were comparable to insulin coma therapy although the patients did not lose consciousness. A series of histamine shocks could be considered a desensitisation procedure that decreased the sensitivity of the brain to "pathogenic" histamine (see Boissier et al., 1971).

Pharmacologists examining the pharmacodynamic profile of chlorpromazine found that in addition to its antihistaminie properties chlorpromazine blocks both the sympathetic and the parasympathetic branches of the autonomous nervous system (ANS). Prior to chlorpromazine there were drugs which blocked one or the other branche of the ANS; chlorpromazine was the first substance that blocked both (Chauchard and Mazouè, 1956). In view of this it seemed appropriate to refer to chlorpromazine as a "neuroplegic."

The action of chlorpromazine on subcortical structures created difficulties for the introduction of the drug into clinical use in my country. In the late 1950s and early 1960s Czechoslovakia, a country with a liberal democratic tradition, was living through the worst attrocities of Stalinism. The atmosphere of terror was manifest also in the field of medicine. In the ideological battle whether *nervous* or *humoral* factors dominate in the regulation of the organism, the followers of Pavlovian "nervism" prevailed (Ivanov-Smolenski, 1952). This was unfavourable to the search for chemical substances serving neurotransmission. We were compelled to apply the Pavlovian doctrine whenever possible – or impossible. Fortunately, the ideology inadvertenly helped to consider conditioned reflexes as a good method for the investigation of the effects of psychotropic drugs. Yet, as conditioned reflexes and the second signalling system (verbal system), are functions of the cerebral cortex, it was predicated that psychotropic drugs are substances which act on the cerebral cortex. The phylogenetically and ontogenetically younger and higher functions of the cerebral cortex had to have a dictatorial control over the older and lower functions in the same way as the young proletariat should have control over the bourgeoisie in the society. We had to adjust to a model in which mental functions are perceived as a product of interaction between cortical excitation and inhibition in the brain; and in which mental disorders are explained on the lines of the experimental neuroses displayed by Pavlov's dogs, that could be effectively treated with caffeine and/or bromide (Pavlov, 1951). Under such circumstances it was difficult to defend the necessity of importing Western drugs acting on the old subcortical structures which are regulating autonomous functions. We had to answer the question why to treat the subcortex when the disorders of "higher nervous activity" are localized in the cortex, and persuade the political authorities that schizophrenia is a disorder with strong subcortical activity in which by blocking the ANS and decreasing subcortical activity we liberate the cerebral cortex to provide "protective inhibition" that was considered to be important for effective treatment (Pavlov, 1951).

Surprisingly, psychoanalysis helped. Psychoanalysis was accepted by old pre-war marxists. Many of them were still influential in Czechoslovakia even in the 1950s although psychoanalysis was officially rejected in the Soviet Union. The reasoning that chlorpromazine is a drug that weakens the *id*, residing in the subcortex, was compatible with their hidden belief that schizophrenia is a narcissistic withdrawal and regression, the result of a losing battle of a weakened *ego*, residing in the cortex, with the *id*. (Freud, 1924). The neurotransmitters of the ANS, adrenaline and acetylcholine, were not known to be significant for cortical functions but it was an acceptable proposition that it could serve well the disturbance of higher nervous activity in schizophrenia if one blocks their effects. It has to be emphasized that this philosophizing is far from attempts to interprete drug treatment in psychoanalytic terms (Sarwer-Foner, 1957).

The presumption of the negative role of acetylcholine, the substance regulating the parasympathetic system, was strengthened by findings that imipramine and amitriptyline, the first antidepressant drugs introduced into clinical use, had strong anticholinergic effects. The "Czech Pharmacological School," represented by O.Benesova, Z.Votava, and K.Nahunek, was among the first to consider anticholinergic properties important in the therapeutic effect of these drugs (Benešová and Trinerová, 1964; Náhunek, 1962).

In 1961 Czech pharmacologists and psychiatrists organized an international symposium on psychopharmacological methods in Prague (Votava et al., 1963). The focus of all papers, irrespective whether their authors were from the West or the East, was on conditioned reflexes and on electrophysiology. Adrenaline and noradrenaline were the subject matter of two papers; and tryptophan of one. Havlíček (Votava et al., 1963) discussed the effects of adrenaline on conditioned reflexes in rabbits and cats. In his review of the literature he noted that chlorpromazine has adrenolytic effects and that some of the derivatives of adrenaline, e.g., adrenochrome, have a similar effect to halllucinogens. Floru (Votava et al., 1963), reported his findings in his research in which he studied the effects of noradrenaline on conditioned reflexes in dogs and cats with implanted electrodes in several brain areas. Ettlinger (Votava et al., 1963), described the effects of tryptophan on the behavior of monkeys (because of the high cost prohibited the use of human subjects), in a study that was supported financially by Sandoz, a Swiss pharmaceutical company.

An important exception to the predominantly "dry" behavioral and electrophysiological presentations were the contributions of a group of researchers (E. Kuhn, K.

Ryšánek, V. Vítek, M. Vojtěchovský and Stanislav Grof) working in the Institute of Human Nutrition in Prague. They reported on the excretion of the serotonin metabolite 5-hydroxyindolacetic acid (5-HIAA) in urine, and on the response of the pituitary-adrenal axis by measuring 3-methoxy-4-hydromandelic acid. The terminology they used indicates that before Schildkraut's publication (Schildkraut, 1965) catecholamines were considered to be hormones rather than neurotransmitters produced in the brain. Most of the reserach of the group from the Institute of Human Nutrition was done in healthy volunteers, but in some instances it was done in patients treated with psychotherapy in combination with hallucinogens such as lysergic acid diethylamide (LSD-25), psilocybine, mescaline, adrenochrome, or other substances, e.g., benactyzine, phenmetrazine, alcohol. Unfortunatley this pioneering research was stopped in Czechoslovakia after several members of the group, e.g., V. Vítek, a biochemist, and Stan Grof, a psychiatrist, who was to become the founder of transpersonal psychology (Grof, 1996), immigrated to the West. Continuing the cooperation across the Iron Curtain was impossible. The virtual lack of presentations on biochemical methods which were of major importace for psychopharmacological research was surprising because the publications of Woolley and Shaw (1954) and Gaddum and Hameed (1954) about the role of serotonin in mental disorders were well known and frequently discussed by Czechoslovakian psychopharmacologists in Jesenik at the annual meetings of the national psychopharmacology society.

Chlorpromazine had an important competitor in reserpine, one of the alkaloids of Rauwolfia serpentina, at the time of its introduction to psychiatry. Used for centuries in India as a sedative, reserpine was rediscovered in the early 1950s for modern medicine as an antihypertensive drug (Litin et al., 1956). Its mechanism of action was known by the late 1950s: depletion of catecholamines and serotonin from their storage granules (Carlsson, 1957). When it turned out that reserpine induced severe depression in some patients treated for hypertension (Litin et al., 1956), the use of the drug was abandoned by internists. Yet, the use of reserpine as an antipsychotic continued. For several years we prefered to use reserpine to chlorpromazine in the treatment of acute mania because of the specific "depressogenic," antimanic effect of the drug (Luby, 1968). We surmised that a brain depleted from catecholamines and serotonin was better protected from the recurrence of mania than a brain where the effects of some of the monoamines were blocked. (We did not speak about receptors at the time). Later on we used reserpine mainly in patients who were in need for continued antipsychotic treatment after recovering from malignant neuroleptic syndrome.

In the former Czechoslovakia we had good access to ergot alkaloids and it was easy to synthesize LSD-25 at the Institute of Pharmacy and Biochemistry in Prague. Z.Votava and his coworkers were among the first to report that LSD-25 has antiserotoninergic e ffects (Votava, 1961). The findings that drugs with antipsychotic effects, such as chlorp romazine and reserpine, and a substance like LSD-25, a psychotomimetic, both have antiserotoninergic effects, indicated that something in our simplistic reasoning about the biochemistry of psychosis was incorrect.

In the gold rush for new psychotropic drugs it was important to have a simple model of schizophrenia in which the antipsychotic action of drugs could be tested. It was already known that chlorpromazine blocked LSD-induced mental states (see Grof et al., 1960) and I was able to demonstrate that it was prophylactic when given as pre-treatment to LSD- induced psychosis. I decided to test the reliability of the LSD-model of schizophrenia with reserpine the other available antipsychotic at the time. I did not use reserpine following LSD administration because it was known that the onset of the antipsychotic effect of the drug was delayed for several days. Therefore I administered LSD-25 to a volunteering nurse after pretreatment with reserpine. The result was awful. She developed extremely disagreeable hallucinations and delusions; became extremely anxious and felt deeply depressed for 36 hours. She also had flashbacks for several weeks (Vinař, 1958a, b). Understandably, I stopped to proceed with these experiments immediately. It became apparent to me that LSD-induced state was not a good model of schizophrenia. I wondered why a drug with antiserotoninergic effects had such a terrifying effect in a subject whose brain was depleted from serotonin (5-HT). When in 1966, I attended the 5th congress of the Collegium Internationale Neuro-Psychopharmacologicum in Washington I told Nathan Kline, a prominent American psychopharmacologist, about my experience with the combination of reserpine and LSD. He interpreted it as further evidence that reserpine is not an antipsychotic that was confirmed by findings in compartive clinical investigations with chlorpromazine (Barsa and Kline, 1956). Only in 1989 could I free myself – at least to certain extent – from feelings of guilt about my LSD-reserpine interaction experiments. By that time LSD was shown to be a partial $5HT_{2A}$ antagonist.

In 1989 I received a supply of ritanserin, a relatively specific $5\text{-}HT_{2A}$ antagonist, developed by Janssen Pharmaceuticals, from Paul Janssen himself. I organised a multicenter clinical trial in which ritanserin was added to haloperidol. As a result we found that antipsychotic action was increased and extrapyramidal effects were suppressed (Vinař et al., 1989). Our clinical trial with the haloperidol–ritanserin combination preceded the rise of risperidone and other second generation antipsychotic drugs.

In 1958 we began to treat a group of depressed and schizophrenic patients with cyanacetic acid hydrazide, a monoamine oxidase inhibitor (MAOI). We found amelioration of depression and worsening of schizophrenia. We also compared the clinical effects of cyanacetic acid hydrazide with iproniazid, a MAOI antidepressant in clinical use at the time but did not discuss the action of these drugs on biogenic amines (Vinař et al., 1960).

In the early 1960s with the discovery of the mode of action of imipramine, the first tricyclic antidepressant introduced into clinical use (Kuhn, 1957), neurotransmitter theory obtained fresh and persuasive support. The equilibrium between a sufficient concentration of catecholamines and serotonin on the one hand and the deficiency on the other became in our opinion a decisive factor in the regulation of mood and it seemed to be a perfect explanation of the mechanism of action of antidepressants and of the depressogenic effects of reserpine.

Reserpine induced ptosis in mice served as a reliable and inexpensive tool in the screening of new compounds for antidepressant effects. A plethora of original antidepressants, synthesized in the laboratory of M.Protiva in Czechoslovakia, which were to be tested in clinical trials, owed their existence to this test (Maxwell, 1964). Clinically only dosulepine (dothiepine, Prothiaden) was successful among these drugs (Rees and Marsh, 1975).

In 1970, nine years after the symposium on psychopharmacological methods, the 7th CINP Congress was organized in Prague. By then the interest shifted from conditioned reflexes to neurotransmitters, and the effects of psychotropic drugs on neurotransmitters were in the foreground at this congress. D. Eccleston, spoke about the role of biogenic amines in affective disorders. He attributed the long latency in the onset of therapeutic action of antidepressants to changes in receptor activity. He expanded neurotransmitter theory within the framework of contemporary knowledge and suggested that "receptor changes may reflect an increased protein synthesis which should produce changes on a much longer time base than that indicatied by the half life of 5-hydrosytryptamine itself." (Eccleston, 1971). He left open the question whether serotonin or noradrenaline plays a role in the aetiology of affective disorders.

Czech and Slovak psychopharmacologists did not consider the role of serotonin (5-HT) and noradrenaline as mutually exclusive of each other (Brodie et al., 1955; Schildkraut, 1965). We discussed issues relevant to the role of 5-HT and noradrenaline in depression at our annual meetings in Jeseník with Herman van Praag, Brian Leonard and Norbert Matussek and considered both of these monoamines important in the pathogenesis of depression. For us it was a matter of choosing the right drug – noradrenergic or serotoninergic - for the right patient.

We were impressed by the findings of dopamine deficit in Parkinson's disease (Hornykiewicz, 1971). Since we were operating on the the assumption that only those drugs which induce extrapyramidal signs were antipsychotic, we were well prepared to accept the dopamine hypothesis of schizophrenia (Snyder, 1976). We made an attempt to test this hypothesis statistically. But when we examined whether the symptomatic improvement correlated with severity of extrapyramidal signs with the employment of our rating scales, the FKP, the rating scale we developed for the quantification of psychotic symptoms in pharmacotherapeutic research, and the DVP, the side effect scale we developed for the detection of treatment emergent symptoms, we did not find statistically significant correlations (Vinař, 1966; Vinař et al., 1963, 1966).

We were more successful when correlating the potency of 11 antipsychotic drugs in 19 pharmacological tests in animal to their clinical action as measuered by the therapeutic response in 18 psychotic symptoms. We found a total of 27 statistically significant rank correlations between symptomatic improvement and catalepy in mice. Since catalepsy was related to antidopaminergic effects, our findings were in keeping with and contributed to the dopamine hypothesis of schizophrenia (Vinař and Kršiak, 1974). I believe that our approach was closer to the thinking of clinicians than the reported correlations between therapeutic dose requirements and affinities to the dopamine₂ (D₂) receptor (Creese et al., 1976; Seeman et al., 1976). In the early 1980s we employed a similar methodology using data obtained in a clinical investigation with 715 schizophrenic patients treated with 17 antipsychotic drugs under double blind conditions. 18 symptoms were rated with the FKP scale. Correlations were sought among the decrease of pathology in the symptoms and the affinity of the drugs to different receptors. I was surprised to find negative correlations between D_2 receptor affinity and therapeutic effects in the majority of symptoms (Vinař, 1986). Instead of correlating with affinities to the D_2 receptors, theraputic efficacy correlated with affinities to the histamine α_1 and α_2 receptors. I considered this work as a contribution to neurotransmiter theory. If it would be corroborated in other large patient samples it could help in the prediction of the therapeutic profile of newly synthesized drugs. First, I thought that our results were contrary to the dopamine hypothesis of schizophrenia. Later on however, I re-analysed our data using the classification of symptoms into positive and negative ones and found that affinities to D_2 receptors correlated negatively to theraputic effects in negative symptoms. These findings were in-keeping with reports that D_2 receptor blockade can worsen "negative symptoms" (Vinař, 1987).

In so far as the role of dopamine in depression is concerned, we found lisuride a dopamine agonist, equally effetive in the treatment of depression to combined treatment with amitriptyline and nortriptlyine (Vinař et al., 1985).

For me, the following questions related to the neurotransmitter theory of mental disorders have remained to be answered:

1. The very rapid onset of action of selective serotonin reuptake inhibitors (SSRIs) in pathological crying after a stroke shows that an increase in 5-HT concentration in the synaptic cleft is sufficient to induce therapeutic effect without long-term modification of the state of receptors and/or of induction of events "beyond the receptor". Why is crying susceptible to this rapid change in contrast to other symptoms related to affectivity?

2. If low activity of the 5-HT transporter gene is a risk factor for depression as Caspi and his associates found (Caspi et al., 2003) why are SSRIs effective in the prophylactic treatment of depression. They should worsen the risk of recurrence!

3. Why does tianeptine a substance that increases 5-HT re-uptake have antidepressant effects?

4. If therapeutic effects are dependent on the changes in the hippocampus and other brain structures would this imply that it is irrelevant what antidepresSants do in the synaptic cleft?

CONCLUSION

When I began to work as a psychiatrist in 1949, I wondered what practical use is there in the minute knowledge of brain anatomy with all the *nuclei*, *ganglia*, *tracts* and *fibres.* Aside of patientS with brain tumour or simptoms of Parkinson's disease, I could diagnose and treat psychiatric patients without this knowledge. The neurotransmitter era changed the situation only a little. It turned my attention to the nuclei of dorsal raphé and the locus coeruleus in the brain.

Currently, thanks to modern brain imaging techniques, organic changes have been found in almost all mental disorders. Changes in the level of glucose or oxygen metabolism in different brain areas are seen in patients and healthy volunteers during various everyday activities, e.g., decision making, watching a video film, etc. Brain anatomy is gaining importance. Unfortunately and paradoxically, especially for younger colleagues, as these developments attract attention to brain morphology, they decrease interest in the role of neurotransmitters in psychopathology, although neurotransmitters are the driving force in activating or inhibiting the functioning of brain structures. This is the reason why I would like to emphasize that the study of neurotransmitters does not relate only to the past . Also recently, the study of neurotransmitters has led to new discoveries, When it was discovered for example that tetrahydrocannabinol (THC) has its own receptors, it opened the path for the discovery of anandamine, its endogenous ligand. Currently we are discovering new neurotransmitter systems and new drugs are being developed which act on their receptors.

The study of neurotransmitters has remained important even at a time, when organic and morphologcal changes are found in the majority of mental disorders. Neurotransmitter theory is the best starting point in the education of non-psychiatrists about neuropsychopharmacology. Instead of relating the effecct of drugs to symptoms in a simplistic way, the new generation of physicians can be guided by the understanding that even if drugs detectably affect the brain, changes in mental states take place only when humoral changes occur in the central nervous system.

With the advent of molecular biology and genetics, I expected a breakthrough in our knowledge about the etiology and pathogenesis of mental disorders in directions which would lead to new realms. For about four years, while the human geonome sequence has been made public (International Human Genome Sequencing Consortium, 2001) we have learned much, but surprise has not transpired. Genetic changes found in schizophrenia and depression are related to genes involved in the function of dopamine and serotonin as well. There is nothing that could constitute a better corroboration of neurotransmiter theory.

REFERENCES
1. Andreasen, N.C., Olsen, S.A., 1982. Negative vs. positive schizophrenia: Definition and validation. Arch.Gen.Psychiat. 39, 789-794.
2. Barsa, J.A., Kline, N.S., 1956. A comparative study of reserpine, chlorpromazine and combined therapy. A.M.A.Arch.Neurol.Psychiat. 76, 90-97.
3. Benešová, O., Trinerová, I., 1964. The comparative study of three prothiadene derivatives III. Antiadrenergic and anticholinergic action in mice. Activ.Nerv.Super. (Prague) 6, 175-176.

4. Bleuler, E., 1911. Dementia Praecox oder Gruppe der Schizophrenien. Deuticke, Leipzig.
5. Bleuler, E. 1930. Physiogenic and psychogenic symptoms in schizophrenia. Amer. J. Psychiat. 87, 203-211.
6. Boissier, J.R., Tillement, J.P., Simon, P., 1971. Histamine et cerveau: approaches biochemiques et pharmacologiques. In: Vinař, O., Votava, Z., Bradley, P.B. (Eds.), Advances in Neuro-Psychopharmacology. North-Holland Publ.Comp./Avicenum, Amsterdam/Prague, pp. 525-540.
7. Brodie, B.B., Pletscher, A., Shore, P.A., 1955. Evidence that serotonin has a role in brain function. Science 122, 968.
8. Carlsson, A., 1957. Effects of reserpine on the metabolism of catecholamines. In: Garattini, S., Ghetti, V. (Eds.), Psychotropic Drugs. Elsevier, Amsterdam, Milan.
9. Caspi, A., Sugden, K., Moffitt, T.E., Tailor, A., Craig, W.A., Harrington, H.L., 2003. Influence of life stress on depression. Moderation by a polymorphism in the 5-HTT gene. Science 301, 386-389.
10. Chauchard, P., Mazouè, H., 1956. Recherches sur le mode d'action centroplégique de quelquels substances psychotropes. Comptes rendues Soc. biol. 150, 158-160.
11. Courvoisier, S., 1956. Sur les propriétés pharmacodynamiques de la chlorpromazine en rapport avec son emploi en psychiatrie. L'encéphale 45, 1248-1257.
12. Creese, I., Burt, D.R., Snyder, S.H., 1976. Dopamine receptor binding clinical and pharmacological potencies of antischizophrenic drugs. Science 192, 481-483.
13. Eccleston, D., 1971. Biogenic amines and the affective disorders. In: Vinař, O., Votava, Z., Bradley, P.B. (Eds.), Advances in Neuro-Psychopharmacology. North-Holland Publ. Comp./Avicenum, .Amsterdam/Prague, pp. 79-89.
14. Freud, S., 1924. Collected Papers. Hogarth Press, London.
15. Gaddum, J.H., Hameed, K.A., 1954. Drugs which antagonize 5-hydroxytryptamine. Brit. J. Pharmacol. 9, 240-248.
16. Grof, S., 1996. Planetary survival and consciousness evolution: Psychological roots of human violence and greed. World Futures 47, 243.
17. Grof, S., Vojtěchovský, M., Votava, Z., 1960. Lysergic acide diethylamide. Cas.lék.čes. 97, 180-187.
18. Hornykiewicz, O., 1971. L-Dopa and parkinsonism. Davis, Philadelphia.
19. International Human Genome Sequencing Consortium, 2001. Initial sequencing and analysis of the human genome. Nature 409, 860-927.
20. Ivanov-Smolenski, A.G., 1952. Ocherki patofyziologii vysshei nervnoi deiatelnosti, Medgiz, Moscow.
21. Kuhn, R., 1957. Über die Behandlung depressiver Zustände mit einem Iminodibenzylderivat (G22355). Schweiz. Med.Wchschr. 87, 1135-1140.
22. Laborit, H., Huguenard, P., 1951. L'hibernation arteficielle par moyens pharmacodynamiques et physiques. Presse Medicale 59, 1329.
23. Litin, E.M., Fawcett, R.L., Achor, R., 1956. Depression in hypertensive patients treated with Rauwolfia Serpentina. Proc. Mayo Clin. 31, 233-237.
24. Luby, E., 1968. Reserpine-like drugs - clinical efficacy. In: Effron, D.H., Cole, J.O., Levine, J., Wittenborn, J.R. (Eds.), Psychopharmacology, A Review of Progress 1957-1967. Public Health Service Publication No. 1836, Washington, pp. 1077-1082.
25. Maxwell, D.R., 1964. The relative potencies of various antidepressant drugs in some laboratory tests. In: Bradley, P.B., Flugel, F., Hoch, P.(Eds.), Neuropsychopharmacology. Elsevier, Amsterdam, pp.501-506.
26. Náhunek, K., 1962. Die Behandlung endogener Depressionen mit Perphenazin und Trihexyphenidyl. Beziehung zur extrapyramidalen Symptomatologie. Acta Psychiatr. Scandinavica 38, 108-116.
27. Pavlov, I.P., 1951. Dvadcatiletnyi opyt obiektivnogo izuchenia vysshei nervnou dejatelnosti (povedenia) zhivotnych, Medgiz, Moscow.
28. Rees, J., Marsh, B., 1975. The outcome of dothiepine treatment in 1900 depressed patients. Int. Pharmacopsychiat.10, 54-57.
29. Sackler, M., Sackler, R.R., Sackler, A.M. van Ophuijsen, J.H.W. Mortimer, D., 1952. Recent biochemotherapeutic developments in psychiatry. Amer. J. Psychiat. 108,669-675.
30. Sarwer-Foner, G.J., 1957. Pasychoanalytic theories of activity-passivity conflicts and the continuum of ego defense: experimental verification using reserpine and chlorpromazine. AMA Arch. Neurol.Psychiat. 78, 413.

31. Schildkraut, J.J., 1965. The catecholamine hypothesis of affective disorders. A review of supporting evidence. Amer. J.Psychiat. 122, 509-522.
32. Seeman, P., Lee, T., Chau Wong, M., Wong, K., 1976. Antiopsychotic drug doses and neuroleptic/dopamine receptors. Nature 261, 717-719.
33. Snyder, S.H., 1976. The dopamine hypothesi of schizophrenia. Focus on the dopamine receptor. Am. J. Psychiat. 133, 140-144.
34. Vinař, O., 1958a. Clinical effects of ataractic drugs in patients and in experimental psychosis. In: Vencovský, E. (Ed.), Chlorpromazine and Reserpine in Psychiatry. Proceedings of the. 5ᵗʰ National Psychiatric Meeting, Plzeň, pp. 81-90.
35. Vinař, O., 1958b. Analogien zwischen schizophrenen Erkrankungen und der LSD-Psychose. Psychiatr. Neurol. med. Psychol. (Leipzig) 10, 162-166.
36. Vinař, O., 1966. Scale for rating side-effects during psychiatric pharmacotherapy. Activ. Nerv.Super. 8, 411-412.
37. Vinař,, O., 1986. Different role of dopamine and noradrenaline in schizophrenia. Activ. Nerv. Super. 28, 298-300.
38. Vinař, O., 1987. The affinity of neuroleptic drugs to their binding sites for neurotransmitters and their therapeutic action: How to interpret the relationship? Activ. Nerv. Super. 29, 214-215.
39. Vinař, O., 1998. My memories of early psychotropic drug development. In: Ban, T.A., Healy, D., Shorter, E. (Eds.), The Rise of Psychopharmacology and the Story of CINP. Animula, Budapest, pp. 229-234.
40. Vinař, O., Kršiak, M., 1974. Prediction of neuroleptic effects from anímal data. In: Forrest, I.S., Carr, C.J., Usdin, E. (Eds), The Phenothiazines and Structurally Related Drugs. Raven Press, New York, pp. 675-683.
41. Vinař, O., Vinařová, M., Gross, J., Hgosák, L., Dlabač, A., Trčka, V., 1960. Possibility of the use of hydrazide of cyanacetic acid in psychiatry. Czechoslovak Physiology 8, 96-97.
42. Vinař, O., Grof, S., Váňa, J., Matoušek, M., 1963. Is there a relation between the extrapyramidal symptoms induced by thioproperazine and its therapeutic effects? Activ. Nerv. Super.(Prague) 5, 201-203.
43. Vinař,, O., Váňa, J., Grof, S., 1966. FKP rating scale Activ. Nerv. Super. (Prague) 8, 405-408.
44. Vinař, O., Zapletalek, M., Kazdová, E., Náhunek, K., Molčan, J., 1985. Antidepressant effets of lisuride are not different from effects of amitriptyline and nortriptyline. Activ., Nerv. Super. 27, 249-251.
45. Vinař, O., Molčan, J., Náhunek, K., Švestka, J., Zapletálek, M., 1989. Ritanserin in schizophrenic patients. Activ. Nerv. Super. 31, 107-109.
46. Votava, Z., 1961. Antiserotoninergic activity of lysergic acide diethylamide. In: Rothlin, E. (Ed.), Neuropsychopharmacology. Elsevier, Amsterdam.
47. Votava, Z., Horváth, M., Vinař, O., 1963. Psychopharmacological methods. State Medical Publishing House/Pergamon Press, Prague/Oxford, pp. 1- 360.
48. Woolley, D.W., Shaw, E.A., 1954. A biochemical and pharmacological suggestion about certain mental disorders. Proc. Nat. Acad. Sci. USA 40, 228-231.

THE NEUROTRANSMITTER ERA IN NEUROPSYCHOPHARMACOLOGY
REFLECTIONS OF A PHARMACOLOGIST

Joseph Knoll

The golden sixth decade of the 20th century with its memorable series of brea k-throughs in the pharmacology of the central nervous system (CNS) changed in a revolutionary manner general views about the principles of behavior and radically altered human attitude toward derangements of psychic functions. Neuropsychopharmacology, an offspring of the neurotransmitter era in biology and medicine, significantly contributed also to the discovery of previously unknown brain mechanisms.

Research over a period of 30 years on the mechanism of action of (-)-deprenyl, a drug registered world-wide for the treatment of Parkinson's disease, led to the recognition of enhancer regulation in the mesencephalic catecholaminergic neurons. (-)-Deprenyl, has also played a catalytic role in the development of a new interpretation about "The Brain and Its Self" (Knoll, 2005).

We developed (-)-deprenyl in the early 1960s when monoamine oxidase inhibitors (MAOIs) were in the center of interest in neuropsychopharmacology (Knoll et al., 1965). As experimental tools and as therapeutic agents MAOIs had an important role on the development of two widely accepted hypotheses that (1) depression is associated with diminished monoaminergic tone in the brain, and (2) patients treated with antidepressants become elated because of enhanced biological activity of monoamine transmitters in their CNS (van Praag, 1978).

The discovery of the mood-elevating effect of MAOIs is a classic example of serendipity in drug research. In 1951 isoniazid and its isopropyl derivative, iproniazid, were introduced in the treatment of tuberculosis (see Fox, 1953) and iproniazid was found to produce undesirable stimulation in some tubercular patients (see Kety, 1976). Within a year it was discovered that one of the two substances, iproniazid, have monoamine oxidase (MAO) inhibiting properties (Zeller and Barsky, 1952). In 1956 Crane analysed the psychiatric side-effects of iproniazid and suggested that the drug might be beneficial in the treatment of depression (Crane, 1956). In 1957 Kline introduced iproniazid as a *psychic energizer* (Kline, 1958) and Kuhn (1957) discovered the antidepressant effect of imipramine.

In the late 1950s there was a keen interest in MAOIs, and several MAOIs were introduced in the treatment of depression. There was a rapid turnover in the introduction and withdrawal of these drugs because of side effects. In 1963 *hypertensive (crises) attacks* we re reported in patients treated with MAOIs after the ingestion of cheese that contains high amounts of tyramine (see Knoll et al., 1968). Blackwell suggested that "the cheese effect" is the result of the inhibition of tyramine breakdown and the consequent increase of the substance in the brain (Blackwell, 1963). The hypothesis was supported by findings that cheese and many other tyramine containing foods provoked hypertensive episode in patients treated with MAOIs (see Knoll et al., 1968).

Deprenyl, the racemic compound (E-250) was shown to be a *psychic energizer*. It differed in our pharmacological studies from other MAOIs by inhibiting the blood pressure increasing effect of amphetamine, a releaser of norepinephrine (Knoll et al., 1965). In variance with other MAOIs it inhibited the hypertensive effect of tyramine (Knoll et al., 1968).

In 1968 Johnston described clorgyline, a substance that inhibits the deamination of serotonin (5-HT). He proposed that there are two forms of monoamine oxidase (MAO): *type A*, that is selectively inhibited by clorgyline, and *type B*, that is not (Johnston, 1968). In 1972 we discovered that (-)-deprenyl is a highly selective inhibitor of MAO-B (Knoll and Magyar, 1972). Our paper was to become a citation classic in 1982 (This Week's Citation Classic, January 15, 1982). For several years (-)-deprenyl's selective MAO-B inhibiting effect was in the center of interest. It delayed the discovery of the drug's enhancer effect.

With the hope that reduction of the dose of levodopa will decrease the severity of side effects of the drug, Birkmayer and Hornykiewicz (1962) combined levodopa with MAOIs in the treatment of Parkinson's disease. They had to abandon the combination because of frequent hypertensive crises. Since (-)-deprenyl was an MAOI free of "cheese effect" (Elsworth et al., 1978; Knoll et al., 1968), Birkmayer and his co-workers (Birkmayer et al., 1977) and Sandler and his co-workers (Sandler et al., 1978) decided to try a levodopa and (-)-deprenyl combination. It decreased the dose required from levodopa without causing hypertensive attacks.

The therapeutic effects of (-)-deprenyl in recently diagnosed Parkinson's disease were established in the Deprenyl and Tocopherd Antioxidative Therapy of Parkinsonism (DATATOP) study in the U.S.A. (Parkinson Study Group, 1989, 1993; Tetrud and Langston, 1989). The substance delayed the progress of the disease by slowing the rate of functional deterioration in nigrostriatal dopaminergic neurons. Findings of the DATATOP study were corroborated in several multicenter studies (Allain et al., 1991; Larsen et al., 1999; Myttyla et al., 1992).

Age-related deterioration of the striatal machinery is on a continuum and any segment of this continuum is sufficient to measure the rate of decline in the presence or absence of (-)-deprenyl. In the DATATOP study of the Parkinson Study Group the effect of (-)-deprenyl was compared with placebo on the time elapsed from the diagnosis of Parkinson's disease until the need for levodopa therapy (Parkinson Study Group, 1989). It was found that deprenyl significantly delayed the need. The average number of days elapsed before levodopa was needed was 312.1 days for patients in the placebo group, and 548.9 days for patients in the (-)-deprenyl group. These findings indicate that (-)-deprenyl can keep the surviving dopamine neurons on a higher level of activity for a longer period of time.

The design of the DATATOP study was similar to the design we used in our pharmacological experiments. By measuring sexual activity, a rapidly aging (declining) dopaminergic function, in male rats, and comparing the effect of (-)-deprenyl and saline on the age-related decline of copulation, we found that (-)-deprenyl significantly slowed age-related decay of sexual performance (Knoll et al., 1989). To demonstrate that the effect of (-)-deprenyl on age-related copulatory activity was unrelated to MAO inhibition we developed (-)-1-phenyl-2-propylaminopentane, [(-)-PPAP], a (-)-deprenyl analogue that differs structurally from its mother compound by the replacement of the propargyl group that blocks MAO-B because it binds irreversible to the flavin group of the enzyme, with a propyl group. (-)-PPAP enhanced dopaminergic activity in the brain like (-)-deprenyl, but did not change the activity of MAO-B (Knoll et al., 1992).

If one selects a measurable dopaminergic function and determines its age-related decline to a particular level in functionig (end-point), the enhancing effect of a drug on dopaminergic activity can be shown by the delay in time reaching the end point. Male rats lose their ability to ejaculate, a natural end-point, because of physiological aging of the striatal dopaminergic system. We found that saline-treated rats lost their ability to ejaculate at the age of 112±9 weeks, whereas their (-)-deprenyl-treated peers lost their ability only at the age of 150±12 weeks (*P<0.001*) (Knoll, 1992).

In the DATATOP study the end-point chosen for early untreated patients with Parkinson's disease, was the level of functioning when they required levodopa treatment. Since both MAO activity and the formation of oxygen radicals contribute to the pathogenesis of nigral degeneration, it was hypothesised that the combination (-)-deprenyl, a MAOI, and α-tocopherol, an antioxidant will delay the time levodopa is needed by slowing the clinical progression of the disease. It was a comparative study in which 401 patients were administered α-tocopherol or placebo, and 399 patients (-)-deprenyl alone or in combination with α-tocopherol. From the α-tocopherol or placebo treated patients 176 and from the (-)-deprenyl treated patients 97 patient reached the (decerased) level of functioning that required levodopa treatment, i.e., (-)-deprenyl reduced the risk of reaching the end point in about 12 months by 57%. There was also a significant reduction in the risk to give up full-time employment in the (-)-deprenyl treated group (Parkinson Study Group, 1989). The Parkinson Study Group (1993) had shown that it was (-)-deprenyl, and not α-tocopherol, that delayed the need of levodopa treatment. (-)-Deprenyl did not reduce the occurence of levodopa's adverse effects (Parkinson Study Group, 1996). A pharmacological study of α-tocopherol and (-)-deprenyl showed that α-tocopherol was devoid of enhancer effect; it did not change the impulse-evoked release of norepinephrine, dopamine and 5-HT (Miklya et al., 2003).

Tetrud and Langston (1989) were first to present evidence in humans that (-)-deprenyl keeps the nigrostriatal dopaminergic neurons on a higher activity level. The highly significant effect of (-)-deprenyl and the ineffectiveness of α-tocopherol during the first year of the DATATOP study indicate that (-)-deprenyl acts by enhancing the activity of the nigrostriatal dopaminergic neurons. Patients with early, untreated Parkinson's disease were ideal for demonstrating this effect. They still had a sufficient number of dopaminergic neurons to be enhanced by (-)-deprenyl in a manner that the need for levodopa therapy was delayed. As Parkinson's disease is incurable, drug effects are necessarily transient in nature. With further decay of the striatal dopaminergic system, responsiveness to (-)-deprenyl decreased (Parkinson Study Group, 1996).

Availability of high-pressure-liquid-chromatography (HPLC) allowed us to measure catecholamines and 5-HT in physiological quantities. An analysis of the dose-dependent effect of (-)-deprenyl on the release of catecholamines and 5-HT from isolated, discrete rat brain regions, i.e., dopamine released from the striatum, substantia nigra and tuberculum olfactorium, norepinephrine from the locus coeruleus, and 5-HT from the raphé, focused attention on enhancer regulation in the mesencephalic neurons. We treated rats once daily with 0.01, 0.025, 0.05, 0.1 and 0.25 mg/kg of (-)-deprenyl for 21 days and measured the biogenic amines released during a 20-minutes period from freshly isolated discrete brain regions 24 hours after the last injection. The increase in the amount of dopamine released from the dopaminergic neurons indi c a t- ed that these neurons worked on a significantly higher activity level in rats treated even with the lowest, 0.01 mg/kg dose of (-)-deprenyl. Since such a small dose of (-)-deprenyl leaves MAO-B activity and the uptake of amines practically unchanged, findings of this study has provided evidence of a hitherto unknown enhancer mechanism in dopaminergic neurons stimulated by (-)-deprenyl (Knoll and Miklya, 1994). Further studies clarified the operation of mesencephalic enhancer regulation. We established that phenylethylamine (PEA), the parent compound of (-)-deprenyl is primarily an endogenous mesencephalic enhancer substance (Knoll et al., 1996). Since PEA, in higher concentrations, is a highly effective releaser of catecholamines from their intraneuronal stores, the catecholamine releasing effect of PEA has covered up the enhancer effect of the substance (Knoll, 2003).

PEA derivatives with a long lasting effect, such as amphetamine and methamphetamine, share catecholamine releasing properties with their parent compound. (-)-Deprenyl is the first PEA/methamphetamine derivative that *has maintained the enhancer effect and lost the catecholamine releasing property* of its parent compound. The difference in the pharmacological profile of (-)–deprenyl made it possible for us to discover enhancer regulation in the mesencephalic neurons, since the enhancer effect of the substance was not covered up by the release of catecholamines.

In the light of our present knowledge clinicians were mistaken if they believed that the therapeutic benefits observed with (-)-deprenyl were due to selective MAO-B inhibition. Most of the clinical benefits are due to the enhancer effect of the drug (Knoll, 2005).

REFERENCES
1. Allain, H., Gougnard, J., Naukirek, H.C., 1991. Selegiline in de novo parkinsonian patients: the French selegiline multicenter trial (FSMP). Acta Neurol. Scand. 136, 73-78.
2. Birkmayer, W., Hornykiewicz, O., 1962. Der L-dioxyphenyl-alanin-effekt beim Parkinson syndrom des Menschen. Arch. Psychiat. Nervenkrh. 203, 560-564.
3. Birkmayer, W., Riederer, P., Ambrozi, L., Youdim, M.B.H., 1977. Implications of combined treatment with Madopar and L-deprenyl in Parkinson's disease. Lancet i, 439-443.
4. Blackwell, B., 1963. Hypertensive crisis due to monoamine oxidase inhibitors. Lancet ii, 849-851.
5. Crane, G.E., 1956. Psychiatric side effects of iproniazid. Am. J. Psychiatr. 112, 494-499.
6. Elsworth, J.D., Glover, V., Reynolds, G.P., Sandler, M., Less, A.J., Phuapradit, P., Shaw, K.M., Stern, G.M., Kumar, P., 1978. Deprenyl administration in man; a selective monoamine oxidase B inhibitor without the "cheese effect". Psychopharmacology 57, 33-38.
7. Fox, H.H., 1953. The chemical attack on tuberculosis. Trans. N.Y. Acad. Sci. 15, 234-242.
8. Johnston, J.P., 1968. Some observations upon a new inhibitor of monoamine oxidase in human brain. Biochem. Pharmacol. 17, 1285-1297.
9. Kety, S.S., 1976. Introduction. In: Monoamine Oxidase and its Inhibition. Ciba Foundation Symposium 39 (new series). Elsevier/Excerpta Medica/ North-Holland, Amsterdam,/Oxford/ New York, pp. 1-4.
10. Kline, N.S., 1958. Clinical experience with iproniazid (Marsilid). J. Clin. Exp. Psychophathol. 19, 72-81.
11 Knoll, J., 1992. Pharmacological basis of the therapeutic effect of (-)deprenyl in age-related neurological diseases. Med. Res. Rev. 12, 505-524.
12. Knoll, J., 2003. Enhancer regulation/endogenous and synthetic enhancer compounds: A neurochemical concept of the innate and acquired drives. Neurochem. Res. 28, 1187-1209.
13. Knoll, J., 2005. The Brain and Its Self. A Neurochemical Concept of the Innate and Acquired Drives. Springer, Berlin/Heidelberg/New York, pp 1-176.
14. Knoll, J., Magyar, K., 1972. Some puzzling effects of monoamine oxidase inhibitors. Adv. Bioch. Psychopharmacol. 5, 393-408.
15. Knoll, J., Miklya, I., 1994. Multiple, small dose administration of (-)deprenyl enhances catecholaminergic activity and diminishes serotoninergic activity in the brain and these effects are unrelated to MAO-B inhibition. Arch. int. Pharmacodyn. Thér. 328, 1-15.
16. Knoll, J., Ecseri, Z., Kelemen, K., Nievel, J., Knoll, B., 1965. Phenylisopropylmethyl propinylamine (E-250) a new psychic energizer. Arch. int. Pharmacodyn. Thér. 155, 154-164.
17. Knoll, J., Vizi, E.S., Somogyi, G., 1968. Phenylisopropylmethylpropinylamine (E-250), a monoamine oxidase inhibitor antagonizing the effects of tyramine. Arzneimittelf. 18, 109-112.
18. Knoll, J., Dalló, J., Yen, T.T., 1989. Striatal dopamine, sexual activity and lifespan. Longevity of rats treated with (-)deprenyl. Life Sci. 45, 525-531.
19. Knoll, J., Knoll, B., Török, Z., Timár, J., Yasar, S., 1992. The pharmacology of 1-phenyl-2-propylaminopentane (PPAP), a deprenyl-derived new spectrum psychostimulant. Arch. int. Pharmacodyn. Thér. 316, 5-29.
20. Knoll, J., Miklya, I., Knoll, B., Markó, R., Rácz, D., 1996. Phenylethylamine and tyramine are mixed-acting sympathomimetic amines in the brain. Life Sci. 58, 2101-2114.
21. Kuhn, R., 1957. Über die Behandlung depressiver Zustände mit einem Imonodibenzilderivat. Schweitz. Med. Wschr. 36, 1135-1139.
22. Larsen, J.P., Boas, J., Erdal, J.E., 1999. Does selegiline modify the progression of early Parkinson's disease? Results from a five-year study. The Norwegian-Danish Study Group. Eur. J. Neurol. 6, 539-547.
23. Miklya, I., Knoll, B., Knoll, J., 2003. A pharmacological analysis elucidating why, in contrast to (-)-deprenyl (selegiline) a-tocopherol was ineffective in the DATATOP study. Life Sci. 72, 2641-2648.
24. Myttyla, V.V., Sotaniemi, K.A., Vourinen, J.A., Heinonen, E.H., 1992. Selegiline as initial treatment in de novo parkinsonian patiens. Neurology 42, 339-343.
25. Parkinson Study Group, 1989. Effect of (-)deprenyl on the progression disability in early Parkinson's disease. New Engl. J. Med. 321, 1364-1371.

26. Parkinson Study Group, 1993. Effect to tocopherol and (-)deprenyl on the progression of disability in early Parkinson's disease. New Engl. J. Med. 328, 176-183.
27. Parkinson Study Group, 1996. Impact of deprenyl and tocopherol treatment of Parkinson's disease in DATATOP patients requiring levodopa. Ann. Neurol. 39, 37-45.
28. Praag, H.M.van, 1978. Amine hypothesis of affective disorders. In: Iversen, L.L., Iversen, S, D., Snyder, S.H. (Eds.), Handbook of Psychopharmacology, Vol. 13. Plenum Press, New York, pp.187-297.
29. Sandler, M., Glover, V., Ashford, A., Stern, G.M., 1978. Absence of "cheese effect" during deprenyl therapy: some recent studies. J. Neural. Transm. 43, 209-215.
30. Tetrud, J.W., Langston, J.W., 1989. The effect of (-)deprenyl (selegiline) on the natural history of Parkinson's disease. Science 245, 519-522.
31. Zeller, E.A., Barsky, J., 1952. In vivo inhibition of liver and brain monoamine oxidase by 1-isonicotinyl-2-isopropylhydrazine. Proc. Soc. Exp. Biol. Med. 81, 459-468.

PART SIX

HISTORICAL PERSPECTIVE

THE NEUROTRANSMITTER ERA IN NEUROPSYCHOPHARMACOLOGY IN THE PERSPECTIVE OF NEUROSCIENCE

Kjell Fuxe and Luigi Agnati

Golgi (1844-1926) and Cajal (1852-1934) paved the road for the scientific investigation of the brain by giving the first accurate description of the cellular organization of the central nervous system (CNS) (see, e.g., Jacobson, 1993). These studies also marked the dawn of neuropathology since neurological deficits could be associated to specific lesions either in brain areas and/or in the pathways connecting them. At the time one could only speculate about the messages that neurons used for their cross talk. Against this background one can fully appreciate that the discovery of some neurotransmitters in the 1950s has moved neuropathology to the investigation of deficits or excesses of some of the neurotransmitters in disease states, and in analogy with endocrinology, to the study of treatments that can restore the physiological balance of neurotransmitters. In other words the discovery of neurotransmitters led to modern neuropsychopharmacology. At the beginning research in this area of investigations was restricted to biochemical studies on samples of brain tissue with the employment of the powerful analytical techniques that were becoming available in the 1950s. However, in the 1960s a new approach was opened by the introduction of chemical neuroanatomical techniques capable of visualizing in great details neurotransmitters at the cellular level.

The first neurotransmitters discovered were monoamines. The neurotransmitters that have had the greatest impact on neuropsychopharmacology are: noradrenaline (NA) discovered by the Nobel laureate Ulf v. Euler (see Von Euler, 1971), dopamine (DA) discovered by the Nobel laureate Arvid Carlsson (Carlsson et al., 1958) and 5-hydroxytrypamine (serotonin, 5-HT) discovered in the CNS by Twarog and Page (1953). Carlsson was the first to have indications that classical antipsychotic drugs act by blocking DA receptors (Carlsson and Lindquist, 1963). The breakthrough in our understanding of brain monoamines came with chemical neuroanatomy, adding to the investigative power of classical hodology the information offered by biochemistry. A highly sensitive, specific and powerful histochemical fluorescence method was developed in the 1960s for the demonstration of cellular catecholamines (CA) and 5-HT (Falck et al., 1962). The Falck-Hillarp technique was based on the fact that CA and 5-HT are condensed with formaldehyde into fluorescent compounds with emission spectra of a green and yellow related fluorescence respectively. With the employment of this technique it became possible "to map out" the central DA, NA and 5-HT neurons of the brain in various species of animals (Dahlström and Fuxe, 1964, 1965; Fuxe 1965 a,b).

This chapter will review developments in cellular organization in each decade of the neurotransmitter era starting from the 1960s. It will be focused on monoamine neurons not only because they are major targets for antipsychotic, antidepressant and antiparkinsonian drugs, but also because they have served as model neurons for the understanding of neuronal structure and function at both molecular and network levels in the CNS.

THE NEUROTRANSMITTER ERA: 1964-1974

It was vital for neuropsychopharmacology to have the central DA, NA and 5-HT neurons mapped because only by visualizing these central neuronal systems has it become possible to understand how the various therapeutic drugs decrease the severity of symptoms of schizophrenia, depression and Parkinson's disease (PD) by affecting brain function at the neurotransmitter level. In the first paper based on research with the employment of the Falck-Hillarp technique the NA nerve terminal networks of the hypothalamus and their innervation of the supraoptic and paraventricular nuclei was demonstrated (Carlsson et al., 1962), opening a new field of investigations on the central control of the pituitary gland, contributing substantially to the new field of neuroendocrinology (Fuxe, 1964).

DA NEURONS

The discovery of mesolimbic DA neurons (Anden et al., 1966) from the ventral tegmental area A10 group to the nucleus .accumbens and olfactory tubercle (Fuxe 1965b) was made with the employment of the Falck-Hillarp technique in combination with lesions and biochemical analysis of DA (Dahlström and Fuxe, 1964). These neurons are a target for the action of antipsychotic drugs. In view of its innervation of the subcortical limbic structures the activity of the mesolimbic DA neuronal system should affect the mental state (Fuxe, 1970). With the discovery of the mesocortical DA neurons (Thierry et al., 1973) another target for the action of antipsychotic drugs was discovered.

The discovery of the nigrostriatal DA neurons (Anden et al., 1964) from the substantia nigra to the caudate-putamen (Fuxe 1965b) was made with the same combination of technologies as the discovery of the mesocortical DA neurons. Its discovery was of fundamental importance for the demonstration that the major lesion in PD was a degeneration of the nigrostriatal DA pathway, for explaining the reduction of DA and its metabolites found by Hornykiewicz (1966) in the brains of PD patients and for the understanding of the therapeutic action of L-dopa (Cotzias, 1968). In fact, selective, reserpine resistant accumulation of DA could be observed in the DA neurons after L-dopa treatment (Lidbrink et al., 1974). Of substantial importance was the discovery of the islandic DA nerve terminal system in the neostriatum of postnatal and adult rat (Olson et al., 1972; Tennyson et al., 1972). It was the first evidence for the compartmentalisation of the neostriatum that was first reported in 1970 by Fuxe (1970) at the 4th Bel-Air symposium in Geneva, Switzerland.

The search for DA receptor agonists in the treatment of PD already began in the late 1960s. These drugs were expected to produce a compensatory reduction of DA turnover, as part of an inhibitory feedback mechanism. In the search for DA agonists rat and monkey models of PD were used together with analysis of stereotyped behaviour in rats as well as biochemical and histochemical analyses of changes in DA turnover (Fuxe, 1979). With the employment of combined behavioural, biochemical and histochemical analyses, apomorphine, an "rigid" analogue of DA (Anden et al., 1967; Ernst, 1967), and piribedil, a non-catechol analogue of DA (Corrodi et al., 1971), were found to be potent DA receptor agonists. The findings with DA agonists in the monkey models of PD were particularly interesting; anti-tremor activity was coupled with an increase of involuntary movements due to exaggerated activation of the supersensitive DA receptors (Goldstein et al., 1973). The most important DA receptor agonist developed in this period was the peptide containing ergot alkaloid bromocriptine (Corrodi et al., 1973). It was initially used as a tool to study the role of the tubero-infundibular DA neurons (Fuxe, 1964) in prolactin secretion and in this analysis it was found to reduce DA turnover in the ascending DA pathways. It gave rise to prolonged contralateral rotational behaviour in the rat model of PD, indicating sustained activation of supersensitive DA receptors (Corrodi et al., 1973).

NA NEURONS

The discovery of the ascending NA pathways from the NA cell groups in the pons and medulla oblongata (Dahlström and Fuxe, 1964) to the telencephalon and the diencephalon was presented in a number of papers by the Swedish group, and especially in the paper of Anden et al. (1966) in which they described the global monosynaptic NA innervation of the entire diencephalon and telencephalon. The NA cell group of the locus coeruleus (Dahlström and Fuxe, 1964) from which the entire global cortical NA innervation arises (Ungerstedt, 1971) has a role in maintaining cortical arousal (Jouvet, 1969; Lidbrink and Fuxe, 1973). The blockade of the NA receptors of this system may explain the sedation produced by many classical antipsychotic drugs, e.g., chlorpromazine (Anden et al., 1970). It seems that the enhancement of NA transmission by the NA uptake blockade in limbic NA terminals caused by several antidepressants such as desimipramine and protriptyline contribute to the antidepressant activity of these drugs (Carlsson et al., 1966) once the inhibitory adrenergic α_2-autoreceptors have become desensitised by chronic antidepressant treatment with restoration of neuronal activity in the NA system of the locus coeruleus. This work was built on the discovery of the Nobel Laureate Julius Axelrod that classical antidepressants such as imipramine and desimipramine are NA uptake blocking agents in the peripheral adrenergic nerves.

5-HT NEURONS

The ascending 5-HT neuron systems were discovered in the same period of time as the ascending NA pathways and by the same investigators (Dahlström and Fuxe, 1964). The origin of these systems is mainly in the raphé 5-HT nuclei of the midbrain (Dahlström and Fuxe, 1964) wherefrom they give rise to a global monosynaptic 5-HT innervation of the entire diencephalon and telencephalon (Anden et al., 1965, 1966; Steinbusch 1981). Qualitative and quantitative findings with the employment of microspectrofluorimetry underline the view that the vast majority of these neurons are 5-HT neurons (Jonsson et al., 1975). This global 5-HT innervation was shown to play a role in the maintenance of Slow Wave Sleep (SWS) (Jouvet, 1972) as it was subsequently supported by selective lesions of the ascending 5-HT pathways using the 5-HT neurotoxin 5,7 dihydroxytryptamine (Kiianmaa and Fuxe, 1977).

In 1967 with intraventricular injections of 5-HT it was possible to demonstrate with the employment of the Falck-Hillarp technique the existence of a plasma membrane uptake-concentration mechanism for 5-HT in the 5-HT neurons (Fuxe and Ungerstedt, 1967). The next year it was shown by Carlsson, et al. (1968) that imipramine could block this uptake mechanism. The same was shown to be true also for other antidepressants (Carlsson et al., 1969). Overall two groups of antidepressants could be distinguished, one which preferentially blocked the 5-HT uptake mechanism and one which preferentially blocked the NA uptake mechanism. This was the beginning of the development of new antidepressants based on their selective ability to block the 5-HT uptake mechanism that led to a new era in antidepressant therapy with the introduction of fluoxetine. These novel antidepressants produce a therapeutic action with chronic drug administration, probably when the inhibitory 5-HT$_{1A}$ autoreceptors in the raphé cell bodies have become desensitised with restoration of their firing rate, by enhancing 5-HT neurotransmission in the limbic and prefrontal 5-HT terminal networks.

In 1968 the hallucinogen d-lysergic acid diethylamide (LSD) was shown to potently reduce 5-HT turnover and activate postjunctional 5-HT receptors. This led to the suggestion that d-LSD can cause hallucinations by activating postjunctional 5-HT receptors (Anden et al., 1968). The same year Aghajanian and colleagues (Aghajanian et al., 1968) found that d-LSD potently reduces the firing of 5-HT neurons in the dorsal raphé and suggested that that the substance may cause hallucinations by activating presynaptic 5-HT receptors and reducing 5-HT neurotransmission. In 1970-1972 the hallucinogenic indolamines psilocybine, dimethyltryptamine (DMT) and 5-methoxy-DMT were also shown to reduce 5-HT turnover, activate postjunctional 5-HT receptors and decrease firing of the dorsal raphé (Aghajanian et al., 1970; Anden et al., 1971; Fuxe et al., 1972). It seems that to all these hallucinogens the prejunctional 5-HT receptors are more sensitive than the postjunctional ones, and that all these substances produce a reduction of 5-HT transmission in low doses and an increase of 5-HT transmission in high doses (Fuxe et al., 1976). However, there are no indications that hallucinogens have biphasic effects, and that high doses of hallucinogens by activating postjunctional receptors counteract the hallucinogenic effects of low doses that should be the case if activation of presynaptic 5-HT receptors are responsible for the hallucinations. Furthermore, antidepressants blocking 5-HT uptake reduce the firing rate in the dorsal raphé without causing hallucinations (Aghajanian, 1972). It seems that activation of certain postjunctional 5-HT, as for example the 5-HT$_{2A}$ receptors that are found concentrated in layer 4 of the visual cortex may substantially contribute to the ability of these compounds to produce hallucinations (Cummins et al., 1987).

DEVELOPMENT OF TURNOVER METHODS AND QUANTIFICATION OF MONOAMINES

In the 1960s methods for the inhibition of tyrosine and tryptophane hydroxylase were developed for the study of changes in DA, NA and 5-HT turnover with biochemical and histochemical methods (Falck-Hillarp technique) in discrete monoamine cellbody groups and terminal networks of the brain (Anden et al., 1969). The degree of disappearance of monoamines was highly correlated with the activity of the discrete systems analysed and the method was frequently used to characterize the dynamic changes in discrete DA, NA and 5-HT neurons in various physiological and pathological states, and after treatment with neuropsychopharmacological agents such as the hallucinogens and DA receptor (D) agonists.

A further important step in this development was the move from subjective evaluation of the fluorescence to quantitative data. Thus, microfluorimetric techniques were introduced to quantify the fluorescence of amines in cell bodies and terminals together with microspectrofluorimetric analysis (Fuxe et al., 1975a; Jonsson, 1971). For the first time a method was introduced that allowed the quantitative comparisons of amine fluorescence in NA terminals. It was based on counts in photographs using different transmittance gratings (Agnati and Fuxe, 1974). This made it possible to base the comparisons not only on fluorescence intensity but also on the number of NA varicosities in the sampled fields. It was the beginning of morphometrical and microdensitometrical analysis of transmitter identified neurons. Thus, we were moving into the quantitative analysis of monoamine neurons, which has proved very helpful in the analysis of the mechanism of action of neuropsychopharmacological drugs. Furthermore, this new way of dealing with chemical neuroanatomy (Agnati and Fuxe, 1985) was the beginning of computer-assisted image analysis in neuropathology and neuropsychopharmacology, an experimental approach that is still in progress (Agnati et al., 2005a).

NEUROTRANSMITTER ERA: 1975-1984

A large number of peptides were discovered especially by professor V. Mutt at the Karolinska Institutet in this period and identified as neurotransmitters (see Mutt,

1990). This was followed by the mapping out of large numbers of peptide neurons in the nervous system including the CNS using immunohistochemistry (Hökfelt et al., 1980). Prolactin-like immunoreactivity was discovered in nerve terminals of the hypothalamus, suggesting a role of such a protein in neurotransmission (Fuxe et al., 1977a). It is of interest to note that gut hormones like secretin and glucagons, and opioid peptides were found to induce discrete changes in DA and NA turnover in the median eminence and the rest of the hypothalamus (Fuxe et al., 1979). It might be the case that gastrointestinal peptides when released into the circulation via activation of their receptors in the hypothalamus and the median eminence can cause changes in neuroendocrine function and food intake. The complexity of neurotransmission was increased by the demonstration of the coexistence of neuronal transmitters like peptides, monoamines, adenosine triphosphate (ATP) and classical transmitters, indicating the existence of multiple transmission lines (Burnstock, 1982; Hökfelt et al., 1985). Computer-assisted image analysis was shown to be a powerful tool to study simultaneously several discrete brain regions (Agnati and Fuxe, 1985). However, in spite of intense research and promising results it has so far not been possible to introduce a drug that targets peptide receptors for the treatment of mental and neurological disorders. This illustrates how difficult it is to introduce novel drugs in the neuropsychopharmacological field.

The Nobel Laureate professor P. Greengard and his colleagues pioneered the field of protein phosphorylation in the nervous system. They made many seminal discoveries of protein kinases and of key proteins phosphorylated by these kinases, like DARPP-32, present mainly in the efferent striatal GABAergic neurons (Greengard et al., 1988), which becomes a potent protein phosphatase (PP)-1 inhibitor upon thr-34 phosphorylation that takes place after the activation of D_1 receptors. DARPP-32 plays a key role in intracellular information handling by being a node for integration of a large number of intracellular signals including those formed upon activation of plasma membrane receptors. There is no doubt that DARPP-32 represents an important target for drug action with a modulation of its PP-1 inhibitory activity that will change the metabolic and ion channel activity of neurons.

This period also saw the first indications of receptor diversity that had a strong impact on drug development leading to the synthesis of receptor subtype specific drugs. Thus, it was shown that the antidepressant drugs amitriptyline and nortriptyline have hardly any affinity for the high affinity ^{3}H-5-HT binding sites in cortical membrane preparations, while they had a high affinity for the ^{3}H-LSD binding sites. These findings together with the finding of a blockade of 5-HT dependent behaviours indicate that these antidepressant drugs may block certain postsynaptic 5-HT receptors. However, the reviewer of our paper in which we described these findings did not allow us to publish the speculation that we may be dealing with two types of 5-HT receptors of which only one is blocked by these antidepressant drugs (Fuxe et al., 1977b). Later on Peroutka et al. (1980) obtained evidence that this may in fact be true and called one of these receptors 5-HT$_1$ receptor and the other receptor 5-HT$_2$ receptor. Another important event was the demonstration of two types of DA receptors one coupled to adenylate cyclase (AC) and the other not. They were called D_1 and D_2 receptors, respectively (Kebabian and Calne, 1979). The antiparkinson DAergic ergot drug bromocriptine (Fuxe, 1979) was shown to act at DA receptors not linked to AC (Schwarcz et al., 1978) as proposed by Calne (Kebabian and Calne, 1979). Thus, the therapeutic effects of bromocriptine in PD (Calne et al., 1974; Lieberman et al., 1976) are due to the activation of D_2 like receptors located mainly in the striatopallidal γ-aminobutyric acid (GABA) pathway that leads to removal of motor inhibition. Various ergot drugs act at a number of DA receptor sites in the brain as partial agonists with the ratio of agonist-antagonist activity varying from one DA receptor population to the other (Fuxe et al., 1978).

DISCOVERY OF INTRAMEMBRANE RECEPTOR-RECEPTOR INTERACTIONS

In the end of the 1970s we had the idea that transmitter signals delivered to a cell were not only integrated at the cytoplasmatic level but also at the membrane level via physical interactions between receptors (receptor-receptor interactions). In this way an already integrated signal could be delivered to the intracytoplasmatic machinery of the cell. Of substantial interest was the evidence obtained by Lefkowitz and colleagues (Limbird et al., 1975) for negative interaction between β-adrenergic receptors. In the first biochemical binding experiments indirect evidence was obtained for the existence of neurokinin1/5-HT_1 receptor-receptor interactions in membrane preparations from the CNS by demonstrating that substance P could modulate the binding characteristics of ^{3}H-5-HT binding sites (Agnati et al., 1980). In 1981 it became possible to obtain with the same techniques evidence for cholecystokinin (CCK)/D_2 receptor-receptor interactions in striatal membrane preparations based on the ability of CCK8 to modulate the binding characteristics of the D_2 receptors (Fuxe et al., 1981). Subsequently indications for antagonistic neurotensin/D_2, glutamate/D_2, and neuropeptide Y receptor (NPYR)/α_2 receptor-receptor interaction were found with this methodology. Biochemical results correlated with results in functional models (Fuxe and Agnati, 1985; Fuxe et al., 1983a). A novel important integrative mechanism appeared to be present at the membrane level with different types of G-protein coupled receptors (GPCRs) interacting directly with each other. This mechanism led to theoretical progress in the modelling of chemical transmission as schematically illustrated in Figure 1A-D. A novel understanding for the existence of receptor subtypes opened up by the proposed existence of intramembrane receptor-receptor interactions. There is a new perspective in the neuropathology of neurotransmission and in therapeutic approaches by modulating the recognition/decoding process via receptor-receptor interaction. Receptor-receptor interactions could also be a pathway to modulate peptide receptors via actions on the monoamine receptors with which these receptors interact at the membrane level.

Fig1A-D. Scheme on the development of our knowledge on the process of cell activation with GPCRs. From the black box model where the receptor was an hypothetical entity (A) to the characterization of receptor recognition and second messenger decoding (B) and the model of the process as a linearly organized process (C) and, finally, to the receptor mosaic concept and the model of the process as a branched decoding process (D).

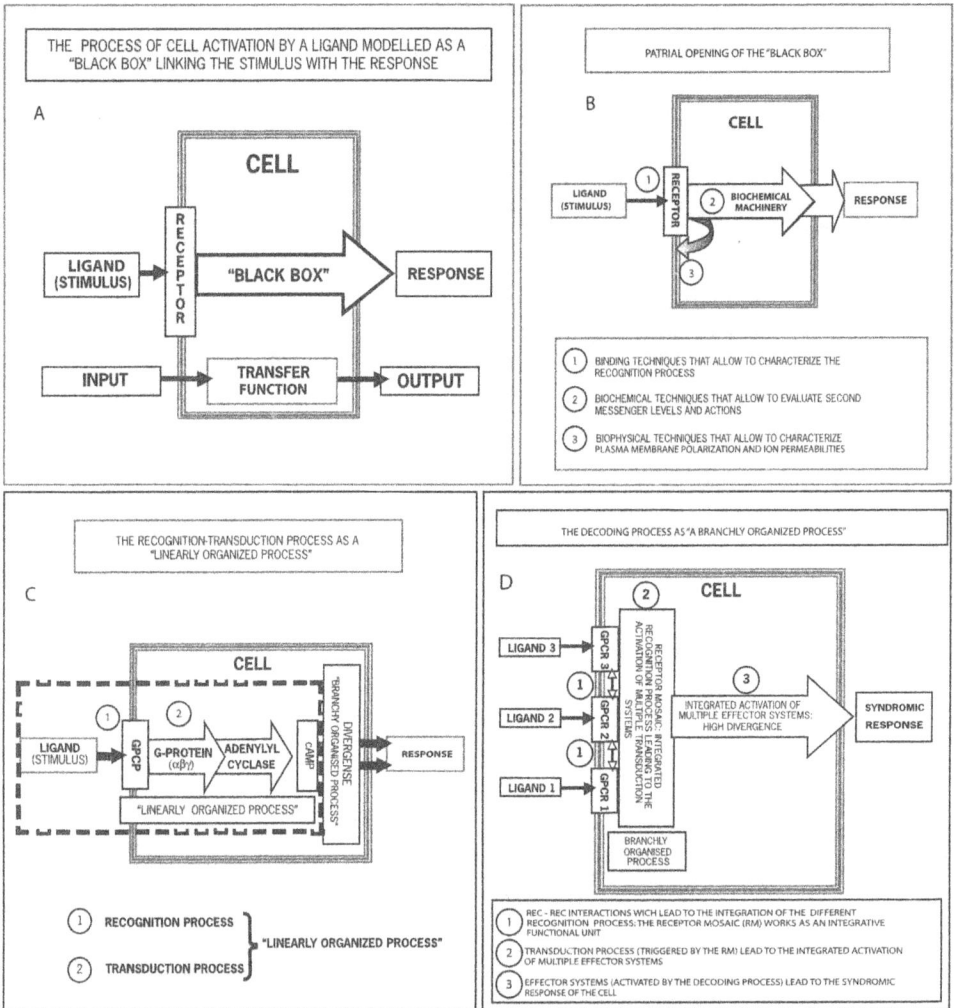

In 1982 we introduced "the receptor mosaic hypothesis of the engram," and postulated the formation of receptor clusters through multiple intramembrane receptor-receptor interactions (Agnati et al., 1982a). It was proposed that these receptor mosaics represent a molecular substrate for the storage of memory traces in the membranes. This was a proteomic approach to the learning process and the opening of investigations on molecular networks located not only inside the cell but also at the membrane level. By now these concepts have been further developed (Figure.2) (Agnati et al., 2005b) and it is reasonable to state that receptor-receptor interactions have turned out to be the beginning of a new field of integrative neuroscience at the membrane level that offer new strategies for the understanding of brain function and dysfunction and hence for drug development (Agnati and Fuxe, 2005).

Figure 2. Development of various proposals for the molecular basis of receptor-receptor interactions among GPCRs. From two interacting receptors to different classes of receptor mosaics acting as input units to horizontal molecular networks (HMN) of proteins at the plasma membrane level.

PROPOSAL (AGNATI AND FUXE)	THEORETICAL IMPLICATIONS	IMPLICATIONS FOR DRUG DEVELOPMENT
RECEPTOR-RECEPTOR INTERACTIONS (RRI)	CROSS-TALK AMONG RECEPTORS (REC) AT PLASMA MEMBRANE LEVEL	IT IS POSSIBLE TO AFFECT REC AFFINITY & DECODING VIA RRI
RECEPTOR MOSAICS (RM)	AGGREGATES OF REC THAT WORK AS AN INTEGRATIVE UNIT AND CAN STORE INFORMATION	THERAPEUTIC ACTIONS AIMED TO FAVOUR OR INHIBIT OR DISRUPT RM
RM AS INPUT UNITS OF HORIZONTAL MOLECULAR NETWORKS (HMN: molecular networks localised at membrane level)	IN SPECIAL MEMBRANE MICRO-DOMAINS ARE LOCALISED HMN THAT INTERACT WITH VERTICAL MOLECULAR NETWORKS	THERAPEUTIC ACTIONS AIMED TO AFFECT THE PLATAFORM (MICRO-DOMAINS) WHERE THE HMN ARE LOCALISED AND/OR THE COMPOSITION OF THE HMN
RELEVANCE OF RM TOPOLOGY FOR SIGNAL INTEGRATION	FROM THE SAME REC (BUILDING BLOCKS) IT IS POSSIBLE TO HAVE DIFFERENT INTEGRATED OUTPUT (EMERGENT PROPERTIES)	THERAPEUTIC ACTIONS AIMED TO ADDRESS THE ASSEMBLING OF THE RM
ON THE EXISTENCE OF DIFFERENT CLASSES OF RM	RM FORMED BY THE SAME REC OR BY ISO-REC CAN SHOW COOPERATIVITY	THERAPEUTIC ACTIONS AIMED TO FAVOUR OR INHIBIT COOPERATIVITY

GABA-DA INTERACTIONS

In the search for non-dopaminergic treatments of schizophrenia a GABAergic approach was introduced in view of the existence of a GABA innervation of the A10 DA cell group wherefrom the mesolimbic DA neurons arise. The evidence obtained with GABAergic drugs like lioresal and aminooxyactic acid indicate the existence of a strong preferential inhibitory GABA control of the mesolimbic DA neurons but not of the nigrostriatal DA neurons (Fuxe et al., 1975b, 1977c). This opened up the possibility to improve treatment of schizophrenia by counteracting the compensatory activation of the mesolimbic DA neurons caused by the DA receptor blocking activity of neuroleptics with combined treatment of a neuroleptic and a GABAergic drug. So far this approach has not been tested in the clinic.

The first indications that benzodiazepines may act by enhancing GABA transmission were obtained in 1974-1975 (Fuxe et al., 1975c ; Mao et al., 1975 ; Polc et al., 1974). Treatment with chlordiazepoxide and diazepam, drugs with preferential effects in low doses in the limbic regions, reduced DA turnover in the caudate, nucleus accumbens and olfactory tubercle (Fuxe et al., 1975c). The action of these benzodiazepiines is similar to the action of GABAergic drugs. Diazepam also reduced GABA turnover possibly by an inhibitory feedback elicited by increased GABA receptor activity caused by the drug (Fuxe et al., 1975c). It seems that these actions of benzodiazepines may contribute to their antianxiety effects, because the mesolimbic DA neurons also innervate the amygdala, where a reduced DA drive may reduce the exaggerated fear output from the central amygdala (Fuxe et al., 2003).

COMPUTER ASSISTED MORPHOMETRY AND MICRODENSITOMETRY OF TRANSMITTER IDENTIFIED NEURONS

In 1982 the principles for the morphological characterization of the transmitter identified cell groups were introduced (Agnati et al., 1982b). It was followed by the introduction of a method for rostrocaudal integration of the morphometric information (Agnati et al., 1984a,b). The same year quantitative morphological methods were developed, the overlap method and the occlusion method, for the evaluation of the coexistence of transmitters (Agnati et al., 1984a). These methods together with quantitative microfluorimetry made it possible to study quantitatively the impact of psychotropic drugs on neurotransmitters and on the morphology of the monoamine systems at the cellular level (Fuxe et al., 1983b).

NEUROTRANSMITTER ERA: 1985-1994

THE VOLUME TRANSMISSION CONCEPT AND EVIDENCE FOR ITS EXISTENCE

Volume transmission (VT) represents a widespread mode of intercellular communication that occurs in the extracellular fluid of the brain and in the cerebrospinal fluid. VT signals are molecules like neurotransmitters, trophic factors, ions and gases, e.g., nitrous oxide (NO) and move from the source cells to the target cells as a consequence of energy gradients leading to diffusion and convection. In 1986 on the basis of the lack of correlation in the regional distribution of central enkephalin and ß-endorphin terminals, and opiate receptors in the rat brain, and on prior observations by us and other groups, it was suggested that there are two main types of communication in the CNS: volume transmission and wiring transmission (Agnati et al., 1986) (Figure 3). In the late 19th century Golgi proposed that communication in the nervous tissue takes place via electronic currents (Golgi, 1891). With the employment of the Falck-Hillarp technique it had been shown in 1968-1969 that after a microinjection of monoamines into the brain, monoamines spread in the cerebral tissue (Routtenberg et al., 1968; Ungerstedt et al., 1969). It was also shown that amphetamine releases DA into the extracellular space (Fuxe and Ungerstedt, 1970). Descarries had discovered the existence of nonjunctional 5-HT varicosities (Descarries et al., 1975). Nicholson had obtained evidence that the microenvironment of the brain cell is a communication channel for ion currents (Nicholson, 1979). Vizi had obtained evidence for non-synaptic interactions between neighbouring nerve terminals (Vizi, 1984) and Kuhar had observed transmitter-receptor mismatches in the CNS (Kuhar, 1985). Prior concepts focused on interneuronal communication and dealt with the hypothesis of paracrine secretion, non-classical neuronal communication, non-synaptic interactions and parasynaptic systems (Fuxe and Agnati, 1991). The essence of Agnati and Fuxe's new concept is that there are two major modes of communication in the brain, the fast (milliseconds) well-known wiring transmission (WT) with private communication channels which connect nerve cells with each other via synapses (chemical or electrical) or via close membrane juxtapositions, and the slow (from seconds to minutes) intercellular communication in the fluid filled extra-cellular space in the brain representing non-private channels where migration of VT signals takes place via diffusion or flow caused by energy gradients. These are two highly complementary modes of brain communication interacting via receptor-receptor interactions (Agnati et al., 1992) and via the glioneuronal networks of the brain immersed in the volume of the extracellular space (ECS). The VT is a one to many transmissions with a high divergence in the channels of the ECS with its main targets being the extrajunctional GPCR with a high affinity for the migrating transmitter. The properties of the ECS have been described by Nicholson and Sykova (1998) in terms of volume fraction, tortuosity and clearance (Fuxe and Agnati, 1991), whereas region-

al heterogeneities have been described for the extracellular matrix as to hyaluronic acid, heparan sulfate proteoglycan immunoreactivity, and for its co-localization
with neural cell adhesion molecule immunoreactivity (Fuxe et al., 1994,1997). This
may influence the local migration of VT signals. In 1991 nonjunctional relationships
we re described and summarised for all monoamine terminals in the cerebral cortex (Descarries et al., 1991).

Figure 3. Summary of the known features of VT and WT and the historical role of Golgi and
Cajal for these two modes of communication.

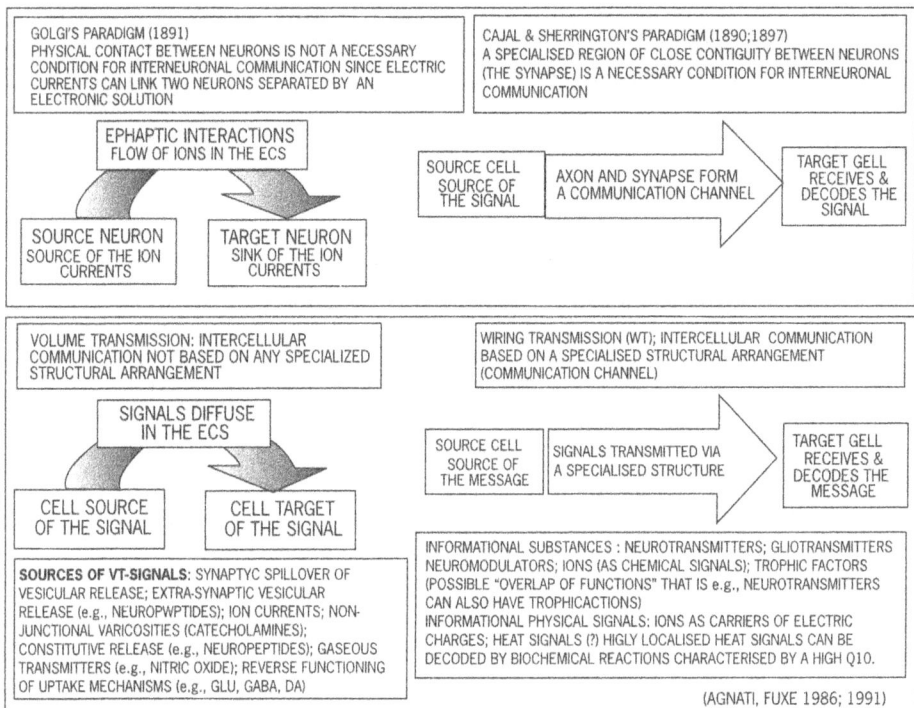

In 1988-1989 further evidence was obtained for VT by analysis of host-graft interactions using intrastriatal adenohypophyseal transplants (Bjelke et al., 1988, 1989).
New transmitter-receptor mismatches were discovered by the Fuxe and Agnati
groups, namely for DA/D_1, and NPY/NPYR and in the pre and postjunctional features
of angiotensin transmission (Bunnemann et al., 1991; Fuxe et al., 1988a; Zoli et al.,
1989). These findings provide further support for the existence of VT, since transmitter-receptor mismatches is the architecture of VT. In 1993 a detailed analysis of the
cerebellar cortex indicated that the 5-HT, NA and DA nerve terminals operate via the
VT mode of communication and that Purkinje cells are important integrators of WT
and VT signals (Fuxe et al., 1993). It was proposed that the therapeutic effects of L-

5-hydroxytryptophan (HTP) treatment of cerebellar ataxias might be related to an enhancement of endogenous compensatory responses in the 5-HT nerve terminal networks with 5-HT formed in the monoamine terminals and then released to diffuse in the ECS to activate distant high affinity 5-HT receptor subtypes (Trouillas et al., 1988).

Since the first international Wenner-Gren symposium on "VT in the brain" organized by Fuxe and Agnati in 1990 in Stockholm VT is considered to be a major mode of communication in the brain that is complementary to WT and the possibility is entertained that neuropsychoactive drugs act as exogenous VT signals (Agnati and Fuxe, 2000; Agnati et al., 1995a; Zoli et al., 1989).

RECEPTOR-RECEPTOR INTERACTIONS CONTINUED

Novel intramembrane receptor-receptor interactions such as the the galanin receptor (GalR)/5-HT$_{1A}$, the adenosine$_{2A}$ (A$_{2A}$)/D$_2$ and the A$_1$/D$_1$ interactions were discovered (Ferré et al.,1991; Ferré et al., 1994a, b; Fuxe et al., 1988b) and it was postulated that heterodimers are the molecular basis for the receptor-receptor interactions (Zoli et al., 1993). The possibility of interactions between extracellular loops, transmembrane domains and intracellular loops of receptors was raised (Agnati et al., 1995b). The GalR/5-HT$_{1A}$ interaction is a bidirectional intramembrane interaction where 5-HT$_{1A}$ activation increases the affinity of the GalR and GalR activation reduces the affinity of the 5-HT$_{1A}$ receptor (Fuxe et al., 1988b; Hedlund et al., 1991). In this way an intra-membrane feedback loop is formed. The GalR/5-HT$_{1A}$ interaction is a novel integrative mechanism in 5-HT transmission. Based on this interaction it was postulated that GalR antagonists are novel antidepressant drugs that remove the inhibitory action of the GalR on postjunctional 5-HT$_{1A}$ receptor recognition and transduction (Fuxe et al., 1991).

The antagonistic intra-membrane A$_{2A}$/D$_2$ receptor interaction with A$_{2A}$ that reduces D$_2$ recognition and G protein coupling is located mainly in the striato-pallidal GABA pathways. Its discovery led to the development of A$_{2A}$ antagonists in the treatment of PD (Ferré et al., 1991; Fuxe et al., 1998). The basis for this new non-dopaminergic strategy in the treatment of PD is the removal of the A$_{2A}$ brake on D$_2$ recognition and G protein coupling. It allows a decrease in the dose of L-dopa and of D$_2$ agonists with a reduction of the side effects of these drugs. In view of the presence of these antagonistic A$_{2A}$/D$_2$ interactions in the ventral striato-pallidal GABA pathways it was postulated that A$_{2A}$/D$_2$ antagonists are antipsychotic drugs (Ferré et al., 1994a; Fuxe et al.,1998).

The antagonistic intramembrane A$_1$/D$_1$ receptor interaction with A$_1$ uncoupling the D$_1$ receptors exists mainly in the direct striatonigral GABA pathways but possibly also in the cerebral cortex (Ferré et al 1994b; Fuxe et al., 1998). These biochemical events may underlay the ability of A$_1$ agonists to counteract D$_1$ induced motor activity, dyskinesias and electroencephalographic (EEG) arousal.

The pioneering work of Lefkowitz and colleagues on the isolation and molecular characterization of the adrenergic receptors (Lefkowitz and Caron, 1988) made it possible to begin the molecular analysis of the direct intramembrane receptor-receptor interactions.

NICOTINIC RECEPTORS

The pioneering work of Changeux and colleagues (Changeux, 1990) in the identification of the nicotinic acetylcholine receptor as an allosteric ligand gated ion channel and in the characterization of its functional architecture and dynamic properties must be recognised.

In an extensive analysis of the effects of nicotine and exposure to cigarette smoke on the nigrostriatal and mesolimbic DA neurons evidence has been obtained that the euphoric action of these substances may be linked to nicotine induced increases of DA turnover in the DA terminals of the anterior parts of the nucleus accumbens and possibly also in the anterior olfactory tubercle (Andersson et al., 1981; Fuxe et al., 1986, 1990a). Thus, these DA terminal systems in the forebrain are preferentially sensitive to nicotine. In view of the evidence that the mesolimbic DA systems and especially those projecting to the nucleus accumbens a re reward systems, the DA neurons from the meso-accumbens to the anterior part of the nucleus accumbens may at least in part mediate nicotine induced euphoria and dependence. Nicotinic receptors exist in both the cell bodies and terminals of the ascending DA pathways.

In an extensive analysis over many years marked effects of nicotine and exposure to cigarette smoke on neuroendocrine functions have been discovered in the male and female rat with inhibition of the luteinising hormone (LH), thyrotropin stimulatig hormone (TSH) and prolactin secretion and activation of corticosterone secretion (Anderson et al., 1982; Fuxe et al., 1977d, 1989). Nicotine induced activation of the tubero-infundibular DA neurons appear to be responsible for the nicotine induced inhibition of LH and prolactin secretion. It is not known whether nicotinic receptors exist on the tubero-infundibular DA neurons or an indirect activation of these structures takes place. This work had shown for the first time how nicotine might target different types of DA neurons to produce its euphoric and neuroendocrine actions. It was also suggested that the increased corticosterone secretion caused by nicotine could modulate nicotine's mood elevating activity by activating glycocorticoid receptors in the mesolimbic DA systems and thereby lead to the development of nicotine dependence (Fuxe et al., 1990a).

An inverse association between cigarette smoking and PD has been reported. In 1988 the first evidence was obtained that chronic nicotine treatment can exert protective effects against surgical lesion and 1-methyl-4-phenyl-1,2,3,6-tetrahydropyridine (MPTP) induced degeneration of the nigrostriatal DA neurons (Fuxe et al., 1990b; Janson et al., 1988a,b). This opened up a new treatment strategy for neurodegenerative diseases based on the development of nicotine receptor sub-type specific agonists. Sustained increase in the synthesis of astroglial basic fibrob-last growth factor (FGF-2) was also seen around degenerating nigral DA cells, indi-cating that astrocytic FGF-2 may cause neuroprotective effects and increased repair in DA nerve cells (Chadi et al., 1994). The concept of astrocyte–kinetic drugs were introduced by the Agnati and Fuxe teams in the treatment of neurodegenerative diseases for drugs which are able to activate astrocytes to secrete trophic factors (Biagini et al., 1994). It was also proposed that there are also microglia-static drugs which are capable of reducing microglia activation (Agnati, 1998). It should be noted that a well known risk factor of neurodegeneration in the elderly is microglia hyperactivation (Agnati, 1998; Blasko et al., 2004).

In 1985 glycocorticoid receptor (GR) immunoreactive neurons and glia began to be mapped out in the brain and spinal cord (Fuxe et al., 1985a,b). It extended the early work of McEwen (McEwen et al., 1968) by showing the accumulation of labelled corticosterone in certain limbic regions. This chemical-anatomical work was completed with an extensive map in combination with computer assisted mor-phometry and microdensitometry of the glycocorticoid immunoreactive neurons and glia (Cintra et al., 1994). Using *in vitro* autoradiography in parallel with this work Reul and de Kloet (1985,1986) characterized two corticosterone receptor sys-tems in the brain, the mineralocorticoid receptor and the GR, the latter having a similar distribution pattern in the brain as GR immunoreactivity. This fundamen-tal work opened up an understanding of how glycocorticoids in stress may tune networks of different regions to obtain optimal integration of information han-dling and thereby increase survival under challenging conditions. It is also pos-sible to see glycocorticoids as modulators of neuronal plasticity assisting in the long-term functional and morphological reconstruction of the glioneuronal net-works. In this remodeling glycocorticoids are organizers of networks that involve both destructive and reconstructive actions (Fuxe et al., 1996). The possible pos-itive role of glycocorticoids is also supported by the demonstration of Agnati's group that corticosterone counteracts lesions induced by neonatal treatment with monosodi-um glutamate in the mediobasal hypothalamus (Zoli et al., 1991). This work underlines that drugs such as GR antagonists may have interesting therapeutic potentials in the different states induced by excessive stress, in which they may reduce the destructive actions of GR activation as well as the development of a depressed state. However, GR agonists may in some instances also have a neuroprotective role, possibly involving a static action on microglia.

NEUROTRANSMITTER ERA: 1995-2005

In 1995 the concept of the trophic unit was introduced and suggested that each nerve cell is part of such a unit (Agnati et al., 1995c). A trophic unit consists of nerve cells, glial cells (astroglia, microglia, oligodendroglia), blood micro-vessels and endothelial cells with extracellular matrix in which the molecules are supporting the survival of each other. Thus, exchange of trophic signals can take place among the different types of cells both via WT and VT. Furthermore, the local microvasculature supports cell metabolism and contributes together with arterioles and venules to the local control of temperature (Agnati et al., 2005a; Yablonskiy et al., 2000). Degeneration may spread from one trophic unit to the other but others may be saved by having partial barriers in the extracellular space or having a strong trophic support that can resist the neurotoxic challenge from neighbouring trophic units. Some trophic units may have high amounts of GR, whereas others have low and will therefore be differentially modulated by glycocorticoids in terms of for example the expression of neurotrophic factors and their receptors. There is no strong evidence for this concept but it can explain heterogeneities in the spread of degeneration and in responses to for example glycocorticoids that have no correlates in neuroanatomical parcellations.

RECEPTOR-RECEPTOR INTERACTIONS CONTINUED

The field exploded in 1998 with the discovery of the first 7 transmembrane (TM) heterodimer, the GABA-B receptor (Marshall et al., 1999). It was composed of two subunits, GABA- B1 and GABA-B2 and the interface between the two may involve TM domains and a coiled-coil interaction of C-terminal tails.

In 2000 with coimmunoprecipation techniques two different 7TM receptors, namely the A_1 and the D_1 receptors were discovered to form a heteromeric receptor complex (Gines et al., 2000), providing the molecular basis for the antagonistic A_1/D_1 interaction observed in the basal ganglia.

In 2000 Liu and colleagues (Liu et al., 2000) discovered that the D_5 receptor may form a complex with GABA-A receptors via a direct protein-protein coupling between the C terminus of dopamine D_5 and the second intracellular loop of the GABA-A receptor γ-2 subunit. It was the first demonstration of a direct protein-protein interaction between a 7TM receptor and an ion-channel neurotransmitter receptor, opening up new avenues for information handling in the brain. This possibility was suggested by Fuxe and Agnati in their opening remarks to the first meeting on receptor-receptor interactions in 1986 (Fuxe and Agnati, 1987).

The demonstration in 1997 that GABA via GABA-A receptors could reduce the affinity of the high affinity component of the D_2 binding site indicates a GABA-A/D_2 receptor- receptor interactions in neostriatal membranes (Perez de la Mora et al., 1997). Future work will reveal whether a direct protein-protein link can be demonstrated also for this interaction. Subsequently a direct interaction was demonstrated between dopamine D_1 and N-methyl-D-aspartic acid (NMDA) receptors (Lee et al., 2002), showing that interactions between 7TM and ionotropic receptors may be a general phenomenon as is the case for the interaction among heptaspanning membrane receptors.

In 2001 Nakata and colleagues elegantly demonstrated a hetero-oligomerization between adenosine A_1 receptors and ATP receptors of the GPCR type (P2Y), leading to an A_1 receptor with P2Y like pharmacology (Nakata et al., 2005; Yoshioka et al., 2001). This might be the basis for the adenine nucleotide mediated inhibition of transmitter release.

On the basis of findings in coimmunoprecipation experiments and BRET and FRET analyses (Canals et al., 2003; Hillion et al., 2002; Kamiya et al., 2003) in 2002-2003 it became evident that A_{2A} and D_2 receptors can form heteromers. A_{2A}/D_2 heterodimers and/or high order A_2/D_2 heteromers exist in the striatopallidal GABA pathways in which A_{2A} receptors reduce D_2 recognition and G protein coupling, and modulate D_2 trafficking. This opens up new ways of treatments for D_2 receptor related disorders. Using mass spectrometry and pull-down assays Woods and colleagues (Ciruela et al., 2004) discovered that A_{2A}/D_2 heteromerization depends on electrostatic events between an arginine (Arg) rich epitope from the third intracellular loop of the D_2 receptor and two adjacent aspartate (Asp) residues, or a phosphorylated Ser residue in the C-terminus of the A_{2A} receptor. Heteromerization is probably an important component of the A_{2A}/D_2 interface. Similar epitopes have been found in D_1/NMDA heteromerization (Woods et al., 2005) and may represent a general mechanism of receptor-receptor interaction.

Receptor-receptor interactions will have a major impact in neuropsychopharmacology, since it opens up a new field of investigations to understand the structural and functional principles in the operation of molecular networks. It will give the molecular basis for pathogenetic mechanisms in the brain and lead to rational approaches for the development of new drugs.

VOLUME TRANSMISSION CONTINUED

Already in the 1994 Agnati and Fuxe described different energy gradients that could have a role in VT-signal migrations (see figure 3) (Agnati et al., 1994). More recently they have pointed out that beside the thermal macro-gradients between active and inactive brain areas (Yablonskiy et al., 2000) micro-gradients could play a role for restricted migration of VT-signals (Agnati et al., 2005c). The uncoupling of proteins (UCPs) could help them in this role (Fuxe et al., 2005). As a matter of fact, UCPs exist in the inner mitochondrial membrane where they partly uncouple oxidative phosphorylation from ATP synthesis by reducing the proton gradient over the membrane, leading to the generation of heat and reduction of oxygen production. UCPs may therefore produce local temperature gradients in the brain that will speed up the migration of neurotransmitters in the extracellular fluid by causing mass movement in the fluid. It was therefore of interest to study the presence of UCP in receptor/transmitter mismatch areas, where there is a need to speed up the VT process. UCP2 IR was increased in the DA terminal rich regions in the nucleus accumbens shell surrounding D_1 rich mismatch areas. UCP2 IR may enhance migration of DA into the mismatch area by creating local temperature gradients and thereby enhancing the activity of DA VT mediated D_1 receptors. There was also strong UCP2 IR in discrete DA and NA terminals in the ventral striatum (DA), cerebral cortex (DA), and neostriatum (NA) with large strongly tyrosine hydroxylase (TH) IR varicosities specialized for VT (Fuxe et al., 2005). This work illustrates the dynamics of VT in the brain and underlines the important role of UCP2 in VT.

The so-called "tide hypothesis" should also be mentioned (Agnati et al., 2004a, 2005c). This hypothesis enlightens two interrelated phenomena: the renewal of the extracellular fluid (ECF), i.e., the homeostasis of the internal milieu of the brain, and the macro-migration of the VT-signals in the ECS. This hypothesis is based on the evidence that when arterial pressure waves reach the sub-arachnoid space (SAS), which is filled with cerebro-spinal fluid (CSF), the dilation of cerebral arteries induces cyclic changes in the hydrostatic pressure inside of the SAS. As each small vessel enters or leaves the brain, it carries with it a sleeve of perivascular space, referred to as Virchow-Robin space. This space extends inward, filled with connective tissue and extra-cellular fluid, to the level at which the vessel becomes a capillary. There are indications that the pia may be left behind on the surface of the CNS. Thus, the SAS is continuous with the Virchow-Robin spaces and with the ECS of the brain parenchyma (Nolte, 2002). Greitz (1993) described the effects that the cardiac pump exerts on the brain mechanics by stating that the brain moves passively like "a piston" due to the alternating pressure gradients created by the heart and this movement affects CSF movement inside the ventricular system of the brain. These pressure waves in the CSF produce a "push and pull" movement, as a "tide" of the fluid filling the Virchow-Robin spaces and possibly the extra-cellular fluid in the pericapillary spaces, especially in the external layers of the cerebral cortex. The tide of the extra-cellular fluid can affect the VT communication in the brain especially the clearance of signals over the brain-blood barrier and the perviousness of the VT pathways. This concept may have an impact on neuropsychopharmacology if it is true that the external layers of the cerebral cortex have a high renewal of extra-cellular fluid. It could also be surmised that drugs, once they have reached the SAS, may have a strong effect in the external layers of the cerebral cortex. A list of the novel proposals for VT and WT is found in figure 4. VT has a special value for neuropsychopharmacology since the VT concept is relevant to pharmacokinetics and to the action of neuropsychoactive drugs (Zoli et al., 1999). According to the VT concept drugs can be considered as exogenous VT signals since they diffuse and/or flow in the cerebral extracellular space. Their diffusion and/or flow is limited by the same factors that influence migration of endogenous VT signals. Neuropsychoactive drugs mimic better and interact more effectively with the rather unconstrained VT than with the more rigid WT such as the synaptic transmission.

Figure 4. Summary of new proposals on the operation of VT and WT.

NEW PROPOSALS (AGNATI, FUXE)	EXPERIMENTAL EVIDENCE
VT AND WT ARE INTEGRATED MODES OF COMMUNICATION AT LOCAL CIRCUIT LEVEL	MISMATCH OF SITES OF TRANSMITTER RELEASE AND RECEPTORS AT THE LEVEL OF LOCAL CIRCUITS
THERE EXIST DIFFERENT CLASSES OF VT-SIGNALS	THERMAL AND PRESSURE GRADIENTS ARE PRESENT IN THE NORMAL BRAIN AND AFFECT NEURONAL FUNCTION
THERE EXIST COMPLEX CELLULAR NETWORKS IN THE BRAIN THAT COMMUNICATE VIA VT AND WT	NEURO DEGENERATION TENDS TO AFFECT VT AND WT INTERCONNECTED CELLS OF DIFFERENT TYPE
VOLUMES OF BRAIN TISSUE WORK AS INTEGRATIVE COMPAR MENTS WHICH CAN ALSO COMMUNICATE VIA VT	DEMONSTRATION OF THE EXISTENCE OF COMPARTMENTS OF PREFERENTIAL TRANSMITTER RELEASE AND OF COMPARTMENTS OF PREFERENTIAL TRANS-MITTER DECODING
LEARNING CAN OCCUR VIA A MODULATION OF THE PREVIUSNESS OF THE DIFFUSION PATHWAYS FOR VT-SIGNALS	DEMONSTRATION OF CHANGES IN THE DIFFUSION PATHWAYS FOR VT-SIGNALS ARE THESE CHANGES SUBJECTED TO A CONTROL?
VT AND WT CAN BE IN OPERATION ALSO AT MOLECULAR NETWORK LEVEL	DEMONSTRATION OF PROT-PROT INTERACTIONS (I.e., WT) AND OF INTRA-CYTOPLASMIC DIFFUSION OF SECOND MESSENGER (I.e., VT)
RELEVANCE OF THERMAL AND PRESSURE GRADIENTS FOR VT-SIGNAL MIGRATIONS	DEMONSTRATION OF INTRACRANIAL PRESURE WAVES PRODUCED BY ARTERIAL PULSES AND OF UCP POSITIVE NEURONS PRODUCING THERMAL GRADIENTS
A GLOBAL MOLECULAR NETWORK ENMESHES THE ENTIRE BRAIN	ECM-MOLECULAR NETWORKS INTERACTY AT MEMBRANE LEVEL WITH INTRA-CELULAR MOLECULAR NETWORKS AND ALSO THEY CONTROL VT-SIGNALS MIGRATION

Finally, it may be mentioned that the VT and WT concept for communication between a source of a signal and its target has been applied also at the molecular network level (Agnati et al., 2003). The same modeling used for cellular networks can be applied to the molecular network and one may search for nodes and channels, and also for hubs or crucial nodes to evaluate communication in the molecular network (Agnati et al., 2004b). This means that we can device drugs that interfere with the integrative actions of the nodes and/or with the communication channels between nodes. Probably of particular interest will be the discovery of hubs and of drugs acting on these crucial nodes.

CONCLUSIONS

This review indicates that understanding the location of transmitters and their receptors in the brain at different network levels, and the release and migration of transmitters in the ECS (i.e., VT), as well as the integration of the transmitter signals at the receptor level (i.e., in receptor mosaics where receptor-receptor interactions takes place) and beyond (i.e., in molecular networks where WT and VT operate) will show how neuropsychoactive drugs work. In fact, this approach has already led not only to a better understanding of brain function in health and disease but also to the development of new drugs for the treatment of mental and neurological disorders.

This paper reviews mainly the work of Fuxe and Agnati during well over 30 years.

Beatrice: *...there's not one wise man among twenty that will praise himself.*

Benedick: *An old, an old instance, Beatrice, that lived in the time of good neighbours.*

(Shakespeare, *Much Ado About Nothing* V.II)

REFERENCES
1. Aghajanian, G.K., 1972. Influence of drugs on the firing of serotonin-containing neurons in brain. Fed. Proc. 31, 91-6.
2. Aghajanian, G.K., Foote, W.E., Sheard, M.H., 1968. Lysergic acid diethylamide sensitive neuronal units in the midbrain raphé. Science 161, 706-708.
3. Aghajanian, G.K., Foote, W.E., Sheard, M.H., 1970. Action of psychotogenic drugs on single midbrain raphe neurons. J. Pharmacol. Exp. Ther. 171, 178-187.
4. Agnati, L.F., 1998. Il Cervello dell'Uomo. Scienza e Letteratura. CEA, Milano, pp.1-338.
5. Agnati, L.F., Fuxe, K., 1974. Quantitative comparisons of amine fluorescence in cortical noradrenaline terminals using smear preparations. J. Histochem. Cytochem. 22, 1122-1127.
6. Agnati, L.F., Fuxe, K., 1985. Quantitative Neuroanatomy in Transmitter Research. Wenner-Gren International Symposium Series. MacMillan Press, London, pp.1-418.
7. Agnati, L.F., Fuxe, K., 2000. Volume transmission as a key feature of information handling in the central nervous system possible new interpretative value of the Turing's B-type machine. In: Agnati, L.F., Fuxe, K., Nicholson, C., Syková, E. (Eds.), Progress in Brain Research. Elsevier, Amsterdam, pp. 3-19.
8. Agnati, L.F., Fuxe, K., 2005. Concluding remarks. J. Mol. Neurosci. 26, 299-302.
9. Agnati, L.F., Fuxe, K., Zini, I., Lenzi, P., Hökfelt, T., 1980. Aspects on receptor regulation and isoreceptor identification. Med. Biol. 58, 182-187.
10. Agnati, L.F., Fuxe, K., Zoli, M., Rondanini, C., Ögren, S.-O., 1982a. New vistas on synaptic plasticity: mosaic hypothesis on the engram. Med. Biol. 60, 183-190.
11. Agnati, L.F., Fuxe, K., Zini, I., Benfenati, F., Hökfelt, T., De Mey, J., 1982b. Principles for the morphological characterization of transmitter-identified nerve cell groups. J. Neurosci. Meth. 6, 157-167.
12. Agnati, L.F., Fuxe, K., Benfenati, F., Zini, I., Zoli, M., Fabbri, L., Härstrand, A., 1984a. Computer assisted morphometry and microdensitometry of transmitter identified neurons with special reference to the mesostriatal dopamine pathway. I. Methodological aspects. Acta Physiol. Scand. (Suppl) 532, 5-36.
13. Agnati, L.F., Fuxe, K., Calza, L., Zini, I., Hökfelt, T., Steinbusch, A., Verhofstad, A., 1984b. A method for rostrocaudal integration of morphometric information from transmitter-identified cell groups. A morphometrical identification and description

of 5-HT cell groups in the medulla oblongata of the rat. J. Neurosci. Methods 10, 83-101.

14. Agnati, L.F., Fuxe, K., Zoli, M., Zini, I., Toffano, G., Ferraguti, F., 1986. A correlation analysis of the regional distribution of central enkephalin and β-endorphin immunoreactive terminals and of opiate receptor in adult and old male rats. Evidence of the existence of two main types of communications in the central nervous system: The volume transmission and the wiring transmission. Acta Physiol. Scand. 128, 201-207.

15. Agnati, L.F., Bjelke, B., Fuxe, K., 1992. Volume transmission in the brain. Do brain cells communicate solely through synapses? A new theory proposes that information also flows in the extracellular space. Am. Sci. 80, 362-374.

16. Agnati, L.F., Cortelli, P., Biagini, G., Bjelke, B., Fuxe, K., 1994. Different classes of volume transmission signals exist in the central nervous system and are affected by metabolic signals, temperature gradients and pressure waves. Neuroreport 6, 9-12.

17. Agnati, L.F., Bjelke, B., Fuxe, K., 1995a. Volume versus wiring transmission in the brain: A new theoretical frame for neuropsychopharmacology. Med. Res. Rev. 15, 33-45.

18. Agnati, L.F., Ferré, S., Cortelli, P., Fuxe, K., 1995b. A brief appraisal on some aspects of the receptor-receptor interaction. Neurochem. Int. 27, 139-146.

19. Agnati, L.F., Cortelli, P., Pettersson, R., Fuxe, K., 1995c. The concept of trophic units in the central nervous system. Prog. Neurobiol. 46, 561-74.

20. Agnati,L.F., Ferre, S, Lluis, C, Franco, R, Fuxe, K., 2003. Molecular mechanisms and thetapeutical implications of intramembrane receptor/receptor interactions among heptahelical receptors with examples from the striopallidal GABA neurons. Pharmacol. Rev. 55, 509-550.

21. Agnati, L.F., Vergoni, A.V., Leo, G., Genedani, S., Franco, R., Bertolini, A., Fuxe, K., 2004a. Energy gradients for VT-signal migration in the CNS: studies on melanocortin receptors, mitochondrial uncoupling proteins and food intake. J. Endocrinol. Invest. 27, 23-34.

22. Agnati, L.F., Santarossa, L., Genedani, S., Canela, E.I., Leo, G., Franco, R., Woods, A., Lluis, C., Ferre, S., Fuxe, K., 2004b. On the nested hierarchical organization of CNS: basic characteristics of neuronal molecular networks. In: Erdi, P., Esposito, A., Marinaro, M., Scarpetta, S. (Eds.), Computational Neuroscience: Cortical Dynamics. Springer, Berlin/ Heidelberg/ New York, pp. 24-54.

23. Agnati, L.F., Fuxe, K., Torvinen, M., Genedani, S., Franco, R., Watson, S., Nussdorfer, G.G., Leo, G., Guidolin, D., 2005a. New methods to evaluate colocalization of fluorophores in immunocytochemical preparations as exemplified by a study on A_{2A} and D_2 receptors in Chinese hamster ovary cells. J. Histochem. Cytochem. 53, 941-53.

24. Agnati, L.F., Tarakanov, A.O., Ferre, S., Fuxe, K., Guidolin, D., 2005b. Receptor-receptor interactions, receptor mosaics, and basic principles of molecular network organization: possible implications for drug development. J. Mol. Neurosci. 26, 193-208.

25. Agnati, L.F., Genedani, S., Lenzi, P.L., Leo, G., Mora, F., Ferre, S., Fuxe, K., 2005c. Energy gradients for the homeostatic control of brain ECF composition and for VT signal migration: introduction of the tide hypothesis. J. Neural. Transm. 112, 45-63.

26. Andén, N.E., Carlsson, A., Dahlström, A., Fuxe, K., Hillarp, N.Å., Larsson, K., 1964. Demonstration and mapping out of nigro-neostriatal dopamine neurons. Life Sci. 15, 523-530.

27. Andén, N.-E., Dahlström, A., Fuxe, K., Larsson, K., 1965. Mapping out of catecholamine and 5-hydroxytryptamine neurons innervating the telencephalon and diencephalon. Life Sciences 4, 1275-1279.

28. Andén, N.-E., Dahlström, A., Fuxe, K., Larsson, K., Olson, L., Ungerstedt, U., 1966. Ascending monoamine neurons to the telencephalon and diencephalon. Acta Physiol. Scand. 67, 313-326.

29. Andén, N.-E., Rubensson, A., Fuxe, K., Hökfelt, T., 1967. Evidence for dopamine receptor stimulation by apomorphine. J. Pharm. Pharmacol. 19, 627-629.

30. Andén, N.-E., Corrodi, H., Fuxe, K., Hökfelt, T., 1968. Evidence for a central 5-hydroxytryptamine receptor stimulation by lysergic acid diethylamide. Br. J. Pharmacol. 34, 1-7.

31. Andén, N.-E., Corrodi, H., Fuxe, K., 1969. Turnover studies using synthesis inhibition. In: Hooper, G. (Ed.), Metabolism of Amines in the Brain. Macmillan, London, pp. 38-47.

32. Andén, N.-E., Butcher, S.G., Corrodi, H., Fuxe, K., Ungerstedt, U., 1970. Receptor activity and turnover of dopamine and noradrenaline neuroleptics. Eur. J. Pharmcol. 11, 303-314.

33. Andén, N.-E., Corrodi, H., Fuxe, K., 1971. Hallucinogenic drugs of the indolealkylamine type and central monoamine neurons. J. Pharmacol. Exp. Ther. 179, 236-249.

34. Andersson, K., Fuxe, K., Agnati, L.F., 1981. Effects of single injections of nicotine on the ascending dopamine pathways in the rat. Evidence for increases of dopamine turnover in the mesostriatal and mesolimbic dopamine neurons. Acta Physiol. Scand. 112, 345-347.

35. Andersson, K., Fuxe, K., Eneroth, P., Agnati, L.F., 1982. Effects of acute central and peripheral administration of nicotine on hypothalamic catecholamine nerve terminal systems and on the secretion of adenohypophyseal hormones in the male rat. Med. Biol. 60, 98-111.

36. Biagini, G., Frasoldati, A., Fuxe, K., Agnati, L.F., 1994. The concept of astrocyte-kinetic drug in the treatment of neurodegenerative diseases: evidence for L-deprenyl-induced activation of reactive astrocytes. Neurochem. Int. 25, 17-22.

37. Bjelke, B., Fuxe, K., Agnati, L., 1988. Survival of adenohypophyseal homologous transplants in the rat striatum associated with prolactin-like immunoreactivity in the surrounding neuropil of the striatum. Neurosci. Lett. 93, 139-145.

38. Bjelke, B., Fuxe, K., Agnati, L., 1989. Increased diffusion of prolactin-like material into the brain neuropil from homologous adenohypophyseal transplants in the rat neostriatum after a 6-OH-dopamine induced degeneration of the mesostriatal dopamine neurons. Neurosci. Lett. 107, 33-38.

39. Blasko, I., Stampfer-Kountchev, M., Robatscher, P., Veerhuis, R., Eikelenboom, P., Grubeck-Loebenstein, B., 2004. How chronic inflammation can affect the brain and support the development of Alzheimer's disease in old age: the role of microglia and astrocytes. Aging Cell 3, 169-76.

40. Bunnemann, B., Fuxe, K., Bjelke, B., Ganten, D., 1991. The brain renin-angiotensin-system and its possible involvement in volume transmission. In: Fuxe, K., Agnati, L. (Eds.), Advances in Neuroscience, Volume 1. Volume Transmission in the Brain, Novel Mechanisms for Neural Transmission. Raven Press, New York, pp. 131-158.

41. Burnstock, G., 1982. The cotransmitter hypothesis, with special reference to the storage and release of ATP with noradrenaline and acetylcholine. In: A.C.Cuello, (Ed.), Co-transmission. Macmillan Press, London, pp. 151-163.

42. Calne, D.B., Teychenne, P.F., Claveria, L.E., Eastman, R., Greenacre, J.K., Petrie, A., 1974. Bromocriptine in Parkinsonism. Br. Med. J. 4, 442-444.

43. Canals, M., Marcellino, D., Fanelli, F., Ciruela, F., de Benedetti, P., Goldberg, S.R., Neve, K., Fuxe, K., Agnati, L.F., Woods, A.S., Ferre, S., Lluis, C., Bouvier, M., Franco, R., 2003. Adenosine A_{2A}-dopamine D_2 receptor-receptor heteromerization: qualitative and quantitative assessment by fluorescence and bioluminescence energy transfer. J. Biol. Chem. 278, 46741-46749.

44. Carlsson, A., Lindqvist, M., 1963. Effect of chlorpromazine or haloperidol on formation of 3methoxytyramine and normetanephrine in mouse brain. Acta Pharmacol. Toxicol. (Copenh.) 20, 140-144.

45. Carlsson, A., Lindquist, M., Magnusson, T., Waldeck, B., 1958. In the presence of 3-hydroxytyramine in brain. Science 127, 471.

46. Carlsson, A., Falck, B., Hillarp, N.A., 1962. Cellular localization of brain monoamines. Acta Physiol. Scand. 56 (Suppl. 196), 1-28.

47. Carlsson, A., Fuxe, K., Hamberger, B., Lindqvist, M., 1966. Biochemical and histochemical studies on the effects of imipramine-like drugs and (+)-amphetamine on central and peripheral catecholamine neurons. Acta Physiol. Scand. 67, 481-497.

48. Carlsson, A., Ungerstedt, U., Fuxe, K., 1968. The effects of imipramine on central 5-hydroxytryptamine neurons. J. Pharm. Pharmacol. 20, 150-151.

49 Carlsson, A., Corrodi, H., Fuxe, K., Hökfelt, T., 1969. Effect of antidepressant drugs on the depletion of intraneuronal brain 5-hydroxytryptamine stores caused by 4-methyl-a-ethyl-meta-tyramine. Eur. J. Pharmacol. 5, 357-366.

50. Chadi, G., Cao, Y., Pettersson, R., Fuxe, K., 1994. Temporal and spatial increase of astroglial basic fibroblast growth factor synthesis after 6-hydroxydopamine-induced degeneration of the nigrostriatal dopamine neurons. Neuroscience 61, 891-910.

51. Changeux, J.P., 1990. The TiPS lecture. The nicotinic acetylcholine receptor: an allosteric protein prototype of ligand-gated ion channels. Trends Pharmacol. Sci. 11, 485-92.

52. Cintra, A., Zoli, M., Rosén, L., Agnati, L., Okret, S., Wikström, A.- C., Gustafsson, J.-Å., Fuxe, K., 1994. Mapping and computer assisted morphometry and microdensitometry of glucocorticoid receptor immunoreactive neurons and glial cells in the rat central nervous system. Neuroscience 62, 843-897.

53. Ciruela, F., Burgueno, J., Casado, V., Canals, M., Marcellino, D., Goldberg, S.R., Bader, M., Fuxe, K., Agnati, L.F., Lluis, C., Franco, R., Ferre, S., Woods, A.S., 2004. Combining mass spectrometry and pull-down techniques for the study of receptor heteromerization. Direct epitope-epitope electrostatic interactions between adenosine A_{2A} and dopamine D_2 receptors. Anal. Chem. 76, 5354-5363.

54. Corrodi, H., Fuxe, K., Ungerstedt, U., 1971. Evidence for a new type of dopamine receptor stimulating agent. J. Pharm. Pharmacol. 23, 989-991.

55. Corrodi, H., Fuxe, K., Hökfelt, T., Lidbrink, P., Ungerstedt, U., 1973. Effect of ergot drugs on central catecholamine neurons: Evidence for a stimulation of central dopamine neurons. J. Pharm. Pharmacol. 25, 409-412.

56. Cotzias, G.C., 1968. L-Dopa for Parkinsonism. N. Engl. J. Med. 278, 630.

57. Cummins, J.T., von Euler, G., Fuxe, K., Ögren, S.O., Agnati, L.F., 1987. Chronic imipramine treatment reduces (+)2-[125I]iodolysergic acid, diethylamide but not 125I-neuropeptide Y binding in layer IV of rat cerebral cortex. Neurosci. Lett. 75, 152-156.

58. Dahlström, A., Fuxe, K., 1964. Evidence for the existence of monoamine-containing neurons in the central nervous system. I. Demonstration of monoamines in the cell bodies of brain stem neurons. Acta Physiol. Scand. 62 (Suppl. 232),1-55.

59. Dahlström, A., Fuxe, K., 1965. Evidence for the existence of monoamine neurons in the central nervous system. II. Experimentally induced changes in the intraneuronal amine levels of bulbospinal neuron systems. Acta Physiol. Scand. 64 (Suppl.247),1-36.

60. Descarries, L., Beaudet, A., Watkins, K.C., 1975. Serotonin nerve terminals in adult rat neocortex. Brain Res. 100, 563-588.

61. Descarries, L., Seguela, P., Watkins, K.C., 1991. Non junctional relationships of monoamine axon terminals in the cerebral cortex of adult rat. In: Fuxe, K., Agnati, L. (Eds.), Volume Transmission in the Brain. Raven Press, New York, pp. 53-62.

62. Ernst, A.M., 1967. Mode of action of apomorphine and dexamphetamine on gnawing compulsion in rats. Psychopharmacologia 10, 316-323.

63. Falck, B., Hillarp, N.-Å., Thieme, G., Torp, A., 1962. Fluorescence of catecholamines and related compounds condensed with formaldehyde. J.Histochem.Cytochem 10, 348-354.

64. Ferré, S., von Euler, G., Johansson, B., Fredholm, B., Fuxe, K., 1991. Stimulation of high affinity adenosine A_2 receptors decreases the affinity of dopamine D_2 receptors in rat striatal membranes. Proc. Natl. Acad. Sci., USA 88, 7238-7241.

65. Ferré, S., O'Connor, W., Snaprud, P., Ungerstedt, U., Fuxe, K., 1994a. Antagonistic interaction between adenosine A_{2a} receptors and dopamine D_2 receptors in the ventral striopallidal system. Implications for the treatment of schizophrenia. Neuroscience 63, 765-773.

66. Ferré, S., Popoli, P., Giménez-Llort, L., Finnman, U.-B., Martinez, E., Scotti de Carolis, A., Fuxe, K., 1994b. Postsynaptic antagonistic interaction between adenosine A_1 and dopamine D_1 receptors. NeuroReport 6, 73-76.

67. Fuxe, K., 1964. Cellular localization of monoamines in the median eminence and the infundibular stem of some mammals. Zeitschrift für Zellforschung 61, 710-724.

68. Fuxe, K., 1965a. Evidence for the existence of monoamine neurons in the central nervous system. 3. The monoamine nerve terminal. Z. Zellforsch. Mikrosk. Anat. 65, 573-596.

69. Fuxe, K., 1965b. Evidence for the existence of monoamine neurons in the central nervous system. IV. Distribution of monoamine nerve terminals in the central nervous system. Acta Physiol. Scand. 64 (Suppl. 247), 39-85.

70. Fuxe, K., 1970. Biological and pharmacological theories, Discussion. In: Bobon, D.P., Janssen, P.A.J., Bobon, J. (Eds), The Neuroleptics. Mod. Probl. Pharmacopsychiat. S.Karger, Basel/Munchen/New York, pp. 121-122.

71. Fuxe, K., 1979. Dopamine receptor agonists in brain research and as therapeutic agents. TINS 2, 1-4.

72. Fuxe, K., Agnati, L.F., 1985. Receptor-receptor interactions in the central nervous system. A new integrative mechanism in synapses. Med. Res. Rev. 5, 441-482.

73. Fuxe, K., Agnati, L.F., 1987. Receptor-receptor interactions. A new intramembrane integrative mechanism. Volume 18. Macmillan Press, London, pp.1-561 .

74. Fuxe, K., Agnati, L.F., 1991. Volume Transmission in the Brain. Novel Mechanisms for Neural Transmission Advances in Neuroscience. Raven Press, New York, pp. 1-602.

75. Fuxe, K., Ungerstedt, U., 1967. Localization of 5-hydroxytryptamine uptake in rat brain after intraventricular injection. J. Pharm. Pharmacol. 19, 335-337.

76. Fuxe, K., Ungerstedt, U., 1970. Histochemical, biochemical and functional studies on central monoamine neurons after acute and chronic amphetamine administration. In: Costa, E., Garattini, S. (Eds.), Amphetamines and Related Compounds. Proc. Mario Negri Inst. Pharmacol. Res., Milano, pp. 257-288.

77. Fuxe, K., Holmstedt, B., Jonsson, G., 1972. Effects of 5-methoxy-N,N-dimethyltryptamine on central monoamine neurons. Eur. J. Pharmacol. 19, 25-34.

78. Fuxe, K., Agnati, L.F., Bolme, P., Everitt, B.J., Hökfelt, T., Jonsson, G., Ljungdahl, A., Löfström, A., 1975a. The use of amine fluorescence histochemistry in the study of drugs, especially morphine on the CNS. Neuropharmacology 14, 903-912.

79. Fuxe, K., Hökfelt, T., Ljungdahl, A., Agnati, L.F., Johansson, O., Perez de la Mora, M., 1975b. Evidence for an inhibitory gabergic control of the meso-limbic dopamine neurons: possibility of improving treatment of schizophrenia by combined treatment with neuroleptics and gabergic drugs. Med. Biol. 53, 177-183.

80. Fuxe, K., Agnati, L.F., Bolme, P., Hökfelt, T., Lidbrink, P., Ljungdahl, Å., Pérez de la Mora, M., Ögren, S., 1975c. The possible involvement of GABA mechanisms in the action of benzodiazepines on central catecholamine neurons. In: Costa, E., Greengard, P. (Eds), Mechanism of Action of Benzodiazepines. Raven Press, New York, pp. 45-61.

81. Fuxe, K., Everitt, B.J., Agnati, L.F., Fredholm, B., Jonsson, G., 1976. On the biochemistry and pharmacology of hallucinogens. In: Kemali, D., Bartholini, G., Richter, D. (Eds.), Schizophrenia Today. Pergamon Press, London, pp. 135-157.

82. Fuxe, K., Hökfelt, T., Eneroth, P., Gustafsson, J.-Å., Skett, P., 1977a. Prolactin-like immunoreactivity: Localization in nerve terminals of rat hypothalamus. Science 196, 899-900.

83. Fuxe, K., Ögren, S., Agnati, L.F., Gustafsson, J.-Å., Jonsson, G., 1977b. On the mechanism of action of the antidepressant drugs amitriptyline and nortriptyline. Evidence for 5-hydroxytryptamine receptor blocking activity. Neurosci. Lett. 6, 339-343.

84. Fuxe, K., Pérez de la Mora, M., Hökfelt, T., Agnati, L.F., Ljungdahl, Å., Johansson, O., 1977c. GABA-DA interactions and their possible relation to schizophrenia. In: Shagass, C., Gershon, S., Friedhoff, A. (Eds.), Psychopathology and Brain Dysfunction. Raven Press, New York, pp. 97-111.

85. Fuxe, K., Agnati, L.F., Eneroth, P., Gustafsson, J.A., Hökfelt, T., Löfström, A., Skett, B., Skett, P., 1977d. The effect of nicotine on central catecholamine neurons and gonadotropin secretion. I. Studies in the male rat. Med. Biol. 55, 148-157.

86. Fuxe, K., Fredholm, B.B., Ögren, S.O., Agnati, L.F., Hökfelt, T., Gustafsson, J.A., 1978. Ergot drugs and central monoaminergic mechanisms: a histochemical, biochemical and behavioral analysis. Fed. Proc. 37, 2181-2191.

87. Fuxe, K., Andersson, K., Hökfelt, T., Mutt, V., Ferland, L., Agnati, L.F., Ganten, D., Said, S., Eneroth, P., Gustafsson, J.-Å., 1979. Localization and possible function of peptidergic neurons and their interactions with central catecholamine neurons, and the central actions of gut hormones. Federation Proc. 38, 2333-2340.

88. Fuxe, K., Agnati, L.F., Benfenati, F., Cimmino, M., Algeri, S., Hökfelt, T., Mutt, V., 1981. Modulation by cholecystokinin of [³H]-spiroperidol binding in rat striatum: Evidence for increased affinity and reduction in the n u m b e r of binding sites. Acta Physiol. Scand. 113, 567-569.

89. Fuxe, K., Agnati, L.F., Benfenati, F., Celani, M.F., Zini, I., Zoli, M., Mutt, V., 1983a. Evidence for the existence of receptor- receptor interactions in the central nervous system. Studies on the regulation of monoamine receptors by neuropeptides. J. Neural Transm. 18, 165-179.

90. Fuxe, K., Agnati, L.F., Andersson, K., Calza, L., Benfenati, F., Zini, I., Battistini, N., Köhler, C., Ögren, S.-O., Hökfelt, T., 1983b. Analysis of transmitter-identified neurons

by morphometry and quantitative microfluorimetry.Evaluation of the actions of psychoactive drugs, especially sulpiride. In: Ackenheil, M., Mattusek, N. (Eds.), Special aspects of psychopharmacology. Expansion Scientifique Francsaise, Paris, pp. 13-35.

91. Fuxe, K., Wikström, A.C., Okret, S., Agnati, L.F., Härfstrand, A., Yu, Z.-Y., Granholm, L., Zoli, M., Vale, W., Gustafsson, J.Å., 1985a. Mapping of glucocorticoid receptor immunoreactive neurons in the rat tel- and diencephalon using a monoclonal antibody against rat liver glucocorticoid receptor. Endocrinology 177, 1803-1812.

92. Fuxe, K., Härfstrand, A., Agnati, L.F., YU, Z.-Y., Cintra, A., Wikström, A.-C., Okret, S., Cantoni, E., Gustafsson, J.Å., 1985b. Immunocytochemical study on the localization of glucocorticoid receptor immunoreactive nerve cells in the lower brain stem and spinal cord of the male rat using a monoclonal antibody against rat liver glucocorticoid receptor. Neurosci. Lett. 60, 1-6.

93. Fuxe, K., Andersson, K., Härfstrand, A., Agnati, L.F., 1986. Increases in dopamine utilization in certain limbic dopamine terminal populations after a short period of intermittent exposure of male rats to cigarette smoke. J. Neural Transm. 67, 15-29.

94. Fuxe, K., Cintra, A., Agnati, L., Härfstrand, A., Goldstein, M., 1988a. Studies on the relationship of tyrosine hydroxylase, dopamine and cyclic AMP-regulated phosphoprotein-32 immunoreactive neuronal structures and D_1 receptor antagonistic binding sites in various brain regions of the male rat - mismatches indicate a role of D_1 receptors in volume transmission. Neurochem. Int. 13, 179-197.

95. Fuxe, K., von Euler, G., Agnati, L.F., Ögren, S.O., 1988b. Galanin selectively modulates 5-hydroxytryptamine_{1A} receptors in the rat ventral limbic cortex. Neurosci. Lett. 85, 163-167.

96. Fuxe, K., Andersson, K., Eneroth, P., Härfstrand, A., Agnati, L.F., 1989. Neuroendocrine actions of nicotine and of exposure to cigarette smoke: medical implications. Psychoneuroendocrinology 14, 19-41.

97. Fuxe, K., Andersson, K., Härfstrand, A., Eneroth, P., Perez de la Mora, M., Agnati, L.F., 1990a. Effects of nicotine on synaptic transmission in the brain. In: Wonnacott, S., Russell, M., Stolerman, I. (Eds.), Nicotine Psychopharmacology. Molecular Cellular and Behavioural Aspects. Oxford Univ Press, Oxford, pp. 195-225.

98. Fuxe, K., Janson, A.M., Jansson, A., Andersson, K., Eneroth, P., Agnati, L.F., 1990b. Chronic nicotine treatment increases dopamine levels and reduces dopamine utilization in substantia nigra and in surviving forebrain dopamine nerve terminal systems after a partial di-mesencephalic hemitransection. Naunyn Schmiedebergs Arch. Pharmacol. 341, 171-181.

99. Fuxe, K., Hedlund, P., Euler, G.v., Lundgren, K., Martire, M., Ögren, S., Eneroth, P., Agnati, L.F., 1991. Galanin/5-HT interactions in the rat central nervous system. Relevance for depression. In: Hökfelt, T., Bartfai, T., Jacobowitz, D., Ottoson, D. (Eds.), Galanin. A new Multifunctional Peptide in the Neuroendocrine System (Wenner-Gren Center Int Series). Macmillan Press, London, pp. 221-235.

100. Fuxe, K., Agnati, L.F., B., B., Hedlund, P., Ueki, A., Tinner, B., Bunnemann, B., Steinbusch, H., Ganten, D., Cintra, A., 1993. Novel aspects on central 5-HT neurotransmission.Focus on the cerebellum. In: Trouillas, P Fuxe, K. (Eds.), Serotonin, the cerebellum and ataxia. Raven Press, New York, pp. 1-37.

101. Fuxe, K., Tinner, B., Gerson, C., Härfstrand, A., Agnati, L.F., 1994. Evidence for a regional distribution of hyaluronic acid in the rat brain using a highly specific hyaluronic acid recognizing protein. Neurosci. Lett. 169, 25-30.

102. Fuxe, K., Diaz, R., Cintra, A., Bhatnagar, M., Tinner, B., Gustafsson, J.A., Ögren, S.O., Agnati, L.F., 1996. On the role of glucocorticoid receptors in brain plasticity. Cell Mol. Neurobiol. 16, 239-258.

103. Fuxe, K., Tinner, B., Staines, W., David, G., Agnati, L.F., 1997. Regional distribution of neural cell adhesion molecule immunoreactivity in the adult rat telencephalon and diencephalon. Partial colocalization with heparan sulfate proteoglycan immunoreactivity. Brain Res. 746, 25-33.

104. Fuxe, K., Ferré, S., Zoli, M., Agnati, L.F., 1998. Integrated events in central dopamine transmission as analyzed at multiple levels. Evidence for intramembrane adenosine A_{2A}/dopamine D_2 and adenosine A_1/dopamine D_1 receptor interactions in the basal ganglia. Brain Res. Reviews 26, 258-273.

105. Fuxe, K., Jacobsen, K.X., Höistad, M., Tinner, B., Jansson, A., Staines, W.A., Agnati, L.F., 2003. The dopamine D₁ receptor-rich main and paracapsular intercalated nerve cell groups of the rat amygdala: relationship to the dopamine innervation. Neuroscience 119, 733-746.

106. Fuxe, K., Rivera, A., Jacobsen, K.X., Höistad, M., Leo, G., Horvath, T.L., Staines, W., De la Calle, A., Agnati, L.F., 2005. Dynamics of volume transmission in the brain. Focus on catecholamine and opioid peptide communication and the role of uncoupling protein 2. J. Neural. Transm. 112, 65-76.

107. Gines, S., Hillion, J., Torvinen, M., Le Crom, S., Casado, V., Canela, E.I., Rondin, S., Lew, J.Y., Watson, S., Zoli, M., Agnati, L.F., Verniera, P., Lluis, C., Ferre, S., Fuxe, K., Franco, R., 2000. Dopamine D1 and adenosine A1 receptors form functionally interacting heteromeric complexes. Proc. Natl. Acad. Sci. USA 97, 8606-8611.

108. Goldstein, M., Battista, A.F., Ohmoto, T., Anagnoste, B., Fuxe, K., 1973. Tremor and involuntary movements in monkeys: effect of L-dopa and of a dopamine receptor stimulating agent. Science 179, 816-817.

109. Golgi, C., 1891. La rete nervosa degh organi centrali del sistema nervoso. Suo significato fisiologico. Rendiconti Regio Istituto. Serie 11, vol.24, Fascicolo VIII, IX. Lombardo. Milano.

110. Greengard, P., Nairn, A.C., Girault, J.A., Ouimet, C.C., Snyder, G.L., Fisone, G., Allen, P.B., Fienberg, A., Nishi, A., 1988. The DARPP-32/protein phosphatase-1 cascade: a model for signal integration. Brain Res. Rev. 26, 274-284.

111. Greitz, D., 1993. Cerebrovascular fluid circulation and associated intracranial dynamics,a radiographic investigation using MR imaging and radionuclide cistemography Department of Neuroradiology. Karolinska Institutet, Stockholm, pp. 1-23.

112. Hedlund, P., von Euler, G., Fuxe, K., 1991. Activation of 5-hydroxytryptamine₁ₐ receptors increases the affinity of galanin receptors in di- and telencephalic areas of the rat. Brain Res. 560, 251-259.

113. Hillion, J., Canals, M., Torvinen, M., Casado, V., Scott, R., Terasmaa, A., Hansson, A., Watson, S., Olah, M.E., Mallol, J., Canela, E.I., Zoli, M., Agnati, L.F., Ibanez, C.F., Lluis, C., Franco, R., Ferre, S., Fuxe, K., 2002. Coaggregation, cointernalization, and codesensitization of adenosine A₂ₐ receptors and dopamine D₂ receptors. J. Biol. Chem. 277, 18091-18097.

114. Hökfelt, T., Johansson, O., Ljungdahl, A., Lundberg, J.M., Schultzberg, M., 1980. Peptidergic neurones. Nature 284, 515-521.

115. Hökfelt, T., Skirboll, L., Everitt, B., Meister, B., Brownstein, M., Jacobs, T., Faden, A., Kuga, S., Goldstein, M., Markstein, R., Dockray, G., Rehfeld, J., 1985. Distribution of cholecystokinin-like immunoreactivity in the nervous system. Co-existence with classical neurotransmitters and other neuropeptides. Ann. N. Y. Acad. Sci. 448, 255-274.

116. Hornykiewicz, O., 1966. Dopamine (3-hydroxytyramine) and brain function. Pharmacol. Rev. 18, 925-964.

117. Jacobson M., 1993. Foundations of Neuroscience. Plenum Press, New York, pp. 1-387.

118. Janson, A., Fuxe, K., Agnati, L., Kitayama, I., Härfstrand, A., Andersson, K., Goldstein, M., 1988a. Chronic nicotine treatment counteracts the disappearance of tyrosine hydroxylase immunoreactive nerve cell bodies, dendrites and terminals in the mesostriatal dopamine system of the male rat after partial hemitransection. Brain Res. 455, 332-345.

119. Janson, A., Fuxe, K., Sundström, E., Agnati, L., Goldstein, M., 1988b. Chronic nicotine treatment partly protects against the 1-methyl-4-phenyl-2,3,6-tetrahydropyridine-induced degeneration of nigrostriatal dopamine neurons in the black mouse. Acta Physiol. Scand. 132, 589-591.

120. Jonsson, G., 1971. Quantitation of fluorescence of biogenic monoamines demonstrated with the formaldehyde fluorescence method. Prog. Histochem. Cytochem. 2, 299-334.

121. Jonsson, G., Einarsson, P., Fuxe, K., Hallman, H., 1975. Microspectrofluorimetric analysis of the formaldehyde induced fluorescence in midbrain raphé neurons. Med. Biol. 53, 25-39.

122. Jouvet, M., 1969. Biogenic amines and the states of sleep. Science 163, 32-41.

123. Jouvet, M., 1972. The role of monoamines and acetylcholine-containing neurons in the regulation of the sleep-waking cycle. Ergeb. Physiol. 64, 166-307.

124. Kamiya, T., Saitoh, O., Yoshioka, K., Nakata, H., 2003. Oligomerization of adenosine A_{2A} and dopamine D_2 receptors in living cells. Biochem. Biophys. Res. Commun. 306, 544-549.

125. Kebabian, J.W., Calne, D.B., 1979. Multiple receptors for dopamine. Nature 277, 93-96.

126. Kiianmaa, K., Fuxe, K., 1977. The effects of 5,7-dihydroxytryptamine-induced lesions of the ascending 5-hydroxytryptamine pathways on the sleep wakefulness cycle. Brain Res. 131, 287-301.

127. Kuhar, M., 1985. The mismatch problem in receptor mapping studies. TINS 8, 190-191.

128. Lee, F.J., Xue, S., Pei, L., Vukusic, B., Chery, N., Wang, Y., Wang, Y.T., Niznik, H.B., Yu, X.M., Liu, F., 2002. Dual regulation of NMDA receptor functions by direct protein-protein interactions with the dopamine D_1 receptor. Cell 111, 219-230.

129. Lefkowitz, R.J., Caron, M.G., 1988. Adrenergic receptors. Models for the study of receptors coupled to guanine nucleotide regulatory proteins. J. Biol. Chem. 263, 4993-4996.

130. Lidbrink, P., Fuxe, K., 1973. Effects of intracerebral injections of 6-hydroxydopamine on sleep and waking in the rat. J. Pharm. Pharmacol. 25, 84-87.

131. Lidbrink, P., Jonsson, G., Fuxe, K., 1974. Selective reserpine-resistant accumulation of catecholamines in central dopamine neurones after dopa administration. Brain Res. 67, 439-456.

132. Lieberman, A., Zolfaghari, M., Boal, D., Hassouri, H., Vogel, B., Battista, A., Fuxe, K., Goldstein, M., 1976. The antiparkinsonian efficacy of bromocriptine. Neurology 26, 405-409.

133. Limbird, L.E., Meyts, P.D., Lefkowitz, R.J., 1975. β–adrenergic receptors: evidence for negative cooperativity. Biochem. Biophys. Res. Commun. 64, 1160-1168.

134. Liu, F., Wan, Q., Pristupa, Z.B., Yu, X.M., Wang, Y.T., Niznik, H.B., 2000. Direct protein-protein coupling enables cross-talk between dopamine D_5 and γ-aminobutyric acid. A receptors. Nature 403, 274-280.

135. Mao, C.C., Guidotti, A., Costa, E., 1975. Evidence for an involvement of GABA in the mediation of the cerebellar cGMP decrease and the anticonvulsant action diazepam. Naunyn Schmiedebergs Arch. Pharmacol. 289, 369-378.

136. Marshall, F.H., Jones, K.A., Kaupmann, K., Bettler, B., 1999. GABA-B receptors - the first 7TM heterodimers. Trends Pharmacol. Sci. 20, 396-399.

137. McEwen, B.S., Weiss, J.M., Schwartz, L.S., 1968. Selective retention of corticosterone by limbic structures in rat brain. Nature 220, 911-912.

138. Mutt, V., 1990. Recent developments in the chemistry of gastrointestinal peptides. Eur. J. Clin. Invest. 20 (Suppl. 1), S2-S9.

139. Nakata, H., Yoshioka, K., Kamiya, T., Tsuga, H., Oyanagi, K., 2005. Functions of heteromeric association between adenosine and P2Y receptors. J. Mol. Neurosci. 26, 233-238.

140. Nicholson, C., 1979. Brain cell microenvironment as a communication channel. In: Schmitt, F., Worden, F. (Eds.), The Neurosciences: Fourth Study Program. The MIT Press, Cambridge,MA, pp. 457-476.

141. Nicholson, C., Sykova, E., 1998. Extracellular space structure revealed by diffusion analysis. Trends Neurosc. 21, 207-215.

142. Nolte, J., 2002. The Human Brain. Mosby, St Louis, pp. 1-650.

143. Olson, L., Seiger, Å., Fuxe, K., 1972. Heterogeneity of striatal and limbic dopamine innervation: Highly fluorescent islands in developing and adult rats. Brain Res. 44, 283-288.

144. Perez de la Mora, M., Ferre, S., Fuxe, K., 1997. GABA-dopamine receptor-receptor interactions in neostriatal membranes of the rat. Neurochem. Res. 22, 1051-1054.

145. Peroutka, S.J., Snyder, S.H., 1979. Multiple serotonin receptors: differential binding of [³H]5-hydroxytryptamine, [³H]lysergic acid diethylamide and [³H]spiroperidol. Mol. Pharmacol. 16, 687-99.

146. Polc, P., Mohler, H., Haefely, W., 1974. The effect of diazepam on spinal cord activities: possible sites and mechanisms of action. Naunyn Schmiedebergs Arch. Pharmacol. 284, 319-337.

147. Reul, J.M., de Kloet, E.R., 1985. Two receptor systems for corticosterone in rat brain: microdistribution and differential occupation. Endocrinology 117, 2505-2511.

148. Reul, J.M., de Kloet, E.R., 1986. Anatomical resolution of two types of corticosterone receptor sites in rat brain with in vitro autoradiography and computerized image analysis. J. Steroid. Biochem. 24, 269-272.

149. Routtenberg, A., Sladek, J., Bondareff, W., 1968. Histochemical fluorescence after application of neurochemicals to caudate nucleus and septal area in vivo. Science 161, 272-274.

150. Schwarcz, R., Fuxe, K., Agnati, L.F., Gustafsson, J.A., 1978. Effects of bromocriptine on ^{3}H-spiroperidol binding sites in rat striatum. Evidence for actions of dopamine receptors not linked to adenylate cyclase. Life Sci. 23, 465-469.

151. Steinbusch, H.W., 1981. Distribution of serotonin-immunoreactivity in the central nervous system of the rat-cell bodies and terminals. Neuroscience 6, 557-618.

152. Tennyson, V.M., Barrett, R.E., Cohen, G., Cote, L., Heikkila, R., Mytilineou, C., 1972. The developing neostriatum of the rabbit: correlation of fluorescence histochemistry, electron microscopy, endogenous dopamine levels, and (^{3}H)dopamine uptake. Brain Res. 46, 251-285.

153. Thierry, A.M., Stinus, L., Blanc, G., Glowinski, J., 1973. Some evidence for the existence of dopaminergic neurons in the rat cortex. Brain Res. 50, 230-234.

154. Trouillas, P., Brudon, F., Adeleine, P., 1988. Improvement of cerebellar ataxia with levorotatory form of 5-hydroxytryptophan. A double-blind study with quantified data processing. Arch. Neurol. 45, 1217-1222.

155. Twarog, B.M., Page, I.H., 1953. Serotonin content of some mammalian tissues and urine and a method for its determination. Am. J. Physiol. 175, 157-161.

156. Ungerstedt, U., Butcher, L., Butcher, S., Anden, N., Fuxe, K., 1969. Direct chemical stimulation of dopaminergic mechanisms in the neostriatum of the rat. Brain Res. 14, 461-471.

157. Ungerstedt, U., 1971. Stereotaxic mapping of the monoamine pathways in the rat brain. Acta Physiol. Scand. (Suppl) 367, 1-48.

158. Vizi, E., 1984. Non-Synaptic Interactions Between Neurons: Modulation of Neurochemical Transmission. John Wiley, New York, pp.1-260.

159. Von Euler, U.S., 1971. Adrenergic neurotransmitter functions. Science 173, 202-206.

160. Woods, A.S., Ciruela, F., Fuxe, K., Agnati, L.F., Lluis, C., Franco, R., Ferre, S., 2005. Role of electrostatic interaction in receptor-receptor heteromerization. J. Mol. Neurosci. 26, 125-132.

161. Yablonskiy, D.A., Ackerman, J.J., Raichle, M.E., 2000. Coupling between changes in human brain temperature and oxidative metabolism during prolonged visual stimulation. Proc. Natl. Acad. Sci. USA 97, 7603-7608.

162. Yoshioka, K., Matsuda, A., Nakata, H., 2001. Pharmacology of a unique adenosine binding site in rat brain using a selective ligand. Clin. Exp. Pharmacol. Physiol. 28, 278-284.

163. Zoli, M., Agnati, L., Fuxe, K., Bjelke, B., 1989. Demonstration of NPY transmitter receptor mismatches in the central nervous system of the male rat. Acta Physiol. Scand. 135, 201-202.

164. Zoli, M., Ferraguti, F., Biagini, G., Cintra, A., Fuxe, K., Agnati, L.F., 1991. Corticosterone treatment counteracts lesions induced by neonatal treatment with monosodium glutamate in the mediobasal hypothalamus of the male rat. Neurosci. Lett. 132, 225-228.

165. Zoli, M., Agnati, L.F., Hedlund, P.B., Li, X.M., Ferre, S., Fuxe, K., 1993. Receptor-receptor interactions as an integrative mechanism in nerve cells. Mol. Neurobiol. 7, 293-334.

166. Zoli, M., Jansson, A., Syková, E., Agnati, L., Fuxe, K., 1999. Volume transmission in the CNS and its relevance for neuropsychopharmacology. TIPS 20, 142-150.

THE NEUROTRANSMITTER ERA IN NEUROPSYCHOPHARMACOLOGY IN A HISTORICAL PERSPECTIVE
PSYCHOPHARMACOLOGY & THE QUANTITIES OF THE BRAIN

David Healy

BACKGROUND

When delegates convened for the first major psychopharmacology meetings in the late 1950s and early 1960s, they came from all over the world – Christian, Hindu, Muslim and Jew, Japanese, and South American as well as Europeans and North Americans. They came because chlorpromazine transcended national frontiers and cultural barriers. Partly because of commonalities of social class and background training, while in the conference halls and wandering around strange cities together, they found – sometimes to their considerable surprise - there was much more that united than divided them despite these national, religious and ethnic differences. Many might have felt swapping children would have made little difference to how these children would have turned out. Yet any one of these foreigners set down alone in London, New York, Delhi or Tokyo in the 1950s would have been severely disconcerted by culture shock.

And if any of today's neuroscientists were to meet up with the earliest British pioneers of neuroscience in 17ᵗʰ century Oxford, they would probably also have much in common. The sense of dislocation, however, for a modern scientist being set down even in a laboratory from the 1950s would likely be immense, and the journey from a 1950s laboratory bench to today's automated and computational systems close to unimaginable. This is the key and the perennial problem of history. Some of the most important things remain the same over millennia and it should be possible to bring out the continuities. People have always fallen in love and been driven by ideals and have entrusted their future to their children. But yet there are equally great discontinuities, not least for instance in the experience of women, and the almost incomprehensible difference in accessibility to material goods for those living now compared with the lot of anyone living previously.

This article attempts to bring out some of these framing issues by considering two pivotal periods of brain research - the years between 1650 and 1660 and between 1950 and 1960, when on the first hand Thomas Willis (1621 - 1675) in Oxford transformed our views of the anatomy of the brain, and then latterly when Arvid Carlsson (1923 -) and others transformed our understanding of the physiology of the brain. Willis' discoveries took place at a time of immense political and cultural upheaval in England and were probably shaped by and shaped those events (Martensen, 2004). The more recent developments that see brain physiology in terms of chemical neurotransmission equally took place at a time of profound socio-political and cultural change and one of the questions to ponder is how much they have been shaped by and shaped the surrounding events in which they we re situated.

WILLIS IN THE 1650s

Before Willis the question of where the human spirit resided, which of the many organs in the body was the seat of thought and decision making, had been the subject of active dispute from the Greeks through to 17th century (Martensen, 2004; Zimmer, 2004). Views of both health and how human beings functioned corporeally were dominated by models which postulated the existence of a set of humors and saw disease as a state in which these humors were out of balance or there was a mismatch between the humors and the humorally tinged constitutional state of the individual or a mismatch between the humoral state of the individual and influences from the environment on those humors.

Blood was a hot and moist humor that seemed closely linked to life itself. The heart was clearly seen as the central point of the economy of blood within the human body – there was no suggestion yet that it was simply pump. It palpitated with changing emotional states. There was therefore a prima facie case to many from Aristotle (384-322 BC) onwards for seeing the heart as the seat of the soul.

Another humor – phlegm – was linked to the brain, from which tears, mucus, and catarrh seeped along with other clear fluids when the head was injured. These were in general wet and cold. Phlegm seemed well designed to help dampen the ardour of the blood. There were however powerful indicators that in some sense the head did the thinking, in that facial expressions and other manifestations of thinking and feeling were visible in the head.

Some of the tensions in efforts to decide just what happened and where were b rought out by humoral views of madness, which in their various forms essentially saw some of the problems of the mad as stemming from a 'rush of blood to the head'. This clearly in some sense located the brain as the organ of thinking but equally it seemed to imply that thoughts came into the brain through the blood (Diethelm, 1971).

With the advance of science in the 16th and 17th centuries, classical notions of human anatomy and physiology were challenged for the first time in a millennium. The new anatomy of Vesalius (Andreas Vesalius 1514-1564), and a series of discoveries from the refractory properties of the lens of the eye through to Harvey's (William Harvey 1578-1657) demonstration of the circulation of the blood, with the consequent realisation that the heart was essentially a pump rather than something that was best seen as the seat of the soul (Zimmer, 2004), opened up a vista of human beings as mechanical. This new vision found its clearest expression in Descartes' [philosophy in books like *Discourse on Method* (Descartes, 1968), and *The Passions of the Soul* (Descartes, 1989)]. But while Descartes (René Descartes 1696-1650) viewed man as almost completely mechanical, he famously reserved the pineal gland as a possible seat for the soul. The new Cartesian view was still an essentially ancient view of the brain, in which the ventricles and the fluid that they contained were critical, and pretty directly open to outside influences from God or the environment. This view did nothing to force people to examine what might be happening within their brains when things became meaningful or they fell in love.

It was this view that Willis overthrew. Willis made it clear that the ventricles were a peripheral manifestation of brain functioning. He opened up a hierarchy of brain tissues from the cerebral cortex through to the midbrain and subcortical areas and on to the cerebellum. A new vision of parts organised into a whole and regulated from a centre took shape. This research took place at the time that the civil war was happening in England, when the king had been dethroned and decapitated and when Willis and colleagues were hoping for a restoration of the monarchy - a restoration of central order. As many have noted, the new vision of brain functioning corresponded well to the new political vision of parliamentary democracy opening up at the time.

The new vision of the brain called for two new sciences – neurology and psychology. Willis himself coined the term neurology and his new discipline laid the basis for the localisation of ancient disorders such as epilepsy and apoplexy. John Locke (1632-1704), one of his students, taking seriously the ideas of brain function put forward by Willis, argued that human beings began life with a *tabula rasa* and through sensory inputs from outside, built up their personalities and thinking styles (Zimmer, 2004). This being the case, a correct education became an increasingly important religious and political tool (Porter, 2003). Psychology had a new basis.

This was a time of great uncertainty. The world was turned upside down (Hill, 1972). While much of the political ferment was driven forward by radical religious sects, a new phenomenon began to appear for the first time - the possibility of a lack of belief in any overarching god or cosmic principle. It had previously been almost impossible to conceive of a desacralized or mechanical world (Febvre, 1982). Against this background, the questions of what to pass on to the next generation became of great importance. What did one tell one's children about what it meant to be human, about what our purpose in life was, about how the human body might shape human behaviour? Even though almost all scientists at the time studied the book of Nature as another path to God (Shapin, 1994), the constant risk that Willis and his colleagues ran was of being accused of laying a basis for atheism and materialism. Their political skill lay in pushing forward the boundaries of science while at the same time persuading a variety of political masters that their new discoveries were consistent with traditional values and with the maintenance of order in society (Martensen, 2004).

CARLSSON IN THE 1950s

Three hundred years later, the situation was in many respects similar. The Western world had just undergone a cataclysm equal to the one that engulfed England in the 17th century. The legitimacy of politics and of an established order was thrown into question. Just as 300 years earlier a new democracy was being born, so also in 1950s and 1960s a new global democratic order was in the process of taking shape, an order in which women, ethnic groups and the young had a part that they had not had previously. Just as in the 1650s, the world was turned upside down and it seemed as though "the people" were capable of subverting the established order.

In the 50 years leading up to the birth of psychopharmacology, Willis' brain was unquestioned as the way brains should be seen. But although the anatomy of this brain was radically different to any brain of the pre-Willis era, there were nonetheless some functional continuities between the new scientific and older humoral brains. When Willis had first outlined the anatomy of the brain, relegating the ventricles to a peripheral place, no one had any idea how a brain might work, how it might think and feel. The 18th and early 19th century brought speculation about the location of different faculties in different brain areas. This was in many ways a deeply disturbing development for those concerned about possible implications for what it meant to be human. In contrast, experimental work in the 19th century led in the later half of the century to the view that the brain conducted its business electrically. Curiously this offered a possibility for many to, in some sense, continue to see humans and their brains as mechanical systems in which an electrical wraith or ghost hovered in the machinery. A ghost that might function independently of the machinery if need be. A ghost that was in some senses immaterial or at least not particulate.

The first intimations of something different came in the years just before the First World War when Henry Dale and others working in England and Germany began to demonstrate that histamine and other agents might pay a role in peripheral neurotransmission (Valenstein, 2005). These early breakthroughs led on to the celebrated work of Otto Loewi (1873-1961) on acetylcholine (Valenstein, 2005), and Walter Cannon on adrenaline and noradrenaline (Valenstein, 2005), in the 1920s and 1930s. But despite an accumulating body of evidence indicating that these neurohumors played a part in peripheral neurotransmission and that drug treatments acted by modulating or blocking the effects of neurotransmitters, the scientific community in general showed an entrenched resistance to the idea of chemical neurotransmission.

Even the scientists who argued for chemical neurotransmission in the periphery found it almost inconceivable that the brain might operate in a similar way (Carlsson, 1996). In a Moses leading his people to the Promised Land moment, Henry Dale, along with Jack Gaddum, Marthe Vogt and Wilhelm Feldberg on the one side, at a

CIBA symposium in London in 1960, found themselves faced with Arvid Carlsson outlining the evidence that serotonin, dopamine and noradrenaline were central neurotransmitters, but chose instead to read the evidence as indicating these chemicals were functioning as poisons when found in the brain (Vane et al., 1960). The resistance to explaining the functioning of the brain in terms of chemical neurotransmission was profound.

While it might be argued that chemical neurotransmission had in some sense been foreshadowed in the 17th century by physicians like Van Helmont (1577-1644), in this case the chemical doctors had seen chemical interactions working in terms of processes such as fermentation that gave rise to vapours and it was these vapours or spirits that did the "business" (Debus, 1991). These vapours were in some senses not much different to the earlier humors or later electrical wraiths. But the emerging chemical physiology of the 20th century was vaporless and spiritless.

In part the resistance displayed by the physiologists of the 1940s and 1950s must have stemmed simply from the complexity of the brain, and difficulties in imagining how a chemical brain might work and the all too imaginable difficulties in manipulating or experimenting on this mass of neurones and their soup of fluids. But the resistance was also partly spiritual.

There is abundant evidence from the participants in the revolution of the 1950s and 1960s that the crisis was a "spiritual" one. For instance Dutch students picketing the lectures of Herman Van Praag did so on the basis that his work was Satanic (Van Praag, 1996). For these students, there were dark aspects to the emerging view of what it meant to be human. One of the mobilising calls of those opposed to neuroscience from the 1960s through to the present day has been that this is an attempt to smuggle into political life social biases against ethnic groups, the poor or others on the basis of a supposed biological taint (Gottesman, 1998).

However while Van Praag and others have recognised the 'spiritual' questions consequent on the brain research that began to open up in the 1950s, others have not. When I interviewed Phillip Bradley (unpublished) and others the idea that spiritual considerations might have played some part in generating an inability or reluctance to embrace chemical neurotransmission seemed completely mystifying to him. There was no suggestion of this as far as he was concerned, and clearly there is not in the records of any CINP meetings or other symposia of the time any explicit statement that a factor like this might have played some part.

This is not surprising in that by the second half of the 20th century, science had become a job rather than a calling. Neuroscientists did not see themselves as exploring a path to God. Science was a secular activity and its practitioners were often atheists. They were concerned with what they found in test tubes and not with whether these discoveries could be reconciled with any moral code. But while they would have been quite dismissive about questions about God, it is still quite reasonable to ask these same scientists about what light if any their findings shed on falling in love or bringing up children. Facts alone can lead to Hiroshima.

And it must be recognised that what was being proposed was a particulate view of brain functioning that broke completely with the electrical view of brain functioning that had existed up till then. While both views might be materialistic, and from this point of view an atheist might readily adopt either, the idea that our personalities and indeed personal functioning and characters might depend on very precise quanta of different chemicals and variations in these chemicals opens up whole new vistas of indeterminacy about what one might say to one's children about what it means to be human. And if it is not now the goal of the scientist to reconcile the ways of God as displayed in Nature to her/his fellow citizens, society still has to be able to accommodate scientific findings and function.

FROM HERE TO HISTORY

There has not been a figure like Willis in modern neuroscience who in his or her own person reconciled the vistas displayed by the new science and the values of the wider society. But the establishment, having appeared to totter during the 1960s, has regained the upper hand. It is a different establishment though in that political power is now much more closely allied to corporate interests than ever before and among the corporations with the greatest influence are the pharmaceutical companies who produce the drugs whose sales depend on a broader acceptance of the new views of brain functioning. Indeed the single greatest concentration of neuroscientists is now within industry rather than academia. As a consequence, among the bodies with the greatest say in mediating between laboratory discoveries and the wider culture are the marketing departments of industry.

One of the astonishing features of recent history has been how quickly words linked to discoveries in brain science have translated out into the wider culture. There is in fact little of great substance that is reliably known about the influence of neurotransmitters on our temperaments, personalities, moods or cognitions but the fact that the drugs clearly operate on neurotransmitters and the fact that these drugs make some difference to some people and a big difference to the balance sheets of major corporations has led to a widespread dispersal of a neurochemical patois. This biobabble is probably in some respects little different to the humoral language of former centuries, with terms being used loosely to express health and physical concerns without these terms having a profound impact on what happens to us when we fall in love, or what we tell our children about what it means to be human, or how we react in the face of sickness or death.

On the other hand it is hard to know how much it is possible to divorce such developments from the growing and intense secularism of modern society. As far as we know there are not likely to be any configurations of neurotransmitters specific to Christian, Muslim, Jewish, Buddhist or Hindu orientations. In so far as a common language or worldview takes hold about how our individual, internal worlds are regulated this would seem to push us toward the generation of a common 'spirituality' or toward a common abandonment of 'spirituality', where by spirituality I mean those things we hold to be of ultimate concern.

In many respects the ultimate concerns of modern societies revolve around health rather than questions of morality. Where once we focussed on future risks, such as gaining heaven, we now focus on a more immediate set of risks – threats to our current physical well-being. Where once we avoided sin we now avoid unhealthy lifestyles. Where once it was almost impossible to be an atheist, it is now almost impossible to get outside of a discourse shaped by health - to be a non-believer in this sense.

But technical knowledge of brain and physical functioning divorced from a vision of what makes life worthwhile has its risks. We celebrate advances in the understanding of stress that might give rise to new treatments for depression, and fail to see that the same understanding yields drugs that are widely used to tranquillise animals as they are industrially processed. Advances in reproductive technologies are promoted on the basis that they will yield therapeutic breakthroughs, but distinctions between husbandry and therapy are human rather than scientific distinctions, and the prospects of a widespread human husbandry grow. The fact that this engineering of human souls will arise from a marketplace rather than in accordance with the dictates of an Engineer of Human Souls is of little comfort.

We need someone to tell us what variations in our neurotransmitters means. Some of this pioneering generation of psychopharmacologists recognised just this point. Fridolin Sulser in 1998 describing his teacher W.R. Hess put it like this: 'Hess explained to his students that single facts mean nothing for CNS physiology unless they are "leistungsbezogen" that is, related to function or to the biological goals of the behavior. For example, when in vitro experiments were conducted in tissue culture, Hess would come by and comment "you are studying mono-layers of cells; how do you think you will learn from such studies why you fall in love with a girl or why you can't remember the name of your grandmother?" Very sarcastic, but he had a point you know. He contrasted his systems-oriented physiology with the fact-oriented British physiology'. (Sulser, 2000).

'I think, we need somebody like him today when the momentum of molecular biology threatens to neglect the very functions so dear to him. Molecular biology per se - no matter how technically sophisticated - operating in a functional vacuum will not contribute substantially to our understanding of emotional and cognitive functions of the brain. I think it is very important to get this philosophy across and I hope someone like W. R. Hess would emerge in the next few years. Otherwise I am afraid we just become technocrats. It worries me when I see today's pharmacology graduate students. They don't know Hess, they don't know the history of Science' (Sulser, 2000).

As the scientists of the 17th and 18th centuries realised, we desperately need a civil order enlightened by science. Without a vision of the human brain and its functioning that connects to love and meaning, fundamentalisms of various hues will carry a much greater appeal to the next generation than either science or the material comforts of a technocracy. It is only when these connections are made and they reveal whatever they reveal that it will be possible to write a history of the modern period that embraces what has happened in neuroscience. Until then all we will have will be a series of monographs on technical developments.

REFERENCES

1. Carlsson, A., 1996. The rise of neuropsychopharmacology: Impact on basic and clinical neuroscience. In: Healy, D. (Interviews), The Psychopharmacologists. Chapman & Hall, London, pp 51-80.
2. Debus, A. G., 1991. The French Paracelsians. Cambridge University Press, Cambridge.
3. Descartes, R., 1968. Discourse on Method and Other Meditations. Penguin Books, Harmondsworth, Middlesex.
4. Descartes, R., 1989. The Passions of the Soul. Hackett Publishing, Indianapolis.
5. Diethelm, O., 1971. Medical Dissertations of Psychiatric Interest Before 1750. S. Karger, Basel.
6. Febvre, L., 1982. The Problem of Unbelief in the Sixteenth Century. Harvard University Press, Cambridge, Massachusetts.
7. Gottesman, I., 1998. Predisposed towards predispositions. In: Healy, D. (Interviews), The Psychopharmacologists. Volume 2. Arnold, London, pp 377-408.
8. Hill, C., 1972. The World Turned Upside Down. Penguin Books, Harmonsworth, Middlesex.
9. Martensen, R.L., 2004. The Brain Takes Shape, An Early History. Oxford University Press, New York.
10. Porter, R., 2003. Flesh in the Age of Reason. Allen Lane, London.
11. Shapin, S., 1994. A Social History of Truth: Science and Civility in Seventeenth Century England. Chicago University Press, Chicago.
12. Sulser, F., 2000. From the presynaptic neuron to the receptor to the nucleus. In: Healy, D. (Interviews), The Psychopharmacologists. Volume 3. Arnold, London, pp. 239-258.
13. Valenstein, E.S., 2005. The War of the Soups and the Sparks. Columbia University Press, New York.
14. Vane, J. R., Wolstenholme, G. E., O'Connor, M., 1960. Adrenergic mechanisms. Ciba Foundation Symposium, J & A Churchill Ltd., London.
15. Van Praag, H., 1996. Psychiatry and the march of folly. In: Healy, D. (Interviews), The Psychopharmacologists. Volume 1. Chapman & Hall, London, pp. 353-380.
16. Zimmer, C., 2004. Soul Made Flesh. William Heinemann, London.

EPILOGUE

ON SPECIFICITY AND COMMUNICATION: REFLECTIONS ON THE PLACE OF LANGUAGES IN PSYCHOPHARMACOLOGY

Joel Elkes

PAST MEMORIES REVISITED

I began to work in our field in the late 1940s in Birmingham, England. From the very beginning, I saw an emerging pharmacology of behavior and subjective experience resting on five footings. They were:

1. Functional Neuroanatomy
2. Regional Neurochemistry (i.e., a chemistry related to regional anatomical differences in the brain)
3. Regional Electrophysiology (related to regional neurochemistry)
4. Animal Behavior Studies
5. The Clinical Trial.

Psychopharmacology, as it grew, demanded interaction between these areas: it called for persons capable of interdisciplinary thinking ("A Team within one head"). I have reviewed my beginnings elsewhere (Elkes, 1998, 1995).

The areas listed above were represented in the department of experimental psychiatry in the University of Birmingham, England. This department was founded in 1951, a year or so before the advent of chlorpromazine.

The idea of specific receptors in the brain derived from my early interest in immunology, particularly my reading of the seminal writings of Paul Ehrlich. His concept of receptor, accompanied by his famous lock and key diagrams and the specificity of side chains ("Seitenketten") implied stereochemical fit. Ehrlich wrote on the elective affinities of dyes for tissues and bacteria; and a fashioning (in our day we would say 'engineering') of drugs that would selectively attach themselves to specific receptors (Himmelweit, 1956). Tissues could learn, and rational chemotherapy was to him an elaborate imitation of the wisdom of nature.

However in my own case, the idea of specificity took a new path when Bradley and I began the study of the effects of drugs on the electrical activity of the brain (Bradley, 1953; Bradley and Elkes, 1953a, b, 1957). The experiments involved a newly developed technique for permanently implanting cortical (and, later, subcortical) electrodes in the cat and repeatedly recording in these "chronic" animals without anesthesia. In those days, in

Britain, acetylcholine was regarded as the principal transmitter in the central nervous system (CNS). So, in defining the desiderata of a neurotransmitter, I duly deferred to its central role. Four desiderata came to mind at the time (Elkes, 1952). Firstly, the substance should be present in the CNS and its concentration should vary with the functional state. It should be identifiable by unequivocal pharmacological means. Secondly, specific enzymes for synthesis and destruction of the substance in question should also be present at the site. Thirdly, inhibition of these enzymes should lead to measurable change in concentration of the neurotransmitter. Fourthly, the application of the substance in question should have demonstrable effects at the site of application and elsewhere.

This 'first order' thinking was an example of the prevailing climate in Britain at the time. While the criteria held for acetylcholine, they were found wanting for other putative neurotransmitters.

In 1948 Feldberg and Vogt published their classical study on the uneven distribution of choline acetylase (the enzyme responsible for acetylcholine synthesis) in the mammalian nervous system (Feldberg and Vogt, 1948). It is well to remember the formidable difficulties and the sheer time and patience required by their method. It involved the dissection and sampling of various regions of the brain; homogenization of each individual sample; the incubation of each individual sample with substrate in the Warburg apparatus for acetylcholine synthesis; and then, as a last and defining step, the assay of the eluate for the amount of synthesized acetylcholine, using the guinea pig ileum preparation for the assay. The results of this rare labor of love were surprising. Apparently large areas of the brain were strikingly low in acetylcholine synthesizing power. This paper influenced me profoundly and made me question the universal transmitter role of acetylcholine. I would add that acetylcholine was a dominant presence in British neurophysiology in the late 1940s and early 1950s and questioning its ubiquitous role did not make me very popular among my colleagues.

Bradley and I however continued with our work on the effects of some drugs related to acetylcholine on the electrical activity of the brain: Atropine, hyoscyamine, physostigmine, neostigmine were tested, followed, later, by amphetamine, lysergic acid diethylamide (LSD-25) and chlorpromazine (Bradley and Elkes, 1953a, b). The experiments showed that putative neurotransmitters had a regional distribution, and that mid-brain regions had a distinctive predilection for amphetamine. At the same time Morruzzi and Magoun's studies (Morruzzi and Magoun, 1949) on the 'waking brain' could be related to our own studies; and Vogt (1954) confirmed the presence of 'sympathin' in the brain. There gradually emerged (and this was my own view) a concept of *families* of neuroregulatory compounds which had arisen in the brain in the course of chemical evolution (Bradley and Elkes, 1957; Elkes, 1958). These compounds seemed chemically related to powerful neurohumoral transmitters familiar to us at the periphery. Three types of transmitters centering around members of choline ester, catecholamine and indole family were proposed (Bradley and Elkes, 1957; Elkes, 1952, 1958).

Implicit in this concept of families of compounds was a notion of the operation of small regional chemical fields and the interaction between molecules found in this field. As we wrote at the time: "It is likely that neurons possessing slight but definite differences in enzyme constitution may be differentially susceptible to neuro-humoral agents. Such neurons may be unevenly distributed in topographically close or widely separated areas in the CNS, that difference extending to the finest level of histological organization. Phylogenetically older parts and perhaps, more particularly the mid-line regions and the periventricular nuclei may, in terms of cell population and chemical constitution be significantly different from parts characteristic of later development... The agents in question may be either identical with or, more likely, derived from neuroeffector substances familiar to us at the periphery. Their number is probably small, but their influence upon integrative action of higher nervous activity profound. The basic states of consciousness, may well be determined by variations in the local concentration of these agents" (Bradley and Elkes, 1957).

The idea of a regional approach to brain chemistry was implicit in these findings. It was later confirmed by the elegant Swedish histochemical techniques that made distinct neuron populations visible (Hökfelt et al., 1976). It is hard to grasp in an age which takes modern ligand techniques and an in vivo positron emission tomography (PET) scan totally for granted, how improbable forty years ago a coherent regional chemistry of the brain seemed. It is warming to recall the first symposium on the regional chemistry of the brain which Seymour Kety and I organized (Kety and Elkes, 1961).

A major transformation of thought occurred when some simple amino acids, primarily partaking in protein synthesis, were found to 'double' as powerful neurotransmitters. Glutamate emerged as a powerful excitatory neurotransmitter, γ-aminobutyric acid (GABA) as the inhibitory one. Glycine played a key inhibitory role in the spinal cord. The differential susceptibilities of neurons, their pharmacological specificity, in even very small cell populations were studied in our laboratory by Salmoiraghi and Bloom using microelectrophoresis and the micropipette (Salmoiraghi and Bloom, 1964). These studies showed conclusively that there was indeed a "differential pharmacology" of individual neurons and that neurons of differential susceptibility could exist side by side in a very small space. The idea of specificity thus moved into very high profile.

However the discovery of the opiate receptor (Snyder, 1975) and enkephalins, ably reviewed in Hökfelt (1991), gave the term neurotransmitter an unwarranted elasticity and the term gradually morphed into a term signifying a total physiological 'state' and 'behavior' rather than a precise and specific synaptic event. The precision of the synaptology gradually gave way to the more general term of 'information.'

F.O. SCHMITT'S 'INFORMATIONAL SUBSTANCES'

In a seminal paper F.O, Schmitt (Schmitt, 1984) proposed as a working hypothesis "informational substances" as molecular regulators of brain function. His list of classical neurotransmitters numbers about ten, comprising the small family of neurotransmitters mentioned above. The list of later members, the neuropeptides and neurohormones, comprises some additional forty members and has grown considerably since. The import of this paper is two fold. First, it traces the evolutionary origin of neurotransmitters suggesting that they may have evolved from being intracellular messengers to a role in rapid intercellular communication. (We will recall that each neuron carries about 200 junctional sites.) Secondly, it argues for a twofold mode of communication: a precise, familiar mode of neuron to neuron synaptic transmission, and a more direct information transmission "in parallel" or alongside, not instead of or in competition with, the neuronal circuitry. This information transfer may take place through release and diffusion of 'informational substances' through the extracellular fluid and the attachment to ligands on the cell surface, the cell thus being 'labelled' by a transponder, coding for particular behavioral repertoire, e.g., in sexual behavior. It is this combination of serial synaptic and parallel parasynaptic communication that makes for the extraordinary flexibility in the repertoire of a particular neural net. Scanning, analysis, recognition, and discharge would seem to depend on a particular molecular configuration. Once again, one is reminded of the immune system.

NEUROTRANSMITTERS AND PEPTIDES IN THE IMMUNE SYSTEM

The awed sense of wonder grows as some of the very informational substances familiar to us in the nervous system turn up in sites widely distributed in the immune system, which more and more is assuming the character of a "liquid brain." Reciprocal immune-neuro-communication is a well-documented reality (Blalock, 1989; Pert, 1997; Roszman and Carlson, 1991). Cells of the immune system can make compounds which were originally identified as neurotransmitters. The cytokine interleukin has been identified in the brain. There is direct and rich innervation of the immune system by the autonomic nervous system, and mounting evidence of a continuous reciprocal signaling between the nervous system and the immune system.

PERT'S 'INFORMATIONAL NETWORK'

In a highly imaginative text written for the lay public Pert (1997) carries Schmitt's ideas a step further. She emphasizes the wide distribution of peptides throughout the body and speaks of an 'information network' spread through the body, and probably, isomorphic with the body itself, i.e., brain, heart, lungs, muscle, gut, bone marrow, spleen, kidney and the lymphoid system. The network is functionally related but not identical with the autonomic nervous system. We will note, in passing, the association, in close proximity, of some of the small-molecular-weight 'classical' neurotransmitters, and the larger neuropeptides. She regards this network as the seat of the homeostatic states, experienced subjectively as 'feelings.' It is these 'feelings' which inform the organism in real time and help it to navigate us safely through life. The outline of her schema is engaging, and gives one much food for thought.

SOME IMPLICATIONS

It is becoming increasingly evident that the three great information systems in the body-mind, the endocrine, nervous, and immune system use common elements in the languages they share. In the society of cells within the skin, chemical signals travel swiftly from one system to the other. We are at the earliest beginnings of understanding this compact, confusing and puzzling traffic, but it is vital that we realize its importance to the advancement of our field. Hitherto, a pharmacology centering on bactericidal and antiviral effects, and preoccupied with the effects of drugs on tissues and organs has reaped rich reward through the relentless pursuit of the precision of 'specificity.' Yet in our field, the pharmacology of total behavior and subjective experience, there is reason to pause, and quietly and consider some less precise and perhaps more probably possibilities. For the disorders we are called on to treat are unlikely to be focal disorders. More likely, they may turn out to be disorders of molecular communication (Elkes, 1990) in an informational network that includes the brain in an ancient partnership with the nervous and endocrine system. Molecular signals of close affinity travel ceaselessly both ways. Partaking in a net capable of responding to a variety of repertoires may be as important as a specific molecular signal at a particular synaptic site. Indeed, we may learn profound lessons from the examination of a single 'specific' system. But it is the cascade, the statistical chatter and conversation in chemically 'labeled' nets that may give us a glimpse –a mere echo– of the resonances of life. We must look to some key ideas that mark the way.

In his contribution to this volume, Fridolin Sulser (See pp 53-64) examines the *noradrenergic-second messenger cascade*, and the effect of chronic administration of the noradrenergic antidepressant desipramine and reboxetine in down-regulating the active form of the nuclear transcription factor CREB-P in the frontal cortex of rats despite the persistent increase in availability of norepinephrine (NE). He also points to the convergence of aminergic and endocrine signals beyond the receptors.

Similarly, Eric Kandel (The molecular biology of memory storage: A dialog between genes and synapses. Nobel Lecture, Stockholm, December 2000) has beautifully analyzed the molecular biology of memory storage, using his classical aplysia preparation as a rare means of understanding a "dialogue between synapses and genes," and the modulatory effect of interneurons on sensory neurons in regulating the release of the excitatory transmitter. Modulation is an ambiguous term; yet, in this very ambiguity there may very well be its virtue. Worth mentioning also are some older experiments on the interaction between neurotransmitters. These experiments, as early as 1941 (Bulbring and Burn, 1941), studied the interaction between epinephrine and acetylcholine on the knee jerk in a double perfusion preparation. They showed that epinephrine distinctly facilitated the action of acetylcholine in this central reflex. Augmentation of the reflex by amphetamine and ephedrine was also observed. Such findings are perhaps the first footprints in the snow. They point to an interaction between receptors hitherto regarded as "specific." We will incidentally recall that chlorpromazine started it journey into psychopharmacology as a peculiar antihistaminic. We might do well to look for such secondary and tertiary affinities in drugs as we pursue the 'holy grail' road towards "true specificity." The universe we are dealing with is more complex and interactive, than our present imagination will allow us to see. Consider the possible sites of action: First, the specificity of the receptor embedded in the neuron membrane; second, the organization of parasynaptic space apposed to the neuron in which many messenger molecules circulate; third, the role of glia; fourth, the traffic between membrane, cytoplasm, the cell organelles and nucleus; fifth, the cross-talk between mobile and fixed memory cells; and, lastly, the whole range of effects of hormones on the binding and release of neurotransmitters (Ramey and Goldstein, 1957). In a word, we have a problem of some magnitude facing us at the very center of our field. It is the problem of *com - munication* between various elements of three deeply interconnected systems and the languages they employ. *Language* and the attributes of language remain central to our problem.

CONTEXT: PSYCHOPHARMACOLOGY AS A ROSETTA-STONE IN PSYCHOBIOLOGY

I have elsewhere examined the function of language in science (Elkes, 1963a) and particularly as it relates to the evolution of physics; but confess readily that the task facing us today is daunting and different. Nonetheless, there are reasons for hope. For as we recognize the importance of *context* in molecular languages and gently shift our focus from *specificity* to *interaction* we may come upon discoveries which may bring us closer to the true state of affairs as it actually operates in the body. Please recall that the drugs we use may impinge not only on the brain but, on similar or identical receptors scattered widely in the soma. Widespread *communication* is the name of the game and remains the backdrop against which familiar phenomena play out.

In psychopharmacology, we have an advantage; for we are in a field peculiarly positioned by history to bridging into adjacent fields. Like the Rosetta-Stone, which carried three languages, (including hieroglyphs) in simultaneous translation and opened up our understanding of the vast treasure trove of ancient Egypt, so modern psychopharmacology mediates between the nervous, the endocrine and the immune system and may lead us to a deeper understanding of the interactive molecular traffic governing these closely related systems (Figure 1).

Figure 1. Like the Rosetta Stone, Psychopharmacology provides a key to three languages: the nervous system (N); the endocrine system (E); and the immune system (I).

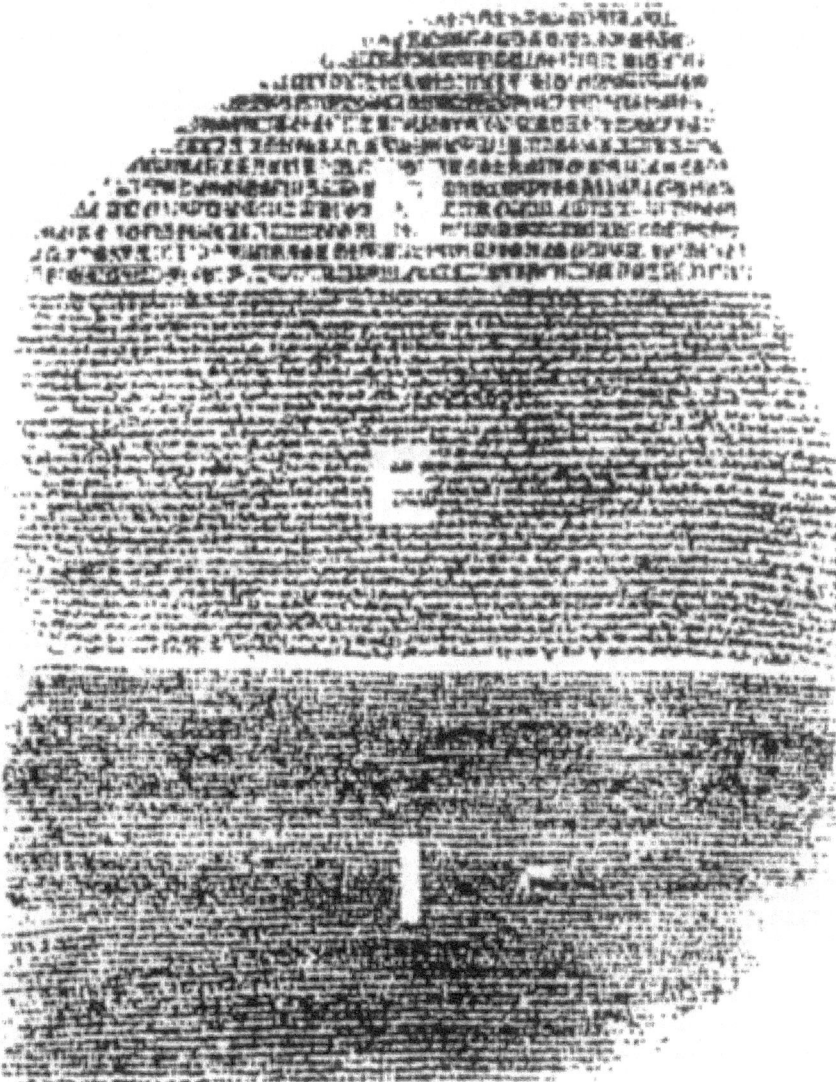

Our field, if used wisely may illuminate not just the chemical traffic of the brain, but the endocrine and immune system as well. The brain itself is emerging as a huge organ of internal secretion; and the far-flung domain of the immune system, endowed with molecular memory, as a widespread information system that as I said before can be likened to a liquid brain. The precise language, the letters and words in the molecular alphabet are shared by three systems. Our 'central' drugs may well exert effects at the 'periphery.' We are working with a widespread molecular network which may provide a molecular basis for the patterns and the fluxes of 'being' of which we may catch a glimpse in 'preconscious' states of mind. The understanding of these molecular languages, the rules by which they operate, their grammar, their syntax, their uncanny effi- ciency and precision in message transmittal presents a huge challenge which we are only beginning to face. As I have said repeatedly in the past, (Elkes, 1963b) it would require close cooperation between chemist, experimental pharmacologist, linguist, information technologist, and computer engineer. However, I am confident that in time - like an image emerging in a photographic negative in the darkroom - the outlines of understanding will emerge. As in physics new mathematical languages will be an absolute necessity. They will be needed to capture, name and describe the patterns, the fluxes of the wave and 'field' phenomena which will be the business of a psychophar- macology of the future. Meanwhile it behooves us to be patient - and wait.

ACKNOWLEDGEMENTS

I wish to express my profound gratitude to Mr. Thomas Beech, President of the Fetzer Institute, and to the Board of Trustees of the Institute for providing me with the time and opportunity to write this paper; to Dr. Fridolin Sulser for his constant encouragement and several very stimulating discussions and for his permission to draw upon his contribution to this volume; and to Mrs. Christee Khan for research assistance and the meticulous typing of the manuscript.

REFERENCES
1. Blalock, J. E., 1989. A molecular basis for bi-directional communications between the immune and neuroendocrine system. Physiological Reviews 69, 1-32.
2. Bradley, P.B., 1953. A technique for recording the electrical activity of the brain in the con- scious animal. Electroencephal. Clinical Neurophysiol. 5, 451.
3. Bradley, P.B., Elkes, J., 1953a. The effect of atropine, hyoscyamine, physostigmine, neostigmine on the electrical activity of the brain in the conscious cat. J. Physiol. (London), 120, 14.
4. Bradley, P.B., Elkes, J., 1953b. The effect of amphetamine and lysergic acid diehylamide (LSD25) on the electrical activity of the brain of the conscious cat. J. Physiol. (London) 120,1.
5. Bradley, P.B., Elkes, J., 1957. The effects of some drugs on the electrical activity of the Brain. Brain, 80, 77-117.
6. Bulbring, E., Burn, J. H., 1941. Observations bearing on synaptic transmission by acetyl- choline in the spinal cord. J. Physiol (London), 337-368.

7. Elkes, J., 1952. Discussion. In: Tanner, J.M. (Ed.), Prospects in Psychiatric Research. Blackwell Scientific Publications, Oxford, pp. 126-135.
8. Elkes, J., 1958. Drug effects in relation to receptor specificity within the brain: Some evidence and provisional formulation. In: Wolstenholme, G.E. (Ed.), Neurological Basics of Behavior. Ciba Foundation Symposium. Butterworth, London, pp. 303-332.
9. Elkes, J., 1963a. The American College of Neuropsychopharmacology: A note on its history, and hopes for the future, ACNP Bulletin 1, 2-3.
10. Elkes, J., 1963b. Subjective and objective observation in psychiatry. In: The Harvey Lectures, Series 57. Academic Press, New York, pp. 63-92.
11. Elkes, J., 1990. On psychobiology, and communication: Psychiatry and the future of medicine. In: Taylor, B.T., Taylor, I.J. (Eds.), Psychiatry: Past Reflections - Future Visions. Elsevier, New York, pp. 75-107.
12. Elkes, J., 1995. Psychopharmacology: Finding one's way. Neuropsychopharmacology 12, 93-111.
13. Elkes, J., 1998. Towards footings of a science: Beginnings in psychopharmacology in the forties and fifties. In: Ban, T.A., Healy, D., Shorter, E. (Eds.), The Rise of Psychopharmacology and the Story of CINP. Animula, Budapest, pp. 15-25.
14. Feldberg, W., Vogt, M., 1948. Acetylcholine synthesis in different regions of the central nervous system.. J. Physiol. (London) 107, 372.
15. Himmelweit, F. (Ed.), 1956. The Collected Papers of Paul Ehrlich. Pergamon Press, London/New York.
16. Hökfelt, T., 1991. Neuropeptides in perspective. Neuron 7, 867-879.
17. Hökfelt, T., Johannson, O., Fuxe, K., 1976. Immunochemical studies on the localization and distribution of monoamine neuron systems in the brain. Medical Biology 54, 427-453.
18. Kety, S., Elkes, J. (Eds.), 1961. Regional Neurochemistry: Proceedings of the Fourth International Symposium in Neurochemistry. Pergamon Press, Oxford.
19. Morruzzi, G., Magoun, H. W., 1949. Brainstem reticular formation and activation of the EEG. Electroenceph. Clin. Neurophysiol. 1, 455.
20. Pert, C., 1997. Molecules of Emotion. Scribner, New York.
21. Ramey, E., Goldstein, M.S., 1957. Adrenal cortex and the sympathetic nervous system. Physiology Review 37, 155.
22. Roszman, T.L., Carlson, S.L., 1991. Neurotransmitters and molecular signaling in the immune response. In: Ader, R., Felten, D.L., Cohen, N. (Eds.), Psychoneuroimmunology. Academic Press, New York, pp. 311-335.
23. Salmoiraghi, G.C., Bloom, F. E., 1964. The pharmacology of individual neurons. Science, 144, 493-498.
24. Schmitt, F. O., 1984. Molecular regulation of brain functions. Neuroscience 13, 991-1001.
25. Snyder, S. H., 1975. Opiate receptors in normal and drug altered brain functions. Nature, 257, 185-189.
26. Vogt, M., 1954. The concentration of sympathin in different parts of the nervous system under normal conditions and after the administration of drugs. J. Physiol. (London) 123, 451-481.

CONCLUDING REMARKS

THE NEUROTRANSMITTER ERA IN NEUROPSYCHOPHARMACOLOGY

Thomas A. Ban and Ronaldo Ucha Udabe

HISTORICAL BACKGROUND

The therapeutic and commercial success of chlorpromazine - first introduced in November 1952 in France - generated interest within the pharmaceutical industry in developing drugs for psychiatric indications. By the end of the 1950s there were at least 12 drugs for the treatment of psychosis; two drugs for anxiety; and seven for depression. There was also one drug for the treatment of mania: lithium carbonate, developed by Mogens Schou and his associates independent of the pharmaceutical industry at the psychiatric hospital in Risskov, Denmark (Schou et al., 1954). The psychiatric establishment received the new drugs incredulously. Yet, with the help of the pharmaceutical industry, pharmacotherapy received a steadily increasing share among the treatments of mental illness, and *psychopharmacology* became part of the teaching curriculum at the universities.

Simultaneously with the introduction of the first set of effective drugs in mental illness, there was a shift in the understanding of the nature of synaptic transmission from a purely electrical to a chemically mediated event. By the end of the 1950s six neurotransmitters had been identified in the central nervous system (CNS): acetylcholine (ACh), dopamine (DA), γ-aminobutyric acid (GABA), norepinephrine (NE), serotonin, i.e., 5-hydroxytryptamine (5-HT), and substance P. Recognition of chemical mediation at the site of the synapse, coupled with the introduction of the spectrophotofluorimeter (Bowman et al., 1955) led to the development of *neuropharma - cology*, the scientific discipline that deals with the detection and identification of structures responsible for the psychotropic effects of centrally acting drugs (Ban, 2001b). The spectrophotofluorimeter is an instrument with a resolution power to measure the concentration of cerebral monoamine neurotransmitters, such as NE and 5-HT involved in neuronal transmission at the synaptic cleft. Spectrophotofluorimetry provides direct access to the detection of biochemical changes that might be responsible for a drug's therapeutic effects (Ban, 2004).

Developments in pharmacotherapy, psychopharmacology and neuropharmacology triggered the development of *neuropsychopharmacology*, the scientific discipline dedicated to the study and treatment of the pathophysiology of mental syndromes with the employment of centrally acting drugs. The new discipline has grown on the premise that neuropsychopharmacological research on the mode of action of psychotropic drugs with well-defined therapeutic indications can generate knowledge about the pathophysiology of mental syndromes that will guide pre-clinical research in developing more selective and thereby more effective pharmacological treatments for mental illness.

By the late 1950s research that led to the *neurotransmitter* era, the first epoch in the history of neuropsychopharmacology, was in progress.

In the neurotransmitter era research in the pathophysiology and treatment of mental illness is guided by knowledge derived from the effect of psychotropic drugs on neurotransmitter dynamics and metabolism.

CINP AND THE NEUROTRASMITTER ERA

Neuropsychopharmacology is a composite discipline. Progress in it depends on interaction among the component disciplines of the field. In 1957, the recognition of the need for a continuous dialogue between clinicians and basic scientists for successful neuropsychopharmacological research led the founding of the Collegium Internationale Neur-Psychopharmacologicum (CINP). It was hoped that CINP, by providing a platform for interaction, would facilitate *translational research* to establish relationships among the various findings (Ban, 2005).

In the early 1960s there was intensive interaction between basic scientists and clinicians at CINP congresses. There were many historical presentations that profoundly affected the development of the field. One such presentation was Arvid Carlsson's, a Swedish pharmacologist who was to receive the Nobel Prize, on selective changes in brain monoamines with psychotropic drugs (Carlsson, 1961). His paper presented in 1960 at the 2nd CINP congress in Basle (Switzerland), signaled the beginning of the neurotransmitter era. In the years that followed interest in findings related to monoamine-neurotransmitter dynamics and metabolism, and the interaction between monoamine neurotransmitters and psychotropic drugs, steadily grew. In 1968, the high point of the 6th CINP congress in Taragona was the presentation of Erminio Costa, a neuropharmacologist at the National Institute of Mental Health (NIMH), of the United States, on the implications of monamine turnover rate for neuropsychopharmacological research (Costa, 2003). The release of monoamines at the synaptic cleft, their breakdown by specific enzymes, their reuptake by the presynaptic neurons, and their binding at postsynaptic sites, were in the center of interest in the late 1960s. It was believed that the alteration of these processes might be the key to the cause and treatment of mental illness (Valdecasas, 1988).

In the early 1980s basic research in neuropharmacology was extended from cerebral monoamines to neurotransmitter modulators, neuropeptides and prostaglandins (Carlsson, 2000). The 12th CINP congress in 1980 in Göteborg (Sweden) was the first meeting to reflect "the shift from neurotransmitter biochemistry at the synaptic cleft to receptor research" (Carlsson, 1988; Radouco-Thomas and Garcin, 1980). Presentations at the 14th congress in 1984 in Florence (Italy) reinforced the belief that employment of molecular neurobiology, an emerging new science, "could lead to research that will transcend the existing boundaries of neuropsychopharmacology" (Kielholz, 1988; Racagni, et. al., 1984). Furthermore, reports at the 15th congress in 1986, in San Juan, Puerto Rico, raised hopes that the study of "receptor site responses to secondary transmitter systems could provide an avenue for the development of new therapeutic substances" (Bunney et al., 1986; Wittenborn, 1988).

In the late 1980s it was recognized that communication in the brain is not restricted to synaptic, *wiring* transmission, based on the neurotransmitter dynamics that connects one neuron directly with another. Rather, there is also another communication system, referred to as *volume transmission* that takes place in the extracellular space (Agnati et al., 1986). With the recognition of two parallel, complementary communication systems in the brain the neurotransmitter era was approaching its end.

CONTRIBUTIONS TO NEUROPSYCHOPHARMACOLOGY

During the neurotransmitter era there have been major changes in psychiatry: the site of psychiatric practice shifted from psychiatric hospitals to the community; the scope of psychiatry was extended from the psychoses and neuroses to dimensional anomalies of abnormal psychology; and pharmacotherapy has become the primary form of treatment in most of the psychiatric disorders. By supplying drugs with demonstrated therapeutic effectiveness, together with information on their pharmacological profile, the pharmaceutical industry has been instrumental in reintegrating psychiatry with the other medical disciplines. Furthermore, by providing support for research, from genetics through neuropharmacology to brain imaging, industry has succeeded in establishing psychopharmacology as the dominant paradigm in psychiatry around the world (Ban, 2004). It is a moot question how much of these changes can be attributed to neuropsychopharmacology, i.e., more selective and effective pharmacological treatments, and how much to interacting social forces.

NEUROPHARMACOLOGY

Neuropharmacological research that led to the neurotransmitter era was based on findings that iproniazid, a monoamine oxidase inhibitor (MAOI) that interferes with the breakdown of monoamines (MAOs), increased cerebral monoamines such as NE and 5-HT and that reserpine, a Rauwolfia alkaloid decreased them (Besendorf and Pletscher, 1955, 1956; Pletscher et al., 1955, 1956). The link between monoamines and mood was based on reports which indicated that treatment with iproniazid induced euphoria, a feeling of well-being in some tubercular patients (Flaherty, 1952; Selikoff et al., 1952), whereas treatment with reserpine induced depressed mood in about 10% of hypertensives (Bunney and Davis, 1965; Freis, 1954; Kline, 1968; Mueller et al., 1955).

In 1956 Brodie et al. postulated a relationship between reserpine-induced deple-tion of monoamines and depression (Brodie et al., 1956); this led to the introduction of the reserpine reversal test in pharmacological screening for antidepressants (Costa et al., 1960). In 1963 Carlsson and Lindquist hypothesized a relationship between DA receptor blockade and antipsychotic effect, based on their findings of an increase in catecholamine turnover in haloperidol or chlorpromazine treated mice (Carlsson and Lindquist, 1963); this led to the extensive use of antagonism to dopamine agonists, such as amphetamine, in the pharmacological screening for neuroleptics (antipsy-chotics) (Janssen et al., 1965). The two screening tests, reserpine reversal and amphet-amine antagonism, had a major impact on the development of pharmacotherapy in depression and schizophrenia in the 1960s and 1970s.

Employment of reserpine reversal in the screening for antidepressants led to the isolation of desipramine, the demethylated metabolite of imipramine, the prototype of tricyclic antidepressants (TCAs). There was special interest in this substance because: (1) the two TCAs in use at the time were found to block the neuronal re-uptake of NE (Axelrod et al., 1961), and (2) desipramine's reserpine reversal was suspended in ani-mals selectively depleted of catecholamines (Brodie et al., 1961; Sulser et al., 1961). Assuming that reserpine reversal corresponds with antidepressant effects, it was hypothesized that NE re-uptake inhibition is the crucial step in the mode of action of antidepressants. It was also on the basis of these findings that it was hypothesized that NE deficiency, and not 5-HT deficiency, is the culprit in the pathophysiology of depression. These hypotheses were not supported by clinical findings; desipramine, a selective NE re-uptake inhibitor was not superior to imipramine, a non-selective re-uptake inhibitor, in the treatment of depression (Ban, 1974, 1981; Klein and Davis, 1969). Yet, on the basis of *neuropharmacological theory* the old non-selective prevail-ingly NE re-uptake blockers were replaced first by selective NE re-uptake blockers and subsequently by selective 5-HT re-uptake inhibitors. Preparation for the shift from NE to 5-HT re-uptake inhibitors began in the early 1970s with the recognition that prefer-entially NE re-uptake blockers become 5-HT re-uptake blockers by halogenation (Carlsson et al., 1972), and with the finding that without an intact 5-HT system ß-adren-ergic receptor down regulation, a common characteristic of TCAs, does not take place. Introduction of selective 5-HT re-uptake inhibitors (SSRIs) began in 1980 after the demonstration of a correspondence between imipramine binding sites and 5-HT bind-ing sites in the human platelet and the hypothalamus of the rat (Langer et al., 1980; Paul et al., 1980). By the early 1990s SSRIs dominated treatment. Yet despite their great success, in the 1990s a non-selective but prevailingly 5-HT re-uptake blocker, venlafax-ine (Costa e Silva, 1998; Thase et al., 2001), and a selective NE re-uptake blocker, reboxetine (Ban et al., 1998) emerged. With the introduction of venlafaxine, a non selective, but prevailingly 5-HT blocker, a full circle of NE and 5-HT blockers was com-pleted; and with the introduction of reboxetine, the circle that opened in the early 1960s with desipramine was reopened in the late 1990s virtually unchanged without offering a more effective antidepressant than imipramine (Ban, 2001a).

In the field of antipsychotics events began with the finding of a linear relationship in the periphery between the sedative and anti-5-HT effect of chlorpromazine and its congeners (Gyermek et al., 1956); as well a debate began about the need to induce extrapyramidal signs (EPS) to obtain therapeutic effects. By the end of the 1950s it was recognized that EPS are not a prerequisite of antipsychotic efficacy. It was also demonstrated that sedative neuroleptics (antipsychotics), such as chlorpromazine (CP2) that produces only mild EPS are just as effective in the treatment of schizophrenia as *incisive neuroleptics* such as haloperidol, that produces marked EPS (Freyhan, 1961). (It was later shown that *sedative neuroleptics* have a low affinity for D_2 receptors). Yet, fueled by neuropharmacological theory - implicating DA receptor blockade in the mode of action of antipsychotics (Carlsson and Lindqvist, 1963; Van Rossum, 1967) - by the late-1960s incisive neuroleptics dominated the field in the treatment of schizophrenia. Their extensive use led to acute and chronic EPS in a high proportion of neuroleptic-treated patients (Ban, 2004). The dominance of *incisive neuroleptics* was perpetuated by the demonstration of DA receptor blockade (Burt et al., 1976; Seeman et al., 1975; Snyder et al., 1975); the finding of an inverse relationship between DA receptor blocking potency and dose requirements to produce therapeutic effects (Seeman et al., 1976); and the formulation of the DA hypothesis of schizophrenia (Snyder, 1976). One widely used neuroleptic, thioridazine was promoted because of its relative absence of EPS. Then, in the early 1970s, clozapine was introduced, a substance with an even lesser propensity to induce EPS than thioridazine (Ackenheil and Hippius, 1977; Angst et al., 1971). Despite numerous side effects, including agranulocytosis (Idanpaan-Heikkila et al., 1975), clozapine became the prototype of *atypical neuroleptics* a series of neuroleptics, which, similar to *sedative neuroleptics* have a lesser propensity to induce EPS than *incisive neuroleptics* now referred to as *typical neuroleptics* Corresponding with the difference in the frequency and severity of EPS are findings with receptor binding assays that indicate that atypical neuroleptics have a higher affinity to the $5\text{-}HT_{2A}$ receptors than to the DA_2 receptors, whereas *typical neuroleptics* have a higher affinity to the dopamine D_2 receptors than to the $5\text{-}HT_{2A}$ receptors. Delineation of the receptor profile of neuroleptics has revealed that *atypical neuroleptics* represent a return to the CPZ-type of neuroleptics after a 20-years detour with *typical, haloperidol-type of neuroleptics* without offering a more effective antipsychotic than CPZ.

Despite lacking evidence of increased therapeutic efficacy in either antidepressants or antipsychotics, neuropharmacological research focused on the mode of action of psychotropic drugs had a major impact on academic psychiatry in the neurotransmitter era. By adopting concepts about the molecular substrate of the brain that is affected by psychotropic drugs used in everyday psychiatric practice, thinking in psychiatry shifted from psychological to biological. In academic departments the old generation of psychoanalysts was replaced by a new generation of biologically oriented psychiatrists, and psychodynamic interpretations about psychogenic etiology were replaced by neuropharmacological interpretations about the molecular substrate of mental illness. By the new generation of psychiatrists, i.e., psychiatrists entering the field during the neurotransmitter era, neuropharmacology is perceived as one of the basic sciences of psychiatry, and psychopharmacology as the bridge between the mode of action and clinical indications of psychotropic drugs.

PSYCHOPHARMACOLOGY

Similar to neuropharmacology, despite the lack of tangible increases in therapeutic efficacy, advances in psychopharmacology had a major impact on treatment in academic psychiatry in the neurotransmitter era.

Introduction of psychotropic drugs in the 1950s focused attention on the differential responsiveness to the same drug within a given diagnosis. The pharmacological heterogeneity within a diagnosis created difficulties for the pharmaceutical industry in demonstrating the therapeutic effectiveness of drugs and for psychiatrists in prescribing drugs in a predictable manner. Academic psychiatry was confronted with the need to resolve the heterogeneity within diagnoses by re-evaluating psychiatric nosology and developing a pharmacologically relevant classification of mental illness. But this did not happen. Instead, a statistical methodology - the randomized clinical trial (RCT) - was adopted for the demonstration of therapeutic effectiveness in pharmacologically heterogeneous diagnostic populations.

The adoption of statistical methodology in psychiatry for the study of therapeutic efficacy had a major impact on academic psychiatry by providing a means of evaluating the effectiveness of various treatment modalities. It was on the basis of findings in these evaluations that pharmacotherapy became the primary form of treatment in schizophrenia and mania in the 1960s, in depression and bipolar disorder in the 1970s, in the anxiety disorders in the 1980s, and in Alzheimer's type of dementia in the 1990s. But the statistical methodology adopted has its limitation. It is capable only to demonstrate therapeutic effectiveness and covers up possible differential effects of treatment. Without a methodology for the demonstration of differential effects, the differential receptor profiles of drugs cannot be translated into therapeutic profiles in a given group of patients. Thus, possible therapeutic advantages of new drugs (apart of side effects) remain hidden (Ban, 1999). Furthermore, an essential prerequisite of neuropsychopharmacological research is the identification of the treatment responsive form of illness. Thus, the statistical methodology that serves the demonstration of therapeutic efficacy virtually blocked the study of the pathophysiology of mental syndromes and the interpretation of findings in biological research in psychiatry.

NEUROPSYCHOPHARMACOLOGY

In neuropsychopharmacological research the effect of a psychotropic drug on mental illness is linked with the effect of the substance on brain structures involved in its mode of action. Hence, learning the mode of action of a psychotropic drug provides clues about the pathophysiology of the mental syndrome affected by the drug, and the identification of a treatment responsive form of illness to a psychotropic drug with a well-defined mode of action provides clues for the development of clinically more selective and thereby more effective psychotropic drugs. By linking the mode of action of a drug with a pharmacologically heterogeneous diagnostic population, neuropsychopharmacological research has provided relevant feedback only to the development of drugs with different adverse effects.

Psychotropic drug development in the neurotransmitter era is driven by neuropharmacological theory and not by neuropsychopharmacological research. Psychotropic drugs are marketed if they meet regulatory requirements of safety and efficacy. To meet efficacy requirements in the United States a drug must show statistically significant superiority to placebo, with a 0.05 or greater level of probability, i.e., with an about a 20% to 25% difference in responsiveness between the drug and the placebo, in two pivotal studies. Such a narrow difference may allow the demonstration of the effectiveness of a drug in more than one diagnostic categories, if the diagnoses share sufficient common features in their pathophysiology, e.g., imipramine, a non-selective monoamine re-uptake inhibitor is proven effective in both depression and panic disorder, fluvoxamine, a SSRI is effective in both depression and obsessive-compulsive disorder, etc. The possible benefit of extending the indications of a drug comes at the price of covering up possibly powerful therapeutic effects. In Frank Fish's study (Fish, 1964), using Karl Leonhard's classification (Leonhard, 1957), 3 of 4 patients with *unsystematic schizophrenia,* responded favorably neuroleptic phenothiazines whereas only about 1 of 4 patients with *systematic schizophrenia* showed a favorable response. Response rate in *affect-laden paraphrenia,* one of the three forms of *unsystematic schizophrenia* was about 85%, whereas in the different forms of *systematic schizophrenia,* response rates were below 25%. With the currently accepted statistical methodology a drug is considered to be effective if 2 of 8 patients show a favorable response to its pharmacological effects. This marginalizes the importance of pharmacological treatments and blurs the difference between pharmacological and other treatments. In the absence of the identification of the treatment responsive form of illness, the potential benefit from drugs are compromised by their indiscriminate use.

There is a great need to resolve the heterogeneity in pharmacological responsiveness within the diagnostic groups. Yet so far attempts to identify treatment responsive forms of illness by linear regression equations, biological markers, pharmacological load tests or biochemical indicators have yielded inconsistent findings (Ban, 1999). It remains to be seen whether this can be achieved by the replacement of the nosological disease model by a reaction-form based disease model as suggested by Van Praag (1997) or by the employment of specially devised instruments for the identification of treatment responsive forms of illness, as for example the composite diagnostic evaluation (CODE) system, that can assign simultaneously a diagnosis from several diagnostic systems, as suggested by Ban (2002).

TOWARDS A GENETIC ERA

As we move forward from the neurotransmitter to a genetic era in neuropsychopharmacology, the need for identifying pharmacologically homogenous populations is increasingly felt. There is gap between a neuropharmacology with the capability to *tailor* drugs to receptor affinities by the employment of a rapidly emerging genetic technology, and a psychopharmacology with a methodology that is restricted to the demonstration of therapeutic efficacy. This gap is becoming so wide that it interferes with progress in the pharmacotherapy of mental illness.

Since all the primary targets of psychotropic drugs in the brain are encoded by genes that have been identified any nosologic entity that corresponds with a treatment responsive population, is suitable for the generation of genetic hypotheses relevant to mental illness. In the new epoch progress will depend on the speed neuropsychopharmacological research can identify suitable populations for molecular genetic research.

REFERENCES

1. Ackenheil, M., Hippius, H., 1977. Clozapine. In: Usdin, E., Forrest, I. (Ed.), Psychotherapeutic Drugs. Applications. Volume 2. Marcel Dekker, Inc., New York, pp. 923-956.
2. Agnati, L.F., Fuxe, K., Zoli, M., Zini, I., Toffano, G., Ferraguti, F., 1986. A correlation analysis of the regional distribution of central enkephalin and β-endorphin immunoreactive terminals and of opiate receptor in adult and old male rats. Evidence of the existence of two main types of communications in the central nervous system: The volume transmission and the wiring transmission. Acta Physiol. Scand. 128, 201-207.
3. Angst, J., Bente, D., Berner, P., Heimann, H., Helmchen, H., Hippius, H., 1971. The clinical efficacy of clozapine. (Investigation with the AMP System). Neuropsychopharmacol 4, 201-211.
4. Axelrod, J., Whitby, L.B., Hertting, G., 1961. Effect of psychotropic drugs on the uptake of ^{3}H –norepinephrine by tissues, Science 133, 383-384.
5. Ban, T. A., 1974. Depression and the Tricyclic Antidepressants, Ronalds Federated, Montreal, pp. 1-74
6. Ban, T.A., 1981. Psychopharmacology of Depression. A Guide for Drug Treatment, S. Karger, Basle. pp. 1-215
7. Ban, T.A., 1999. Selective drugs versus heterogeneous diagnoses towards a new methodology in neuropsychopharmacological research. Psiquiatria Biologica 7, 177-189.
8. Ban, T.A., 2001a. Pharmacotherapy of depression: A historical analysis, J. Neurol. Transm. 108, 707-711.
9. Ban, T.A., 2001b. Pharmacotherapy of mental illness. A historical analysis. Prog Neuro-Psychopharmacol & Biol Psychiat 25, 709-726.
10. Ban, T.A., 2004. Neuropsychopharmacology and the history of pharmacotherapy in psychiatry. A review of developments in the 20th century. In: Ban, T.A., Healy, D., Shorter, E. (Eds.). Reflections on Twentieth-Century Psychopharmacology. Animula, Budapest, pp. 697-720.
11. Ban, T.A., 2005. History of the CINP. Ceska a Slovenska Pssychiatrie 5, 258-264.
12. Ban, T. A., Gaszner, P., Aguglia, E., Batista, R., Castillo, A., Lipcsey, A., Macher, J.-P., Torres-Ruiz, A., Vergara, L., 1998. Clinical efficacy of reboxetine. A comparative study with desipramine, with methodological considerations, Human Psychopharmacology 13, S29-S39.

13. Besendorf, H., Pletscher, A., 1956. Beeinflussung zentraler Wirkungen von Reserpin und 5-hydroxytryptamin durch Isonicotinic–säuerhydrazine. Helv. Physiol. Acta 14, 383-390.

14. Bowman, R.L., Caulfield, P.A., Udenfriend, S., 1955. Spectrophotofluorimetry in the visible and ultraviolet. Science 122, 32-33.

15. Brodie, B.B., Shore, P. A., Pletscher, A., 1956. Limitations of serotonin releasing activity to those Rauwolfis alkaloids possessing tranquilizing action. Science, 123, 992-993.

16. Brodie, B.B., Bickel, M. H., Sulser, F., 1961. Desmethylimipramine, a new type of antidepressant drug. Med. Exp. 5, 454-458.

17. Bunney, W. E., Jr., Davis, J.M., 1965. Norepinephrine in depressive reactions. A review.Arch. Gen. Psychiatry 13, 483-494.

18. Burt, D.R., Creese, I., Snyder, S.,H., 1976. Properties of [³H]haloperidol and [³H]dopamine binding associated with dopamine receptors in calf brain membranes. Mol. Pharmacol. 12, 800-812.

19. Bunney, W., Costa, E., Potkin, S., (Eds.), 1986. Clinical Neuropharmacology. Raven Press, New York, pp. 1-596.

20. Carlsson, A., 1961. Brain monoamines and psychotropic drugs. In: Rothlin, E. (Ed.), Neuropsychopharmacology. Elsevier, Amsterdam, pp. 77-92.

21. Carlsson, A., 1988. The 12th CINP Congress. In: Ban, T.A., Hippius, H. (Eds.), Thirty Years CINP. Springer, Berlin, pp. 42-43.

22. Carlsson, A., 2000. Comments from the president of the 12th CINP Congress. CINP in the 1970s. In: Ban, T.A., Healy, D., Shorter, E. (Eds.), The Triumph of Psychopharmacology and the Story of CINP. Animula, Budapest, pp. 352-354.

23. Carlsson, A., Lindqvist, M., 1963. Effect of chlorpromazine or haloperidol on formation of 3-methoxytyramine and normetanephrine on mouse brain. Acta Pharmacol. Toxicol. 20, 140-144.

24. Carlsson, A., Berntsson, P., Corrodi, H., 1972. Zimelidine. Belgian Patent No. 781.105, March 23, 1972. In : Healy, D., 1997. The Antidepressant Era. Harvard University Press. Cambridge, Mssachusetts, p. 166, p. 201.

25. Costa, E., 2003. An Early Attempt to Foster Neuroscience Globalization. An Autobiography. Good Life Press, Nashville, pp. 1-127.

26. Costa, E., Garattini, S., Valzelli, L., 1960. Interaction between reserpine , chlorpromazine and imipramine. Experientia 15, 461-463.

27. Costa e Silva, J., 1998. Randomized, double-blind comparison of venlafaxine and fluoxetine in outpatients with major depression. Journal of Clinical Psychiatry 59, 352-357.

28. Fish, F., 1964. The influence of the tranquilizer on the Leonhard schizophrenic syndromes. Encephale 53, 245-249.

29. Flaherty, J.A., 1952. The psychiatric use of isonicotinic acid hydrazide: a case report. Delaware med. J. 24, 298-300.

30. Freyhan, F., 1961. The influence of specific and non-specific factors on the clinical effects of psychotropic drugs. In: Rothlin, E (Ed.), Neuropsychopharmacology 2. Elsevier, Amsterdam, pp. 189-203.

31. Freis, E.D., 1954. Mental depression in hypertensive patients treated for long periods with large doses of reserpine. N. Engl. J. Med. 251, 1006-1008.

32. Gyermek, L., Lázár, G.T., Csák, Zs., 1956. The antiserotonin action of chlorpromazine and some other phenothiazine derivatives. Arch. Int. Pharmacodyn. 107, 62-74.

33. Idanpaan-Heikkila, J., Alhave, E., Olkimora, M., Palva, J., 1975. Clozapine in agranulocytosis.Lancet Sept.27, p.611.

34. Janssen, P., Niemegeers, C.J.E., Schellekens, K.H.L., 1965. Is it possible to predict the clinical effects of neuroleptic drugs (major tranquilizers) from animal data? Part I. Neuroleptic activity spectra for rats. Arzneimittelforschung 15, 104-117.

35. Kielholz, P. 1988. The 14th CINP Congress – Florence 1984. In: Ban, T.A., Hippius, H. (Eds.), Thirty Years CINP. Springer, Berlin, pp. 49-50.

36. Klein, D.F., Davis, J., 1969. Diagnosis and Drug Treatment of Psychiatric Disorders. Williams & Wilkins, Baltimore, pp. 1-480.

37. Kline, N.S., 1968. Psychiatric diagnosis and typology of clinical drug effects. Psychopharmacologia 13, 359-386.

38. Langer, S.Z., Moret, C., Raisman, R., Dubokovitsch, M.L., Briley, M., 1980. High affinity ^{3}H-imipramine binding in the rat hypothalamus. Association with uptake of serotonin, but not of norepinephrine. Science, 210, 1133-1135.

39. Leonhard, K., 1957. Aufteilung der endogenen Psychosen. Akademie-Verlag, Berlin.

40. Mueller, J.C., Pryor, W. W., Gibbons, J.E., Orgain, E.S., 1955. Depression and anxiety occurring during Rauwolfia therapy. JAMA 159, 836-839.

41. Paul, S., Rehavi, M., Skolnick, P., Goodwin, F.K., 1980. Demonstration of high affinity binding sites for [^{3}H] imipramine in human platelets. Life Sci. 26, 953-959.

42. Pletscher, A., Shore. P.A., Brodie, B.B., 1955. Serotonin release as possible mechanism of reserpine action. Science 122: 374-375.

43. Pletscher, A., Shore, P.A., Brodie, B.B., 1956. Serotonin as a modulator of reserpine action in brain. J.Pharmacol. Exper. Ther. 116. 84-89.

44. Racagni, G, Paoletti, R, Kielholz, P., 1984. Proceedings of the 14th Collegium Internationale Neuro-Psychopharmacologium. 7 (Suppl.1), 1-990.

45. Radouco-Thomas, C, Garcin, F., 1980. Abstracts of the 12th CINP Congress, Goteborg, Sweden 22-26 June 1980. Pergamon Press, Oxford, pp.1-380.

46. Schou, M., Juel-Nielson, N., Strömgren, E., Volby, H., 1954. The treatment of manic psychoses by the administration of lithium salts. J. Neurol. Neurosurg. Psychiatry 17, 250-260.

47. Seeman, P., Chau-Wong, M., Tedesco, J., Wong, K., 1975. Brain receptors for antipsychotic drugs and dopamine: Direct binding assays. Proc. Nat. Acad. Sci. (USA) 72, 4376,-4380.

48. Seeman, P., Lee, T., Chau-Wong, M. Wong, K., 1976. Antipsychotic drug doses and neuroleptic/dopamine receptors. Nature 261, 717-719.

49. Selikoff, I.J., Robitzek, E.H., Orenstein, G.G., 1952. Treatment of pulmonary tuberculosis with hydrazine derivatives of isonicotinic acid. JAMA 150, 973-987.

50. Snyder, S., 1976. The dopamine hypothesis of schizophrenia. Focus on the dopamine receptor. Am. J. Psychiatry 133, 140-144.

51. Snyder, S.H., Creese, I., Burt, D.R., 1975. The brain's dopamine receptor: labeling with [3H] dopamine and [^{3}H] haloperidol. Psychopharmacol. Commun. 1, 663-673.

52. Sulser, F., Watts, J., Brodie, B.B., 1961. On the mechanism of antidepressant action of imipramine-like drugs. Ann. NY Acad. Sci. 96, 270-296.

53. Thase, M., Entsuah, A., Rudolph, R., 2001. Remission rates during treatment with venlafaxine or selective serotonin re-uptake inhibitors. Br. J. Psychiatry 178, 234-241.

54. Valdecasas, F.G., 1988. The 6th CINP Congress - Tarragona, 1968. In: Ban, T.A., Hippius, (Eds.), Thirty years CINP. Springer, Berlin, pp. 20-22.

55. Van Praag, H.M., 1997. Over the mainstream: diagnostic requirements for biological psychiatric research. Psychiat. Res. 72, 201-212.

56. Van Rossum, J.M., 1967. The significance of dopamine-receptor blockade for the action of neuroleptic drugs. In: Brill, H., Cole, J.O., Deniker, P., Hippius, H., Bradley, P.B. (Eds.), Neuropsychopharmacology. Proceedings of the Fifth International Congress of the Collegium Internationale Neuro-Psychopharmacologicum. (March 1966). Excerpta Medica Foundation, Amsterdam, pp. 321-329.

57. Wittenborn, J.R., 1988. The 15th CINP Congress - San Juan, 1986. In: Ban, T.A., Hippius, H. (Eds.), Thirty Years CINP. Springer, Springer, pp. 51-55.

NAME INDEX

DRUG AND CHEMICAL INDEX

SUBJECT INDEX

www.ingramcontent.com/pod-product-compliance
Lightning Source LLC
Chambersburg PA
CBHW051407200326
41520CB00023B/7147